Football as Medicine

It is beyond dispute that physical activity is good for us, but what are the benefits, challenges and impacts of sport on health? This is the first book to focus on football in the context of health from individual, public and population-level perspectives.

Football as Medicine examines the effects of football training on the three main types of fitness (cardiovascular, metabolic and musculoskeletal) and on specific target populations (for example, children, type 2 diabetes patients, cancer patients, people with mental health conditions, the socially deprived and older people). It discusses the significance of football for public health and assesses the efficacy of football interventions by clubs and community sport development programs.

With its multi-disciplinary approach, this is a valuable resource for students, researchers and practitioners working in physical activity and health, public health, health promotion and medicine, as well as football and sport business management, sport and exercise science, and the sociology of sport.

Peter Krustrup is Professor of Sport and Health Sciences at the University of Southern Denmark, Honorary Visiting Professor of Exeter University, UK, and Guest Professor at Shanghai University of Sport, China. His research interests include the fitness and health effects of football and other sports, physical-tactical-technical match analyses, and fatigue, recovery, training and testing in elite football. He is a UEFA Pro-Licensed football coach and Fitness Coach for the Danish Women's national team. He is also the leader of a Football is Medicine group of 225 researchers in more than 20 countries.

Daniel Parnell is Senior Lecturer in Sport Business at the University of Liverpool Management School, UK. His research interests lie in sport business management and policy, and he has a growing interest in examining social and economic networks in sport. Dan is co-Founder and Editor of The Football Collective, a global network of football scholars. He serves as co-Editor-in-Chief of *Managing Sport and Leisure* and is co-Editor of the Routledge book series 'Critical Research in Football'. He also co-edited the *Routledge Handbook of Football Business and Management.*

Critical Research in Football

Series Editors:
Pete Millward, *Liverpool John Moores University, UK*
Jamie Cleland, *University of Southern Australia*
Dan Parnell, *University of Liverpool, UK*
Stacey Pope, *Durham University, UK*
Paul Widdop, *Manchester Metropolitan University, UK*

The *Critical Research in Football* book series was launched in 2017 to showcase the inter- and multi-disciplinary breadth of debate relating to 'football'. The series defines 'football' as broader than association football, with research on rugby, Gaelic and gridiron codes also featured. Including monographs, edited collections, short books and textbooks, books in the series are written and/or edited by leading experts in the field whilst consciously also affording space to emerging voices in the area, and are designed to appeal to students, postgraduate students and scholars who are interested in the range of disciplines in which critical research in football connects. The series is published in association with the *Football Collective, www.footballcollective.org.uk*.

Available in this series

Football, Fandom and Consumption
Oliver Brooks

Football Fandom, Protest and Democracy
Supporter Activism in Turkey
Dağhan Irak

African Footballers in Europe
Migration, Community, and Give Back Behaviours
Ernest Yeboah Acheampong, Malek Bouhaouala and Michel Raspaud

Football in Fiction
A History
Lee McGowan

Football as Medicine
Prescribing Football for Global Health Promotion
Edited by Peter Krustrup and Daniel Parnell

For more information about this series, please visit: www.routledge.com/sport/series/CFSFC

Football as Medicine

Prescribing Football for Global Health Promotion

Edited by Peter Krustrup and
Daniel Parnell

Routledge
Taylor & Francis Group
LONDON AND NEW YORK

First published 2020
by Routledge
2 Park Square, Milton Park, Abingdon, Oxon OX14 4RN

and by Routledge
52 Vanderbilt Avenue, New York, NY 10017

Routledge is an imprint of the Taylor & Francis Group, an informa business

British Library Cataloguing-in-Publication Data
A catalogue record for this book is available from the British Library

Library of Congress Cataloging-in-Publication Data
A catalog record for this book has been requested

ISBN: 978-0-367-24888-8 (hbk)
ISBN: 978-0-429-28489-2 (ebk)

Typeset in Baskerville
by Apex CoVantage, LLC

Dedication

It is a great pleasure to see this book become a reality. Sport has always played an important part in my life. I started playing football at the age of 5 in Vanløse IF, with my uncle Jan Krustrup as my first football coach, and started my coaching career at the age of 14, coaching under-10 girls. In school and university, I majored in sport, along with math and Danish literature. I became a board member of Vanløse IF at the age of 24 while playing for their first team. Today, aged 48, I have been playing football for 43 years and coaching for 22 years. My coaching experience includes all age groups and most competitive levels, from under-4 to over-70 and from Football Fitness teams to my two daughters in the local club Frederikssund FB and the Danish women's national team. I have also run marathons and played club-based tennis, badminton, table tennis and ten-pin bowling. Danes are generally very active.

I am a fervent believer that sport, not least football, can be enjoyed by everyone. In 1987, I organised family football for the parents and grandparents of my under-14 girls team, and in 1989 I invited the mums supporting my under-16 girls team to join with my mother and her friends in warm-ups, ball drills and small-sided games. I believed that football could be fun fitness training for all groups, and at Vanløse IF I adopted the slogan 'Football is for All'. However, I did not know just how healthy football was and the huge potential it offered in the prevention and treatment of lifestyle diseases. My postgraduate studies at Copenhagen University, from 1996 onward, culminated in a 250-page PhD thesis on the subject of single-fibre metabolism and muscular efficiency during dynamic exercise that did not even mention football once! However, despite the low priority of football science in my department, I was able to conduct several football-related projects, including tracking, training and testing of female footballers and match officials. Furthermore, in 2003, my wife Birgitte and I initiated pioneering studies on the fitness and health effects of football for homeless men, low-level seniors and inactive computer enthusiasts. After 2 years of remarkable results, we knew we were onto something! Then, things really began to change in 2005 when I became associate professor of the theory and practice of ball games at Copenhagen University and was given the opportunity to apply basic and applied methodologies to football and other ball games. In my subsequent professorships at Exeter University, Copenhagen University and the University of Southern Denmark, we conducted numerous feasibility studies, descriptive studies, small-scale randomised controlled trials and large-scale implementation projects, combining methodologies and research expertise in sports science with sports psychology, sociology and pedagogics. This work has examined the cardiovascular, metabolic and musculoskeletal demands of football training and other sports in various groups across the lifespan to understand the effects of different types of exercise training on the risk of lifestyle diseases, and the implementation potential of exercise concepts and their ability to elicit sustainable lifestyle changes.

It is a privilege for me to thank more than 225 collaborators from 22 countries for their valuable contributions to my work, of which 75 authors from 5 continents have contributed to this book. I am grateful to my current and former research institutions for supporting my sport and health work, and many other institutions around the world for supporting my colleagues in their work, and I hope that many more will join in. Special thanks must go to the Danish FA, the Danish Sports Confederation, Team Danmark, FPF, FIFA, UEFA, the IOC and the EU for their willingness to develop and implement evidence-based Sport for All concepts. Also, a special personal thank you to Magni Mohr, Morten B. Randers, Laila Ottesen, Peter Riis Hansen, Eva Wulff Helge, Per Aagaard, Jens Jung Nielsen, Jacob Uth, Anne-Marie Elbe, Birger Peitersen, Anders Ellebæk Madsen, John Rasmussen, Bo Kousgaard, Henrik Holm Andersen, Jørgen Povlsen, Jonas Havelund, Morten Mølholm Hansen, Kenneth Reeh, Bent Clausen, Kenneth Grønlund Rasmussen and Tina Enestrøm. This book brings together many years of research from many fields of expertise and provides a comprehensive up-to-date overview of the health effects of football training and how football can be used as a vehicle for improving world health. I hope it will inspire organisations and policymakers around the globe to work harder to derive the full benefits of sport for health, fitness, wellbeing and learning! Football is Medicine – it is time for patients to play! A heartfelt thanks to my mum Inge, my dad Jørgen, my daughters Sarah and Andrea, my wife Birgitte, who has been with me every step of the way, and my entire family. Finally, I would like to thank Dan Parnell for his excellent collaboration on this book and our previous book *Sport and Health – Exploring the Current State of Play*. I look forward to continuing this important work and to seeing you again in Odense soon!

Peter

I have been delighted to work on the concept of Football as Medicine and this new contribution with Peter Krustrup. Over the past few years of our collaboration, Peter has proven to be a collaborative scholar committed to supporting others within his network, a leader in science and football and a very good friend. This book has been a pleasure to work on and represents the work of many fantastic multi-disciplinary scholars from around the world specialising in the football and health agenda. I am proud to have helped facilitate this work, and I am hopeful this proves a valuable resource for students and researchers alike.

From a personal perspective, this work is a product of efforts dating back to when I began my PhD thesis examining the effectiveness of football-based community interventions at Everton Football Club in 2006. Since then, the football and health agenda has been an incredible personal journey and a truly collective effort. What started at Everton with the creation of the Everton Active Family Centre, which housed the Extra Time (Football Foundation), Fit Fans and Everton Active Families projects, grew into initiatives across Liverpool and the United Kingdom. I have been fortunate to have the support of incredible undergraduate and postgraduate students from Liverpool Johns Moores University, the University of Abertay Dundee, the University of Derby, Leeds Beckett University and Manchester Metropolitan University, some of whom have gone on to carve out successful careers in football, public health and academia. These people have been truly fundamental to these projects, working with myself and colleagues to deliver some genuinely impactful community projects, including a number with Burton Albion Community Trust, the English Premier League, the Football Foundation and the English Homeless FA. Along this journey, I have worked with many quality scholars, practitioners and friends who have kept their support for our work and friendship completely solid. Each knows what they mean to me. I hope I am there for them, too, as and when. These include Paul Widdop, Peter Millward, Ed Cope, Richard Bailey, Anthony May, Danny Fitzpatrick, Jamie Cleland, Joel Rookwood, Alex Bond, Rob Wilson, Ryan Groom, Jordan Peel, Gareth Stratton, Dave Richardson and Barry Drust. In addition, I am thankful to the University of Liverpool Management School for supporting my research endeavours and the Politic Studies Association sport sub group for their ongoing collegiate guidance. I would also like to mention one of my closest collaborators, the Football Foundation, and in particular Mike Rigby, Rory Carroll and Paul Thorogood, who have been continual supportive, critical and analytical leaders in the game. Similarly, I would like to thank Andy Reed of the Sports Think Tank for his constant support, guidance and commitment to critical analysis and knowledge exchange in sport. I am indebted to the Football Collective, a truly unique group of people who are committed to supporting, analysing, enhancing and sharing research. Indeed, this book is part of the *Critical Research in Football* series by Routledge in association with the Football Collective. In this respect, I am especially thankful to Simon Whitmore for his support for this book and the broader football/sport discipline – we are lucky to have you. Additional thanks must go to Rebecca Connor for overseeing the project on behalf of Routledge and to the book series co-editors Peter Millward, Stacey Pope, Jamie Cleland and Paul Widdop. Finally, I am lucky to have a very understanding family that supports my ambitions and research in every way. Thank you Sarah, Niamh, George and Betty.

Dan

Contents

Figures

Photos

Tables

Contributors

Per Aagaard is Professor in Biomechanics at the Department of Sports Science and Clinical Biomechanics, Muscle Physiology and Biomechanics Research Unit, University of Southern Denmark. His research focuses on the adaptive plasticity in neuromuscular function and muscle morphology/architecture with exercise training in young and old adults, including the collateral effects on musculoskeletal health.

Andreina Alfieri is Researcher of Human Movement Sciences at the University Parthenope in Napoli, Italy. Her main research areas are functional analyses of molecular variants associated to human obesity and molecular adaptations of skeletal muscle induced by physical exercise in LHCN-M2 human myoblast cells.

Jesper L. Andersen is Senior Researcher and Head of Laboratory at the Institute of Sports Medicine Copenhagen, Bispebjerg Hospital, University of Copenhagen, Denmark. The overall focus of his research is trying to understand the mechanism behind hypertrophy/atrophy and changes in fibre type composition in skeletal muscle with use and disuse. His current research evolves around changes in myosin heavy chain isoform composition and muscle mass in skeletal muscle due to various types of exercise or inactivity. More specifically, he is looking into the influence of various growth factors in an attempt to understand pathways leading to changes in the size and phenotype of skeletal muscle. He also works with the two major football clubs in Denmark to optimise the physical training for the players, and is an Instructor for the Danish FA, UEFA and the Asian Football Confederation at the Pro License level.

Thomas Rostgaard Andersen is Sports Scientist and Lecturer at the University of Southern Denmark, Department of Sports Science and Clinical Biomechanics. His main research areas are performance changes, health benefits and muscular adaptations following team sports training with emphasis on football at the elite and recreational level. He has since 2006 been Head of Performance in several Danish premier league football clubs and is currently working as physical advisor for the Danish Under-21 national football team.

Roald Bahr is Professor of Sports Medicine in the Department of Sports Medicine at the Norwegian School of Sport Sciences and the Chair of the Oslo

Sports Trauma Research Center, Norway. He is also Chief Medical Officer for Olympiatoppen and Chair of the Medical Department at the National Olympic Training Center, as well as heading the Aspetar Sports Injury & Illness Prevention Programme. He is a fellow of the American College of Sports Medicine and serves as Team Physician for the beach volleyball national teams. He is a member of the IOC Medical Commission – Medical and Scientific Group. His main research area is sports injury prevention.

Svein Barene has a PhD in Exercise and Sports from the University in Copenhagen, Denmark, and is affiliated with the Department of Public Health and Sports Sciences, Inland Norway University of Applied Sciences, Norway. His research interest relates to physical activity and health.

Søren Bennike is Project Lead for Research and Knowledge at the Danish Football Association. His main research areas are rooted in policy and politics, institutions and organisations, implementation and innovation – all related to sport.

Mario Bizzini is Research Associate at the Schulthess Clinic, Zürich, Switzerland, where he works for the Human Performance Lab and the Swiss Concussion Centre. He also spent 12 years (2002–2016) with the FIFA Medical Research and Assessment Centre (F-MARC), and his research interests focus on prevention and rehabilitation of sports injuries.

Klaus Brasso is Professor at the Department of Clinical Medicine, University of Copenhagen, Denmark. He has been working with different aspects of prostate cancer for nearly 30 years and is active in the development of football training in prostate cancer patients in the FC Prostate trial.

João Brito is Physiologist for the Portuguese Football Federation (FPF). He was the exercise physiologist for Portugal during the EURO 2016. He collaborates with several domestic and international academic institutions, and has been involved with coaching education in UEFA A and Pro License courses. His interests are in monitoring training and competition loads, fatigue and recovery, injury prevention and recreational football for health.

Pasqualina Buono is Professor of Human Movement Sciences at the University Parthenope in Napoli, Italy. She is Team Leader of research lines focused on genetic and epigenetic determinants of human obesity, new molecular biomarkers in the fight against GH or DEHA doping, and molecular responses to exercise and sport training. She was P.I. at CEINGE – Biotecnologie Avanzate Scarl, and a Scientific Collaborator of IRCCS SDN Foundation, Napoli, Italy.

Tim Carter is Mental Health Nurse and Cognitive Behavioural Therapist who works as an Assistant Professor at the University of Nottingham, UK and a Therapist within the National Health Service. Tim's PhD examined the effects of a group exercise programme for young people with depression and his research continues to explore the impact of exercise across mental health conditions.

Carlo Castagna is Lecturer and Researcher at the School of Sport and Exercise Science of the University of Rome Tor Vergata, Italy. He is Head Sport Scientist of the fitness and technical department of the Italian Football Referees Association (AIA-FIGC) and Head of the Football Training and Biomechanics Laboratory of the Technical Department of the Italian Football Association (FIGC). His main research interests are physiology of training, match analysis, field-testing and training-load optimisation for elite, young and recreational soccer players and referees of different competitive levels.

Anna M. Cooper-Ryan is Lecturer in Public Health at the University of Salford, UK. Anna has carried out a number of research projects for local community organisations and councils to evaluate their services or explore the current evidence base around a topic they are exploring. Anna's research focuses on behaviour change interventions, with particular interest in the use of digital data collection tools within interventions and during their evaluation.

Kathryn Curran is Senior Lecturer in Physical Activity and Nutrition at Liverpool John Moores University, UK and Non-Executive Director of the European Healthy Stadia Network. Kathryn's research, teaching and consultancy focuses on the design, implementation and evaluation of community physical activity and health interventions. Kathryn is primarily interested in the social role of sport and sport stadia as a vehicle for health promotion with hard-to-reach groups. Kathryn's work and research using football as a vehicle for physical activity and health engagement with socially disadvantaged men has been championed by the World Health Organization as an example of best practices.

Jiri Dvorak is Research Consultant at the Schulthess Clinic, Zürich, Switzerland. He was the founder and the chairman of the FIFA Medical Research and Assessment Centre (F-MARC) for 23 years. He is also Professor at the University of Zurich, and his research interests are focused on the prevention of communicable and non-communicable diseases, and on injury prevention in sports. He is currently focusing on prevention of concussion in sport and prevention of injuries in golf.

Anne-Marie Elbe is Full Professor of Sport Psychology at Leipzig University, Germany. Her research interests focus on motivational and self-regulatory aspects of athletic performance, doping, the health aspects of team sports and the integrative role of sports. Anne-Marie Elbe is President of FEPSAC (The European Federation of Sport Psychology), Associate Editor for *Science and Medicine in Football* and on the editorial board of *Psychology of Sport and Exercise*.

Peter Elsborg is a postdoc researcher at Steno Diabetes Center Copenhagen, Health Promotion Research, Denmark. His research interest is the psychological factors which are important for participation in sport-based recreational physical activities in various target groups during the life-course such as motivation, volition and physical literacy.

Ioannis Fatouros is Professor of Exercise Biochemistry at the Department of Physical Education and Sports Science at University of Thessaly, Greece. His research is in the fields of strength and conditioning, exercise-induced inflammation, sports nutrition, exercise physiology and overtraining, as well as football and basketball conditioning.

Oliver Faude is Senior Researcher at the Department of Sport, Exercise and Health at the University of Basel, Switzerland. His main research areas are exercise physiology, injury prevention, football research and neuromuscular performance in various populations, from children to seniors and clinical populations.

Alex Fenton is Lecturer in Digital Business for Salford Business School, UK. He has won a range of teaching and digital industry awards for his practical digital transformation projects. He undertakes various real-world research projects including Fan Fit and works closely with various organisations including sports clubs.

Emma S. George works with health and sporting organisations to develop innovative, evidence-based community engagement initiatives to improve health and wellbeing. Her research expertise includes health promotion intervention design, implementation and evaluation, mixed methods research, men's health and community engagement. Emma's research aims to promote lifelong physical activity and improve health outcomes.

Marie Hagman is Researcher of Sport and Health Sciences, University of Southern Denmark, Denmark. Her main research areas are team sports and health with a focus on the biological ageing process in young elite football players and lifelong football and handball trained elderly.

Amri Hammami is a PhD student in Exercise Physiology with a focus on physical activity and health and team sport performance at the Laboratory of Physiology, Faculty of Medicine of Sousse in the University of Sousse, Tunisia.

Peter Riis Hansen is Senior Consultant at the Department of Cardiology, Herlev and Gentofte University Hospital, Denmark and Professor of Cardiology with a focus on inflammation and ischaemic heart disease (IHD) at the Copenhagen University Faculty of Health and Medical Sciences. Other research interests include cardiovascular effects of exercise in children and adults, pharmacoepidemiological studies of the interaction between IHD and other chronic inflammatory diseases, and strategies for precision medicine in cardiovascular disease.

Eva Wulff Helge is Associate Professor and Head of Studies in Exercise and Sport Sciences at the University of Copenhagen, Denmark. Her main research interest is health promotion through exercise and sports, with a specific focus on preventing and treating osteoporosis.

Jørn Wulff Helge is Professor in Exercise Physiology and Health at the Department of Biomedical Sciences at University of Copenhagen, Denmark. His key interests are adaptation to physical activity and inactivity with a particular emphasis on skeletal muscle, obesity, type 2 diabetes, and metabolic fitness and flexibility. In addition, he has focused on fat utilisation and the link implications for endurance performance.

Therese Hornstrup is a PhD student currently investigating the physiological and motivational effects of team handball for young, middle-aged and elderly participants. She has extensive experience as a research assistant on football training studies for untrained healthy individuals, hypertensive patients, diabetes patients and prostate cancer patients.

Niklas Rye Jørgensen is Professor and Head of Section of Clinical Biochemistry at Rigshospitalet Glostrup and Professor at Institute of Clinical Research at The University of Southern Denmark. His research focuses on the biochemical markers of bone turnover and on the biological effects of loading on bone and bone cells.

Karim Khan is Editor in Chief of the *British Journal of Sports Medicine* and Professor at the University of British Columbia in Vancouver, Canada. He serves as the Scientific Director for the Canadian Institutes of Health (CIHR) and Institute of Musculoskeletal Health and Arthritis (IMHA).

Don Kirkendall is Exercise Physiologist and Member of F-MARC and sits on the US Soccer Sports Medicine Advisory Committee. Don is also a lifelong football player and licensed coach. He brings a broad perspective on training, nutrition and specific topics in football medicine.

Birgitte Rejkjær Krustrup is Football Development Officer at the Danish Football Association Zealand (DBU Sjælland). She has worked with health promotion through physical activity for 15 years and has taken part in the evaluation and implementation of several football for health concepts. Her main research interest is the development of social capital in team sports.

Malte Nejst Larsen is Teaching Assistant Professor at the Department of Sports Science and Clinical Biomechanics, University of Southern Denmark. Research interests focus on football and other types of exercises in terms of health promotion for all children, as well as the physical and technical demands of youth players.

Felipe Lobelo is Associate Professor in the Hubert Department of Global Health at Emory's Rollins School of Public Health, USA. Dr. Lobelo's interests are in chronic disease prevention, physical activity, obesity and cardio-metabolic diseases in high and low-to-middle income countries. He is a member of ACSM's Exercise is Medicine Initiative advisory board, directing their Global Research and Collaboration Center. Dr. Lobelo has a special interest in global health and health disparities in both non-communicable and infectious diseases. In 2006, he was the recipient of the prestigious ACSM Paffenbarger-Blair Award for Research on Physical Activity Epidemiology, and in 2012 was elected as Fellow of the AHA's Nutrition, Physical Activity and Metabolism Council.

Annamaria Mancini is Researcher of Human Movement Sciences at the University Parthenope in Napoli, Italy. Her main research areas are physical activity and health, and molecular adaptations of skeletal muscle induced by lifelong football training in elderly subjects.

Jannick Marschall is Head of the Physiotherapy programme at University College Copenhagen, Denmark. He is the former Physiotherapist of the homeless national team of Denmark and has for many years been involved in developmental projects, rehabilitation projects and research projects related to the use of football for the socially deprived and homeless.

Paulina S. Melby is a PhD student at the Department of Nutrition, Exercise and Sports at the University of Copenhagen, Denmark. Her primary research areas are physical literacy, diversified physical activity, motor competence proficiency, physical activity and perceived sport competences in children.

Amy E. Mendham is Research Fellow in the Division of Exercise Science and Sports Medicine in the Department of Human Biology at the University of Cape Town, South Africa. Amy investigates the mechanisms underlying insulin resistance in indigenous populations.

Julie Midtgaard is Associate Professor at The Department of Public Health at The University of Copenhagen, Denmark and Senior Researcher at The Copenhagen University Hospital Rigshospitalet. Her areas of special interest include exercise-based rehabilitation, health promotion and tertiary prevention across several medical subspecialties. Her particular interests are on issues related to pragmatic (effectiveness) trials supporting real-world decision-making and implementation.

Zoran Milanović is Assistant Professor at the Faculty of Sport and Physical Education, University of Nis, Serbia and Researcher at the Institute for Kinesiology Research, Koper, Slovenia. His main research areas are training, testing and performance in team sports. He is particularly interested in the health benefits of team sports, especially football.

Magni Mohr is Professor of Tracking, Training and Testing in Football at the University of Southern Denmark, and professor in Exercise Physiology at the University of Faroe Islands. His main research areas are skeletal muscle physiology and human performance with an emphasis on fatigue development during high-intensity intermittent exercise, and the health effects of sports with a primary focus on team sports training. He is part of the Football Fitness research group at the University of Southern Denmark. He has worked as

Fitness Coach and Performance Director for several European top-teams and national teams. He is also an UEFA and FIFA instructor and teaches fitness training at Pro License courses around the world.

George P. Nassis is a Sports Scientist and Exercise Physiologist with research interest and publications in football performance and health. He is academic staff at City Unity College, Athens, Greece, and guest professor at Shanghai University of Sport. George co-founded Panathinaikos FC Performance Lab and served as its head for more than 5 years. He is Fellow of the European College of Sport Science, Senior Associate Editor for the *British Journal of Sports Medicine* and Editorial Board Member for the *Science and Medicine in Football* journal.

Jens Jung Nielsen holds a PhD in exercise physiology, and is working as a member of the academic staff in the research unit of Integrative Physiology at the University of Copenhagen, Denmark. His research interests include fatigue development during dynamic exercise and the training effects of team sports, such as football, team handball and basketball.

Lars Nybo is Professor in Human Physiology at the University of Copenhagen, Denmark. His main research area relates to fatigue mechanisms and performance optimisation with special reference to exercise in the heat. Studies include highly specialised and invasive lab experiments as well as applied field studies. Furthermore, he is involved in the guidance of national and international athletes preparing for competitions in adverse environmental settings.

Stefania Orrù is Associate Professor of Human Movement Sciences at the University Parthenope in Napoli, Italy. Her main research interests are: to define the molecular effects of doping agents on biological systems, to define protein markers related to exercise and healthy ageing and to evaluate physical fitness in young people.

Laila Ottesen is Associate Professor at the University of Copenhagen, Denmark and a member of the steering committee at Copenhagen Centre for Team Sport and Health. Her main research areas are rooted in the sociology of sport and health summed up by the keywords Voluntary Organisations, Implementation, Sport Policy, Health Promotion and Prevention.

Keith D. Parry is Senior Lecturer at the University of Winchester, UK and an Associate Fellow of Western Sydney University, Australia. His research interests are based on the sociology of sport, with a focus on sports fandom and the spectator experience. He is an award-winning writer, receiving a UN Day Media Award for a co-authored media piece 'Pushing casual sport to the margins threatens cities' social cohesion'.

Svein Arne Pettersen is Associate Professor at School of Sport Sciences and Head of Research at Alfheim Research Lab, University of Tromsø, The

Norwegian Arctic University. He is also Project Leader in 'From Elite Sport to Public Health' and member of the Corpore Sano Centre. His main research areas are tracking and testing in football from children to elite athletes and the innovation, implementation and daily use of technology in professional football.

Gertrud Pfister is Full Professor at the University of Copenhagen, Denmark. She was awarded with the Order of Merit of the Federal Republic of Germany, and knighted by the queen of Denmark. Pfister conducted a number of large national and international research projects, many of them focused on gender issues in sport and society. Pfister continues to play a leading role in scientific communities; she was President of the International Society for the History of Physical Education and Sport and of the International Sport Sociology Association.

Matthew Philpott is Executive Director of European Healthy Stadia Network and CEO of the Health Equalities Group. He is responsible for the overall operations and growth of Healthy Stadia, including partnership development and programme management, and liaises directly with key partners at UEFA, EU and European public health agencies.

Alan Pringle is Mental Health Nurse who works as Assistant Professor at the University of Nottingham's School of Health Sciences, UK. Alan's PhD examined the impact on mental health of supporting a small football professional club (Mansfield Town FC), and he has been involved in the design, development, delivery and evaluation of mental health projects in football clubs in various parts of the UK.

Susana Póvoas is Assistant Professor at the University Institute of Maia and member of the Research Center in Sports Sciences, Health Sciences and Human Development, in Portugal. Her research is focused on tracking, testing and performance enhancement of youth and elite-level team sports athletes and on physical activity and exercise, including the effects of recreational team sports on health and physical fitness of different populations across the lifespan. She is the international coordinator of the Handball4Health project and the national Portuguese coordinator of the Football Fitness programme.

Morten B. Randers is Associate Professor at the University of Southern Denmark and a Guest Professor at the University of Tromsø, The Norwegian Arctic University. His research interests lie in the field of football – fitness and health effects for untrained and recreational players, as well as testing and performance enhancement in elite football players. He has worked as a Fitness Coach in a Danish Premier League club and for the Danish elite referees.

Kenneth Grønlund Rasmussen is Head of Project and Analysis at the Danish Football Association and former Project Lead for the implementation of the Football Fitness concept. He is a member of the Danish FA Grassroots

Committee and UEFA Grassroots panel. He is among others working with strategies related to UEFA, the Danish Sports Federation and several other partners including NGOs.

Jessica Richards researches in areas related to sports fandom, gender and stadium geography. Her current research focuses on fan experiences in new sporting stadiums and the rise and visibility of female sport/female athletes in the sportscape.

Knud Ryom is a postdoc researcher at Department of Public Health, Aarhus University, Denmark. His research interest is in the field of sport and exercise psychology and public health. A special interest is inactivity, physical literacy and health behavior. He also serves as Sports Psychologist for the Danish Ice Hockey Federation.

Mikael Rørth is Professor at the Department of Clinical Epidemiology at Aarhus University, Denmark. He has worked with germ cell tumours – pathophysiology, treatment and late effects; and is involved in physical rehabilitation of cancer patients, including football.

André Seabra is Auxiliar Professor with Aggregation at the Faculty of Sport, University of Porto, Portugal. He is also the Director of the Portugal Football School – Portugal Football Association. His research interests are in the field of epidemiology of physical activity and more particularly in the use of football as a strategy to promote active and healthy lifestyles in children and adolescents.

Fabio Serpiello is Senior Lecturer in Sports Physiology and Chair of the Master of Sports Science (Football Performance). His research is in the area of exercise physiology and training adaptations related to team sport training. He is also Head of Academy Performance and Sport Science at Melbourne Victory FC, Australia.

Maysa Vieira de Sousa is a Sports Nutrition Researcher at the Endocrinology Division, School of Medicine of University of Sao Paulo, Brazil. Her research interests focus on the impact of nutritional and physical training interventions on physical performance, hormonal and molecular modulations of highly competitive athletes, and improving health in chronic metabolic disease. She has been working as a licensed Sports Dietitian over 17 years.

Andy Stevens is Senior Lecturer in Sport Management at the University of Winchester, UK. Previously, he was a consultant to the Football Association, specialising in five-a-side football and futsal.

Jacob Uth has nearly 20 years of experience in physiotherapy and rehabilitation for patients with cancer and neurological diseases. His PhD dissertation was related to the health effects of football training for men with prostate cancer and he is currently a postdoc at The University Hospitals Centre for Health Research in Copenhagen, Denmark, focusing on the health effects of football training for women treated for breast cancer.

Cristina M. Vasilica is Researcher and Lecturer in Digital Health & Society. Her research interests focus on digital skills and creating digital tools which embed sustainable engagement strategies in the healthcare and educational context. She explores the expansion of digital/social media and emerging technologies across different contexts, combining technical understanding with theoretical constructs to impact real-life information provision, individual engagement in health and social care.

Michael Viggars is Project Manager at the European Healthy Stadia Network based in the UK. Michael is responsible for the planning, delivery and implementation of several key projects that address a range of lifestyle risk factors across the life course. He also provides policy guidance and consultancy support to key stakeholders including professional sports clubs, their stadia, their community programmes and governing bodies of sport.

Dimitris Vlachopoulos is Lecturer at the Sport and Health Sciences department within Children's Health and Exercise Research Centre (CHERC), UK. His research focuses on musculoskeletal development and exercise during growth. Throughout the years, Dimitris has been awarded with 5 New/Young Investigator Awards at international conferences and received the Neil Mackenzie Public Engagement Award and the Barbara Mawer Travel Fellowship from the Bone Research Society. He was also elected New Investigator Representative (non-clinical) of the Bone Research Society in 2018.

Paul Widdop is Senior Research Fellow at Leeds Beckett University, UK. His research focuses on the consumption, production and social and spatial inequalities of sport and culture in society. Underlying these academic fields, his substantive research area is in the importance of place and networks. In addition, he studies the theory and methodology of Social Network Analysis.

Johan M. Wikman is Assistant Professor at the Academy for Health and Welfare, Halmstad University, Sweden. His research interests are motivation for sport and exercise, psychological aspects of sport and exercise, sport psychological interventions and talent development. He also serves as Editor-in-Chief of the *Scandinavian Journal of Sport and Exercise Psychology*.

Craig A. Williams is Professor and Director of the Children's Health and Exercise Research Centre, UK. He is an internationally recognised expert on paediatric exercise physiology whose research work focuses on the physiological responses of exercise training of young people.

Jincheng Xu, PhD, Associate Professor, graduated from Beijing Sport University in 2015. Worked in China Institute of Sport Science from 2015–2018 and is currently working in the Chinese Winter Sports Administration Center preparing for the 2022 Beijing Winter Olympic Games. Main research fields: Sport and Exercise and Health; training monitoring; performance enhancement.

Mette K. Zebis, MSc, PhD in Exercise Physiology and is working as Senior Associate Lecturer at University College Copenhagen, Denmark. Her main research areas relate to investigations into injury occurrence in various sports, injury prevention and return to play after injuries as well as examinations of the use of various training types for vulnerable subject groups.

Foreword

The idea of sport for health goes back at least as far as Hippocrates' time – Hygea. Football may have predated that, as there are reports of a type of football in China in 2500 BC. The 'Cambridge Rules' and the UK 'Football Association' came to birth in the mid-1800s. The sport has given men and women pleasure as participants and as a fabric of communities for at least several hundred, if not thousands, of years.

We believe football has promoted physical and mental health, and possibly societal happiness, for all those years. To be fair we must report adverse events, too, and football has seen too many mass tragedies, as well as the death of individual players the world over.

The purpose of this book is to increase awareness of the physical health, mental health and societal benefits of football. Professors Peter Krustrup, Daniel Parnell and colleagues have done a remarkable job of capturing the science and locating it in one easy-to-read book. This book is important and unique. It provides a blueprint for Football as Health – also known as Football Fitness.

We fully support the vision of Peter Krustrup and the global breadth of scholars who contribute to the collective effort to harness the power of football to make our world a better one. At first, reading these words may sound like hyperbole – over the top – but they withstand scrutiny as they are accurate. The scientists and clinicians offer evidence which cannot be ignored! Because of the world's appetite for football, the beautiful game can be a force for health and wellbeing. But, like any force – consider fire as an example – football needs to be wielded wisely.

To international governments, sporting organisations/football leaders, health policy makers and clinicians we say, 'Study this book and implement the programs, because when football talks people listen'.

Professors Jiri Dvorak,
Karim Khan and Roald Bahr

Introduction

Football as Medicine

Peter Krustrup and Daniel Parnell

Football has long been a subject of philosophical analysis and has been featured in various historical and cultural narratives, which should come as no surprise given its status as the world's favourite game. In an editorial to the recent *Football is Medicine* special issue of the *Scandinavian Journal of Medicine & Science in Sports*, the concept of football as therapy is illustrated through the French philosopher Voltaire, who describes the potential of football in *The Book of Fate* (1747):

> full-blown and carefully cover'd with the softest Leather. You must kick this Bladder, Sir, once a Day about your Hall for a whole Hour together, with all the Vigour and Activity you possibly can. . . . Ogul, upon making the first Experiment, was ready to expire for want of Breath. . . . In short, our Doctor in about eight Days Time, perform'd an absolute Cure. His Patient was as brisk, active and gay, as One in the Bloom of his Youth.
>
> (De Voltaire, 1747/2008; Krustrup et al., 2018)

From Shakespeare to Shankly, football has been a focus of debate, and it will no doubt continue to be so. Leeds United manager Marcelo Bielsa stated, as shared by our colleague Jon Mackenzie:

> What happens to their team has a great impact on the life of fans. If the game is won, you feel better and it affects your personal life. If the team loses, you become proportionally depressed, it affects everything you do.

Pioneering Professor of the Sociology of Sport John Sugden stated, 'sport is intrinsically value neutral and under carefully managed circumstances it can make a positive if modest contribution to peace building' (Sugden, 2010) and that 'sport alone will not change the world . . . but doing nothing may no longer be an option' (Sugden, 2005).

Indeed, in certain sections of society football has a kind of capital – not too dissimilar to political and social capital – in that it has power to change, constitutes a resource for hope and can offer many health benefits to those who have access to it. Furthermore, it is arguable that when football capital is combined with social capital, its social benefits can diffuse through the network and act as a social learning tool and genuine positive social activity. If, therefore, we draw on Voltaire and extend the quote of Albert Camus, who outlined something slightly different during his interview in the 1950s – 'What little I know on morality, I learned it on football pitches and theater stages. Those were my true universities'. – we propose that this book brings together evidence on what we have learnt from the football pitches, our universities, on whether football can work as a form of medicine, and then provides considerations for future research and applied practice.

We have been working on the football and health agenda for 17 and 12 years, respectively. Peter began his research in this area in 2003 through observational pilot studies on the movement patterns, exercise intensity and fitness benefits of football training in Danish low-level senior and veteran players, homeless men and sedentary computer enthusiasts. In the latter study, 16 computer enthusiasts came together as FC Zulu, and the pilot results demonstrated an average increase in VO_2max from 35 to 52 mL/min/kg over 2 years. This led to the first randomised controlled trials (RCTs) in 2006–2009 comparing football training with other popular exercise regimes like jogging, interval running and strength training for sedentary young men (Krustrup et al., 2009; Krustrup et al., 2010a) and women (Krustrup et al., 2010b; Krustrup, Helge, Hansen et al., 2018; Ottesen et al., 2010) and schoolchildren (Krustrup et al., 2014). Later, Peter conducted numerous RCTs incorporating football training in patient groups with hypertension, type 2 diabetes, osteopenia, prostate cancer and breast cancer (Krustrup et al., 2010a; Krustrup et al., 2013; Milanović et al., 2015; Uth et al., 2016; Krustrup, Williams, Mohr et al., 2018; Krustrup, Helge, Hansen et al., 2018; Skoradal et al., 2018; Milanović et al., 2019). Based on the results of these investigations, which combined physiological, medical, psychological and sociological methodologies, Peter and his wife Birgitte developed a holistic Football is Medicine model (Krustrup & Krustrup, 2018) (Figure 0.1).

This model describes the cardiovascular, metabolic and musculoskeletal training components of recreational football training; training-induced adaptations in fitness and health variables; and use of football training in the prevention, treatment and rehabilitation of non-communicable diseases. The model also describes the psychosocial elements of acute recreational football training as well as the long-term psychosocial training-induced effects and the possibility of creating adherence to an active lifestyle. Over the past decade, Peter and his team have also been heavily involved in the practical application of their football for health research, specifically the development, testing, adjustment and implementation of evidence-based concepts using football as a tool for increasing fitness, health profile, well-being and learning for children (FIT FIRST and 11 for Health), young and older sedentary adults (Football Fitness), patients (Football Fitness ABC [After Breast Cancer], FC Prostate and Football for the Heart) and socially deprived people. This has been done in close collaboration with the Danish FA, the Danish Sports Confederation, Danish charities, and international football and sports governing bodies.

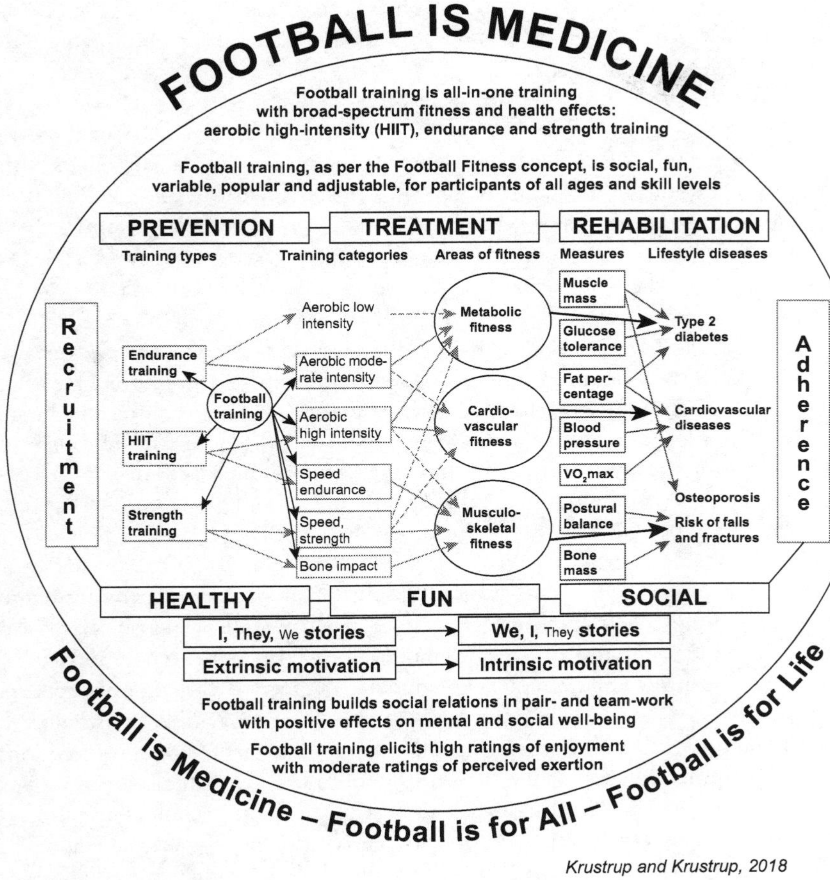

Figure 0.1 The Holistic Football is Medicine model.
Source: Adapted from Krustrup & Krustrup, *British Journal of Sports Medicine*, 2018.

Dan began his research in 2006 examining the effectiveness of a football-based community intervention delivered by an English Premier League football club, Everton FC. The intervention examined the impact of a 16-week football programme in primary-school children using a multi-method evaluation which included pedometers, physical activity diaries, writing and drawing exercises, interviews, focus groups and the principles of ethnography. The findings pointed to a number of opportunities for strategic and operational changes to improve the effectiveness of interventions (Parnell et al., 2013a). This intervention, part of a broader action research project within the club, entailed Dan shifting his focus from intervention evaluation towards helping manage positive change in practice at Everton FC. Some of the areas of attention and focus over the remaining years of his PhD were developing a clear strategic purpose and objectives; recruiting appropriately skilled staff; providing relevant, continued professional development opportunities to the coaching staff and practitioners; promoting a culture of research and evaluation (i.e. understanding what works and making practice more effective); and creating meaningful partnerships with relevant higher-education departments with a clear focus on helping practitioners improve their practice (i.e. engaging in action research) (see Parnell et al., 2013a). Dan's research then evolved in a collaborative partnership at Everton FC through the creation of a community-facing facility to support activity for the local community within the Everton Active Family Centre (Curran et al., 2014; Bingham et al., 2014). He went on to establish a number of partnerships, working with many clubs and organisations on initiatives primarily focused on evaluation (Parnell et al., 2015), but also on providing genuine partnerships and professional development for clubs and the staff involved (Parnell et al., 2013a). His current interests include the impact of policy and politics on football, and the role of corporate social responsibility in professional football (Parnell et al., 2013b; Parnell, Curran and Philpott, 2016).

We are both fortunate to be able to exercise our passion for football through our coaching practice and engagement with the sport. Moreover, we are committed to understanding the role that football can play in health. As such, this book on Football as Medicine brings together a culmination of extensive research in the field of football and health. The 17 chapters of this edited collection aim to provide sharp, critical analysis of key features and topics that underpin Football as Medicine. Each chapter critically analyses its respective area and provides key considerations and/or recommendations for the prescription of Football as Medicine, as well as future research. The book should be an important addition for politicians, policy-makers and analysts, researchers and academics, sports developers, educationists and coaches, and the general public, who frequently assume that sport is good for us and that participation in sport offers a range of public-health benefits. This book collates the accumulated and extensive evidence to provide both the substance and rationale for Football as Medicine, providing a basis for the role that football can play in promoting health. It provides the most comprehensive analysis of the most recent and contemporary research in the field, with a broad variety of research approaches, including sports physiology, training physiology, sports medicine, sports psychology and sports management.

The first part of the book mostly focuses on the physiological response to various types of recreational football and training-induced fitness adaptations in relation to the cardiovascular, metabolic and musculoskeletal health profile. Similarly, several chapters deal with the training-induced fitness and health effects of football in specific target populations (children, cancer patients, socially deprived, elderly), football training in specific settings (schools, sports clubs and workplaces) and injury-prevention strategies. The book also has several chapters on

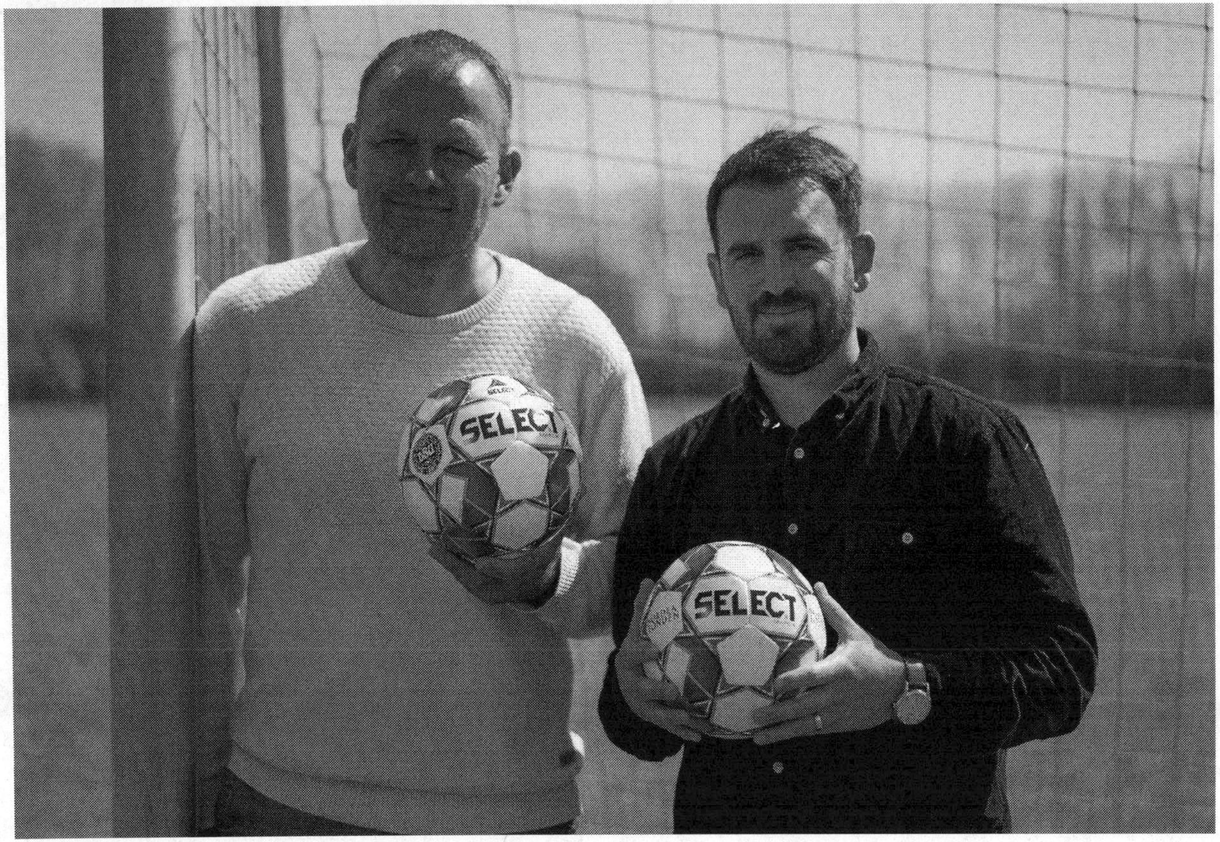

Photo 0.1 The book editors, Peter Krustrup and Dan Parnell.

Source: Photo Credit: Bo Kousgaard, University of Southern Denmark.

the motivational and psychosocial climate during recreational football training and the training-induced psychosocial effects of long-term football in relation to wellbeing and mental health. The last part of the book mostly focuses on the development and implementation of evidence-based football training concepts, and how fan culture and fan programmes can influence population health. Last, but not least, there is a discussion of how the evidence and concepts presented on the potential use of football for global health promotion can be taken up and applied by health workers and policymakers around the world.

References

de Voltaire, F.-M.A., Zadig, ou la Destinée (Zadig, or the Book of Fate, an Oriental History). (1747/2008). *Chapter XV: The Basilisk.* (English translation). Boston, MA: Mobile Reference.

Bingham, D.D., Parnell, D., Curran, K., Jones, R., & Richardson, D. (2014). "Fit fans: Perspectives of a practitioner and understanding participant health needs within a health promotion programme for older men delivered within an English Premier League Football Club." *Soccer & Society* 15(6): 883–901.

Curran, K, Bingham, D.D., Richardson, D., & Parnell, D. (2014). "Ethnographic engagement from within a football in the community programme at an English Premier League Football Club." *Soccer & Society* 15(6): 934–950.

Krustrup, P., Aagaard, P., Nybo, L., et al. (2010a) "Recreational football as a health promoting activity: A topical review." *Scandinavian Journal of Medicine and Science in Sports* 20(Suppl 1): 1–13.

Krustrup, P., Hansen, P.R., Nielsen, C.M., Larsen, M.N., Randers, M.B., Manniche, V., Hansen, L., Junge, A., Dvorak, J., & Bangsbo, J. (2014). "Cardiovascular adaptations to a 10-wk small-sided school football intervention for 9–10-year-old children." *Scandinavian Journal of Medicine and Science in Sports* 24(Suppl 1): 4–9.

Krustrup, P., Hansen, P.R., Randers, M.B., et al. (2010b). "Beneficial effects of recreational football on the cardiovascular risk profile in untrained premenopausal women." *Scandinavian Journal of Medicine and Science in Sports* 20(Suppl 1): 40–49.

Krustrup, P., Helge, E.W., Hansen, P.R., et al. (2018). "Effects of recreational football on women's fitness and health: Adaptations and mechanisms." *European Journal of Applied Physiology* 118: 11–32.

Krustrup, P., Krustrup, B.R. (2018). "Football is medicine: It is time for patients to play!" *British Journal of Sports Medicine* 52(22): 1412–1414.

Krustrup, P., Nielsen, J.J., Krustrup, B.R., et al. (2009). "Recreational soccer is an effective health-promoting activity for untrained men." *British Journal of Sports Medicine* 43: 825–831.

Krustrup, P., Randers, M.B., Andersen, L.J., et al. (2013). Soccer improves fitness and attenuates cardiovascular risk factors in hypertensive men. *Medicine and Science in Sports and Exercise* 45(3): 553–560.

Krustrup, P., Williams, C.A., Mohr, M., et al. (2018). "The 'football is medicine' platform-scientific evidence, large-scale implementation of evidence-based concepts and future perspectives." *Scandinavian Journal of Medicine and Science in Sports* 28(Suppl 1): 3–7.

Milanović, Z., Pantelić, S., Čović, N., et al. (2015). "Is recreational soccer effective for improving VO_2 max a systematic review and meta-analysis." *Sports Medicine* 45: 1339–1353.

Milanović, Z., Pantelić, S., Čović, N., et al. (2019). Broad-spectrum physical fitness benefits of recreational football: A systematic review and meta-analysis. *British Journal of Sports Medicine* 53(15): 926–939.

Ottesen, L., Jeppesen, R.S., & Krustrup, B.R. (2010). "The development of social capital through football and running: Studying an intervention program for inactive women." *Scandinavian Journal of Medicine and Science in Sports* 20(Suppl 1): 118–131.

Parnell, D., Curran, K., & Philpott, M. (2016). "Healthy stadia: An insight from policy to practice." *Sport in Society* 20(2), 181–186.

Parnell, D., Stratton, G., Drust, B., & Richardson, D. (2013a). "Football in the Community schemes: Exploring the effectiveness of an intervention in promoting positive healthful behaviour change." *Soccer and Society* 14, 1, 1–17.

Parnell, D., Stratton, G., Drust, B., & Richardson, D. (2013b). "Implementing 'monitoring and evaluation' techniques within a premier league football in the community scheme: A case study involving Everton in the Community." In Kathy Babiak, Juan Paramio & Geoff Walters (eds.) March 2013. *The Handbook of Sport and Corporate Social Responsibility*. Routledge: London.

Parnell, D., Pringle, A., Zwolinsky, S., McKenna, J., Rutherford, R., Richardson, D., Trotter, L., Rigby, M., & Hargreaves, J. (2015). "Reaching older people with physical activity delivered in football clubs: The reach, adoption and implementation characteristics of the extra time programme." *BMC Public Health* 15: 220. Doi: 10.1186/s12889-015-1560-5. http://www.biomedcentral.com/1471-2458/15/220

Skoradal, M.B., Weihe, P., Patursson, P., Mortensen, J., Connolly, L., Krustrup, P., & Mohr, M. (2018). "Football training improves metabolic and cardiovascular health status in 55- to 70-year-old women and men with prediabetes." *Scandinavian Journal of Medicine and Science in Sports* 28(Suppl 1): 42–51.

Sugden, J. (2005). "Sport and community relations in Northern Ireland and Israel." In Bairner, A. (ed.), *Sport and the Irish: Histories, Identities, Issues*. Dublin: University College Dublin Press, 238–251.

Sugden, J. (2010). "Critical left realisms and sport interventions in divided societies." *International Review for the Sociology of Sport* 45(3): 258–272.

Uth, J., Hornstrup, T., Christensen, J.F., Christensen, K.B., Jørgensen, N.R., Helge, E.W., Schmidt, J.F., et al. (2016). "Football training in men with prostate cancer undergoing androgen deprivation therapy: Activity profile and short-term skeletal and postural balance adaptations." *European Journal of Applied Physiology* 116(3): 471–480.

Chapter 1

Football as Medicine against cardiovascular disease

Magni Mohr, Peter Riis Hansen, Felipe Lobelo, Lars Nybo, Zoran Milanović and Peter Krustrup

Exercise as treatment for cardiovascular disease

Cardiovascular disease (CVD) encompasses multiple pathological conditions for which exercise may be a significant part of the treatment protocol, including cerebrovascular disease, hypertension, coronary heart disease, heart failure and intermittent claudication.

Cerebrovascular disease, including stroke, transient ischemic attack and cerebral bleeding, is clinically defined as a rapid onset disorder of brain function with symptoms lasting more than 24 hours or causing death. The cause is likely to be of vascular origin. Average age of the patients is 75 years, however 20% are younger than 65 years. Parts of brain functions deteriorate, and symptomatic stroke patients mainly have unilateral paresis of extremities. In addition, about one third also experience aphasia. Some stroke patients may also display cognitive and emotional impairment, and around 30% experience post-stroke depression (Paolucci et al. 2006). Patients with prior stroke are therefore likely to be physically inactive (Rand et al. 2009). Physical inactivity is a major cause for atherosclerotic disease and hypertension, which is supported by epidemiological findings demonstrating that physical inactivity is a predictor of apoplexy (Hu et al. 2007; Krarup et al. 2007; Krarup et al. 2008; Sui, LaMonte, and Blair 2007; Boysen and Krarup 2009). In contrast, stroke patients who have a high physical activity level display comparatively fewer severe subsequent strokes and show superior recovery results compared to their inactive counterparts (Krarup et al. 2008).

Hypertension markedly elevates the risk of stroke, coronary artery disease (CAD) such as acute myocardial infarction, heart failure and sudden death. Epidemiological reports indicate that regular physical exercise and a high fitness level prevents hypertension (Fagard 2005; Fagard and Cornelissen 2007, 2005). Lewington and colleagues (2002) demonstrated a linear relationship between a reduced cardiovascular mortality rate and the lowering of arterial blood pressure to a systolic blood pressure of below 115 mmHg and a diastolic blood pressure of below 75 mmHg (Lewington et al. 2002). A decline of 20 mmHg in systolic blood pressure or 10 mmHg in diastolic blood pressure induced a 50% reduction in risk of cardiovascular mortality. Thus, an individual with systolic blood pressure of 120 mmHg has half the cardiovascular mortality risk of a person with systolic blood pressure of 140 mmHg (Pedersen and Saltin, 2015). Despite this, arterial hypertension is still diagnosed as systolic blood pressure >140 mmHg and diastolic blood pressure >90 mmHg. According to this definition, ~20% of the population suffer from arterial hypertension or require blood pressure-lowering medication (Burt et al. 1995). However, the definitions of optimal and normal blood pressure and of mild, moderate and severe hypertension are arbitrary (Burt et al. 1995) and the paradox of optimal and normal arterial blood pressure is highly complex. CAD that impairs the blood flow supply to the myocardium cells will provoke myocardial ischaemia. The principal cause is atherosclerothrombosis-induced obstruction of the coronary arteries, but myocardial ischaemia can also develop in patients with other heart conditions. Physical activity level and aerobic fitness status are positively associated with adverse cardiovascular endpoints in healthy individuals, as well as patients diagnosed with CAD (Myers et al. 2002).

Heart failure patients have attenuated maintenance of blood flow to cover the metabolic demands of the peripheral tissue (Braunwald and Libby 2008). The most common symptoms are fluid retention, breathlessness or tiredness when resting or exercising, and can relate to impaired systolic function of the left ventricle (Pedersen and Saltin, 2015). Heart failure syndrome can be initiated by CAD, but can additionally be provoked by hypertension or valvular heart disease (Braunwald and Libby 2008). Since the capacity for peripheral oxygen delivery and consumption is deteriorated in heart failure patients (Sullivan et al. 1989), they are likely to encompass a low daily physical activity level, which may impair quality of life and induce a negative impact on adaptability to exercise training. This may attenuate myocardial function and peripheral complications in skeletal myocytes (Pedersen and Saltin 2015). Heart failure patients may consequently also develop muscle atrophy, tiredness and low muscle strength (Anker et al. 1997; Harrington et al. 1997). Finally, heart failure patients experience a myriad of homeostasis dysfunctions (Bradham et al. 2002), including insulin resistance (Paolisso et al. 1991). The characteristic symptom of accelerated tiredness is likely to impair physical abilities, creating a vicious circle that patients with heart failure may partly reverse by regular exercise training (Pedersen and Saltin 2015).

Lower limbs arterial insufficiency, such as symptomatic ischaemia in the legs, is a chronic obstructive disease in the aorta below the outlet of the renal arteries, the iliac artery and the arteries in the legs provoked by atherosclerosis (Pedersen and Saltin 2015). Peripheral arteriosclerotic disease increases with increasing age, and since conventional medical treatment of the condition has poor outcome exercise training is a major component in the treatment (TASC 2000). When the condition develops and becomes severe, the patients experience a marked impairment in function level and deterioration of quality of life. Patients often have increasing pain when walking and the exercise anxiety, may gradually cause physical inactivity and social isolation. This further leads to deterioration of physical ability and the progression of atherosclerosis, reduced muscle strength and muscle atrophy.

Thus, exercise training should be applied to counteract this negative spiral and target the pathogenesis of the condition by increasing training status and muscle strength, changing pain perception, reducing the degree of exercise anxiety and preventing the progression of the disease.

Aerobic exercise training for stroke patients has substantiated clear positive effects on walking speed and CV function, and some evidence for reducing mortality (Pedersen and Saltin 2015). In relation to hypertension, meta-analyses have concluded that physical exercise has a positive impact on blood pressure in both normotensive and hypertensive individuals (Fagard and Cornelissen 2007; Cornelissen, Buys, and Smart 2013; Cornelissen and Smart 2013; Huang et al. 2013). Meta-analysis evidence demonstrate an effect of both aerobic and strength training (Pedersen and Saltin 2015). Additionally, there is strong documentation in favour of beneficial effects of exercise training on patients with CAD. Exercise training increases survival rates and may have a direct effect on the pathogenesis of the disease. Aerobic training at moderate intensities is recommended for this patient group (Pedersen and Saltin 2015). Moreover, international guidelines recommend exercise training for patients with heart failure since numerous studies demonstrated the beneficial effect on central and peripheral factors, as well on function abilities and quality of life without significant negative side-effects (Hunt et al. 2005; Swedberg et al. 2005). Indeed, the positive effects of exercise training on patients with heart failure has been assessed in numerous meta-analyses (Hwang and Marwick 2009; Davies et al. 2010; Pedersen and Saltin 2015), interval training is suggested as exercise treatment protocol for heart failure patients (Pedersen and Saltin 2015). Finally, there is strong evidence for the beneficial effect of exercise training on patients with intermittent claudication. In a Cochrane review (Lane et al. 2014) analysing 30 trials and nearly 2000 participants with continuous leg pain showed positive effects of different exercise regimes ranging from strength to aerobic exercise. Collectively, there is clear scientific evidence that exercise training should be deployed to treat a wide range of CVDs, though the training protocols differ. Thus, complex training protocols, such as football training, can be suggested for targeting several of the pathophysiological mechanisms in cardiovascular patients.

Effects of football on cardiac structure and function

CVD, e.g., CAD, stroke, arrhythmias and heart failure, account for approximately 1 in every 3 deaths, and in high-income countries, IHD remains the leading cause of death, albeit IHD mortality has declined over the past decade (Benjamin et al. 2017). Also, CVD rates are increasing on a global scale owing to, for example, the aging population and increased urbanisation, with environmental pollution, nutritional transition to more animal-source, processed and sugar-rich food, lack of physical exercise and other factors fuelling the epidemic rise in major CVD risk factors such as obesity, diabetes and hypertension (Laslett et al. 2012). Although exercise is a safe and effective intervention for primary and secondary prevention of CVD, it is well recognised that it remains poorly implemented in clinical practice. Lack of time is a frequently cited barrier to exercise, and shorter-duration high-intensity interval training may be a time-efficient way to achieve multifaceted health benefits that can lead to reduction of CVD (Karlsen et al. 2017; Weston, Wisloff, and Coombes 2014). Also, there is ample evidence to suggest that team sports, including football, offer a range of positive psychological and psychosocial effects that promote participation in and adherence to the sport irrespective of the subject's age and the presence of chronic somatic or mental conditions (Andersen, Ottesen, and Thing 2018). On several parameters, the physiological load characteristics of football training are similar to high-interval aerobic training, and here we provide a short overview of the effects of football on the cardiovascular system and circulating lipid levels (Iaia, Rampinini, and Bangsbo 2009; Bangsbo et al. 2015; Krustrup et al. 2018).

Effects of football on the cardiovascular system and circulating lipid levels

Myocardial structure and function

Physical inactivity is an important contributor to childhood obesity and is associated with a clustering of cardiovascular risk factors that track into adulthood and are linked with increased subclinical atherosclerosis in young adulthood and increased risk of CVD in adults (Andersen et al. 2011; Pahkala et al. 2011; Baker, Olsen, and Sorensen 2007). There are limited studies of the effects of football training on myocardial structure and function in children, but significant increases in left-ventricular posterior-wall thickness and right-ventricular systolic function have been demonstrated by echocardiography after football training in obese children, and discrete cardiac adaptations were found in normal-weight, school-aged, football-playing boys and children of both genders in response to a school-based football intervention (Barczuk-Falecka et al. 2018; Krustrup et al. 2014; Larsen et al. 2018; Hansen et al. 2013).

In randomised controlled studies with football as the intervention, favourable changes in left-ventricular dimensions and systolic and diastolic functions have also been reported, as well as amelioration of right-ventricular function in untrained premenstrual women, hypertensive men, men with type 2 diabetes and elderly men, respectively, compared to control subjects (Andersen et al. 2010, 2014; Schmidt et al. 2013, 2014). In addition, a cross-sectional study showed that left-ventricular systolic function was increased in veteran football players compared to untrained elderly healthy men (Schmidt et al. 2015). Intriguingly, football was not associated with changes of echocardiographic variables in elderly men with prostate cancer undergoing androgen deprivation therapy, suggesting that the latter may diminish the myocardial effects of football training (Schmidt et al. 2015, 2017).

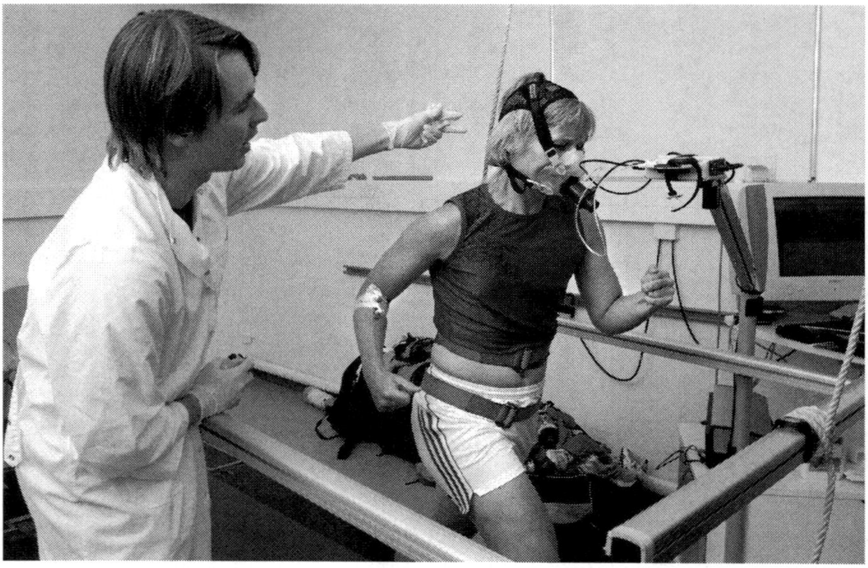

(a)

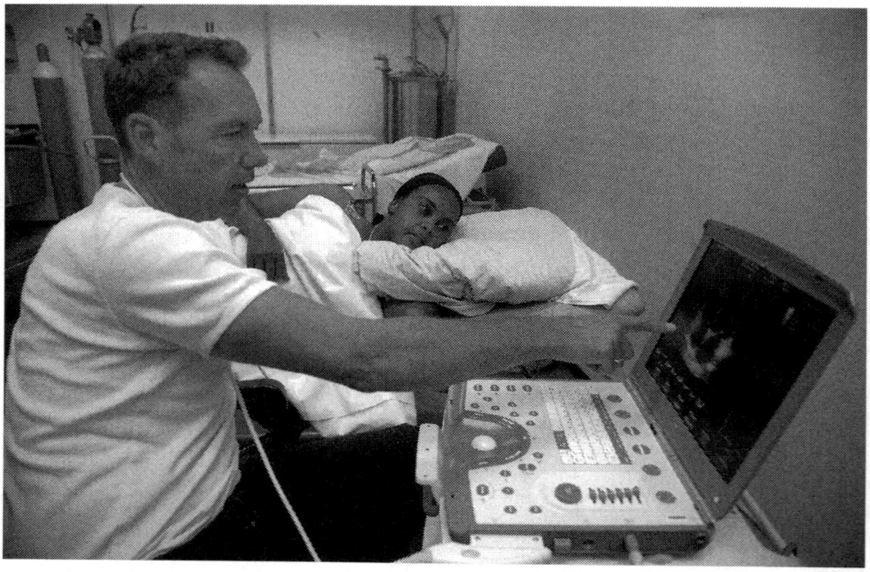

(b)

Photo 1.1 Testing the aerobic fitness (a) and cardiac function and structure (b) before and after 16 and 64 weeks of recreational football training for sedentary 20- to 45-year-old women.

Source: Photo Credit: Lizette Kabre.

While overall changes in myocardial structure and function following football training, e.g., increases in left- and right-ventricular systolic function, may confer reduced risk of CVD and improved prognosis, the long-term consequences of football training for cardiovascular morbidity and mortality await further study and the potential of football training to add to cardiac rehabilitation programmes, e.g., in patients with IHD and heart failure, is unknown. However, it is notable that positive results are accumulating for high-intensity interval training in various patient subsets, and high-intensity training comparable to football is increasingly advocated for the primary and secondary prevention of CVD (Iaia, Rampinini, and Bangsbo 2009; Bangsbo et al. 2015; Krustrup et al. 2018; Price et al. 2016). Moreover, favourable psychosocial effects of team sports that promote the subject's participation and adherence appear to be independent of the presence of a range of chronic diseases, indicating that football may be a winning ticket for cardiac rehabilitation exercise programmes (Andersen, Ottesen, and Thing 2018).

Arterial function

Arterial function and characteristics, e.g., arterial stiffness and flow-mediated endothelial-dependent vasodilatation, contribute importantly to myocardial afterload and regulation of tissue perfusion (Mitchell 2009). It is therefore hardly surprising that measures of arterial function carry prognostic information and are increasingly utilised as preclinical surrogates of CVD (Mitchell 2009; Flammer, 2012). By using peripheral arterial tonometry, we found that, in hypertensive men, the augmentation index (a measure of arterial stiffness that predicts CVD) was lowered after football training, whereas the reactive hyperaemia index (a correlate of endothelial function that is also a predictor of CVD) was unchanged (Krustrup et al. 2013). Similar findings were observed after football training in premenopausal women, and here the decrease in the augmentation index was tied to an 18% increase in leg muscle capillarisation (Krustrup, Hansen et al. 2010). Indeed, a comparable increase in the number of capillaries per muscle fibre was reported after football training in untrained men (Krustrup et al. 2009a). In addition, the reactive hyperaemia index was significantly higher in veteran football players compared to elderly healthy controls (Schmidt et al. 2015). Level of physical activity is also directly associated with flow-mediated vasodilatation and measurable changes of the retinal microvasculature in children and adolescents (Pahkala et al. 2011; Gopinath 2011). Evidence for the effects of football training on vascular function in children is limited, but we found no significant changes in the reactive hyperaemia index measured by peripheral arterial tonometry after a 10-month school-based football intervention compared to controls (Larsen et al. 2018). However, for children, microvascular function develops with age, masking the effects of physical exercise in this age group (Radtke et al. 2012).

Circulating lipid levels

Football training is associated with favourable changes in circulating lipid levels, and a recent meta-analysis of randomised controlled trials of recreational football in men and women with or without hypertension found that football training achieved a reduction in low-density lipoprotein (LDL) cholesterol levels of 0.21 (95% CI, 0.06–0.36) mmol/L compared to non-active control groups (Milanović et al. 2019). This effect size was considered to be 'possibly beneficial' for reducing long-term cardiovascular risk, whereas smaller decreases in total cholesterol and triglyceride levels, as well as minor increases in high-density lipoprotein (HDL) cholesterol levels, were observed and deemed 'likely to be trivial' (Milanović et al. 2019). The influence of football training on less-traditional lipid parameters related to cardiovascular risk, e.g., lipoprotein(a), oxidised LDL and HDL cholesterol function, is unknown at present.

Effects of football on maximal oxygen uptake, blood pressure and resting heart rate

Recreational football training, and in particular the high-intensity periods observed in both small-sided matches/exercises and 11v11 matches, stimulates a broad spectrum of physical fitness components, including maximal oxygen uptake (VO_2max). Previous studies confirmed larger improvements in VO_2max after recreational football compared to continuous moderate-intensity endurance running, strength training and no-exercise groups (Milanović et al. 2015; Krustrup et al. 2009). VO_2max increases by an average of 3.5 mL/kg/min during a recreational football training programme in comparison with other training types (Milanović et al. 2015). Overall improvement is equivalent to a 10.3% increase in VO_2max after short- to medium-term recreational football training, which is enough to prevent a decrease of 5–10% in VO_2max per decade caused by physiological aging (Hawkins and Wiswell 2003). According to current evidence, recreational football is suitable for VO_2max improvement in healthy males and females, regardless of age or fitness level, as well as untrained patients with mild-to-moderate hypertension, type 2 diabetes patients, men with prostate cancer and untrained elderly people.

Interestingly, recreational football and continuous endurance running produced similar increases in VO_2max at the beginning of a training intervention (first month), equivalent to 7% and 6%, respectively (Krustrup et al. 2009). However, further increases during the next 8 weeks were much higher in participants who performed recreational football compared to their peers who were involved in continuous endurance running because the stimulus of factors affecting VO_2max during the running training was not large enough for additional increases (Bangsbo et al. 2006; Midgley, McNaughton, and Wilkinson 2006). In contrast, typical patterns of cardiovascular adaptations and stimuli elicited during recreational football training have similarities to interval training. Marked and frequent changes in exercise intensity when playing recreational football, despite the fact that average heart rate is the same in football and continuous endurance running groups (~80% HRmax), lead to larger improvements in VO_2max. During recreational football, ~20% of the total training time usually comprises activities with intensity above 90% HRmax, compared to only 1% for continuous running (Krustrup et al. 2009).

Lack of time is often given as a barrier to participation in regular physical training. However, investigations involving previously inactive participants completing short-term intervention studies involving 2–3 sessions of recreational football per week demonstrate that the effects are similar to, or even higher than, the improvements in VO_2max observed for a control training group following the recommendation of the American College of Sports Medicine (ACSM) of 5 training sessions per week (Milanović et al. 2015). Recreational football could therefore be considered a time-efficient form of exercise training for VO_2max improvement.

As aforementioned, hypertension is one of the most common CVDs in both men and women, and it is predicted that the prevalence of hypertensive adults will be more than 1.56 billion by the year 2025 (Kearney et al. 2005). However, a short-term recreational football programme (40–60 min, 2–3 sessions per week) is

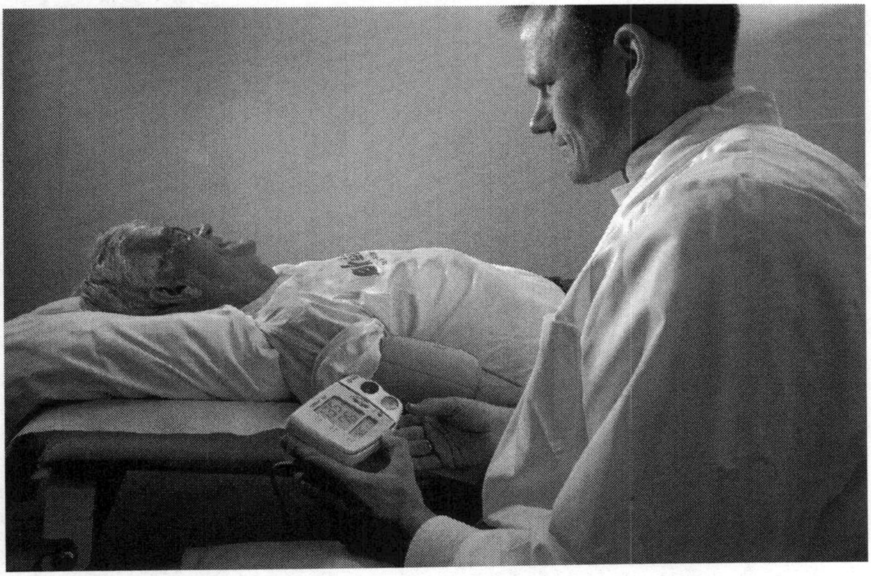

Photo 1.2 Testing the blood pressure before and after 16 and 52 weeks of football training for 65- to 78-year-old men.

Source: Photo Credit: Mikal Schlosser.

most likely beneficial for systolic and diastolic blood pressure, with the magnitude of reduction in pre- to mildly hypertensive adults observed at 11 and 7 mmHg, respectively (Milanović et al. 2019). Moreover, recreational football reduces systolic and diastolic blood pressure by 2.9% and 8.6% in overweight children (Cvetkovic et al. 2018). The aforementioned improvements are comparable to the acute effect of taking one standard dose of a blood pressure-lowering drug (Law, Morris, and Wald 2009) and are of clinical importance given that a blood pressure reduction of such a magnitude corresponds to a lowered risk of sudden cardiac stroke by 20–30% in hypertensive individuals (Law, Morris, and Wald 2009). Recreational football is an adequate stimulus to upregulate a multitude of physiological parameters associated with CVD (Hansen et al. 2013; Andersen et al. 2010). These cardiovascular system adaptations, which are the consequence of frequent high-intensity movements performed during recreational football, also lead to a moderate decrease in resting heart rate, with a magnitude of 4–12 bpm depending on aerobic fitness at baseline (Milanović et al. 2019)

Prescription of football training for cardiovascular patients

Given the well-documented and broad-spectrum beneficial effects of recreational football training on several central and peripheral components of cardiovascular health in patients with cardiovascular deficiencies (Milanović et al. 2015, 2019), we suggest the prescription of this training modality as part of the treatment for this patient group. In the vast majority of the studies presented above, 2–3 weekly sessions lasting 1 hour were applied for 3–6 months (Krustrup, Aagaard et al. 2010; Bangsbo et al. 2015; Krustrup and Krustrup 2018). Thus, clinically relevant beneficial effects on numerous physiological parameters of importance for treating a number of CVDs were attainable within this timeframe when the training was organised and supervised by researchers.

In relation to patients with stroke, aerobic exercise is recommended (Pedersen and Saltin 2015). Football training has been demonstrated to be an aerobic training form, including for weak patient groups, since average heart rate responses of 75–80% HRmax have been determined in patients with hypertension, prostate cancer and type 2 diabetes (Randers et al. 2010; Mohr et al. 2014; Uth et al. 2016; Skoradal et al. 2018). Since stroke patients normally have a poor physical status (King et al. 1989), it is suggested to start the training at low to moderate intensity. In order to control the exercise intensity and avoid excessive workload in the early phase of training during rehabilitation from stroke, the pitch size can be reduced (Randers et al. 2014) or walking football (McEwan et al. 2018) can be deployed.

As previously stated, football training combines aerobic, anaerobic and strength training (Krustrup and Krustrup 2018), and since several training forms are recommended for patients with arterial hypertension, football could be an efficient treatment protocol for mild and moderate hypertension (Pedersen and Saltin 2015). In support of this, meta-analysis evidence confirms that the deployment of

1-hour sessions of football training 2–3 times per week for 12–16 weeks reduces mean arterial pressure by ~8 mmHg (Milanović et al. 2019).

For patients with CAD, aerobic training at moderate intensities should be prescribed (Pedersen and Saltin 2015). Thus, football training with small pitch sizes combined with walking football may be deployed to maintain the intensity at a moderate aerobic level. Football training has been shown to have beneficial effects on central as well as peripheral factors (Krustrup, Aagaard et al. 2010; Krustrup and Krustrup 2018), which is essential for CAD patients.

On the other hand, interval training should be deployed for patients with heart failure (Pedersen and Saltin 2015). As football training is a high-intensity intermittent training form, if may be highly relevant for heart failure patients. These patients have lower fitness statuses, maximal oxygen uptakes and muscle strength, and a greater degree of skeletal muscle atrophy (Pedersen and Saltin 2015), so broad-spectrum training modalities, such as football training, should be deployed for this patient group.

Football training may have some limited application for patients with intermittent claudication, depending on the severity of the disease. Football training has, for example, been shown to increase muscle capillarisation in m. vastus lateralis (Krustrup, Aagaard et al. 2010) in untrained individuals, as well as arterial function in hypertensive subjects (Krustrup et al. 2013), which is beneficial for patients with intermittent claudication. Generally, both strength training and aerobic exercise for upper or lower limbs is suggested (Pedersen and Saltin 2015). Football training is also an alternative form of strength training (Krustrup, Aagaard et al. 2010). It has been shown to improve the oxidative capacity in both arms and legs (Nordsborg et al. 2015), and may therefore be applied to patients in this group. It is recommended that the training should be administered in a progressive and individualised manner, possibly starting with walking football and slowly increasing the volume and intensity.

Since the prevalence of most CVDs increases with age, it is essential to apply exercise as medicine in a manner that can also be used by elderly patient groups. Several studies have tested football training in elderly populations (Schmidt et al. 2014; Schmidt et al. 2015; Bangsbo et al. 2015; Mancini et al. 2017; Skoradal et al. 2018), with similar outcomes to those obtained in younger populations.

In summary, football training can be integrated into the treatment strategy for numerous cardiovascular patient groups due to its broad-spectrum effects with beneficial impact on cardiac and peripheral components. The Football Fitness concept has now been implemented in hundreds of football clubs in Scandinavia, where it is organised to a greater or lesser extent by the clubs in cooperation with the national football associations (Bennike, Wikman, and Ottesen 2014). Furthermore, in 2016 we conducted a national intervention in the Faroe Islands with around 2% of the adult population taking part (Flotum et al. 2016). Several of these clubs and original participants are still active, which from an organisational point of view indicates that this is a sustainable exercise training method.

Directions for future studies of recreational football and cardiovascular patients

The promising health effects of football training both for lowing cardiovascular risk factors (prevention) and improving CVD (treatment) calls for further optimisation and understanding of the associated mechanisms. These may include combination with other health interventions, e.g., nutritional optimisation of diet to support weight loss in obese individuals or further lowering of blood pressure potentially via reduced dietary sodium content, albeit the overall health effects of lowering habitual dietary salt intake are debated (Rust and Ekmekcioglu 2017). This may be relevant for patients with heart failure. Given the average size effect for CVD reduction as a result of lowering blood pressure, it is clear that an overall decrease of 6–8 mmHg would have a marked effect on public health. But, for the individual with severe hypertension, combinations of interventions may of course be required and it will be attractive to evaluate the incremental effects of such strategies in the future. Analogously, for patients with very high plasma lipid levels, combination with pharmacological and nutritional interventions may be required, and in terms of glucose tolerance, the interaction of physical exercise with muscle metabolic adaptations and improved insulin sensitivity in patients with CVD is an area of importance. Also, studies combining football training with the administration of conventional pharmacological agents may provide new treatment perspectives. We encourage future studies to evaluate the size effects of physical exercise interventions on cardiovascular endpoints as well as explorations of the physiological mechanisms involved.

References

Andersen, L. B., C. Riddoch, S. Kriemler, and A. P. Hills. 2011. "Physical activity and cardiovascular risk factors in children." *British Journal of Sports Medicine* 45 (11):871–6. doi: 10.1136/bjsports-2011-090333.

Andersen, L. J., P. R. Hansen, P. Sogaard, J. K. Madsen, J. Bech, and P. Krustrup. 2010. "Improvement of systolic and diastolic heart function after physical training in sedentary women." *Scandinavian Journal of Medicine & Science in Sports* 20 (Suppl 1):50–7. doi: 10.1111/j.1600-0838.2009.01088.x.

Andersen, L. J., M. B. Randers, P. R. Hansen, T. Hornstrup, J. F. Schmidt, J. Dvorak, P. Sogaard, P. Krustrup, and J. Bangsbo. 2014. "Structural and functional cardiac adaptations to 6 months of football training in untrained hypertensive men." *Scandinavian Journal of Medicine & Science in Sports* 24 (Suppl 1):27–35. doi: 10.1111/sms.12237.

Andersen, M. H., L. Ottesen, and L. F. Thing. 2018. "The social and psychological health outcomes of team sport participation in adults: An integrative review of research." *Scandinavian Journal of Public Health* 1403494818791405. doi: 10.1177/1403494818791405.

Anker, S. D., T. P. Chua, P. Ponikowski, D. Harrington, J. W. Swan, W. J. Kox, P. A. Poole-Wilson, and A. J. Coats. 1997. "Hormonal changes and catabolic/anabolic imbalance in chronic heart failure and their importance for cardiac cachexia." *Circulation* 96 (2):526–34.

Baker, J. L., L. W. Olsen, and T. I. Sorensen. 2007. "Childhood body-mass index and the risk of coronary heart disease in adulthood." *The New England Journal of Medicine* 357 (23):2329–37. doi: 10.1056/NEJMoa072515.

Bangsbo, J., P. R. Hansen, J. Dvorak, and P. Krustrup. 2015. "Recreational football for disease prevention and treatment in untrained men: A narrative review examining cardiovascular health, lipid profile, body composition, muscle strength and functional capacity." *British Journal of Sports Medicine* 49 (9):568–76. doi: 10.1136/bjsports-2015-094781.

Bangsbo, J., M. Mohr, A. Poulsen, J. Perez-Gomez, and P. Krustrup. 2006. "Training and testing the elite athlete." *Journal of Exercise Science Fitness* 4 (1):1–14.

Barczuk-Falecka, M., L. A. Malek, H. Krysztofiak, D. Roik, and M. Brzewski. 2018. "Cardiac magnetic resonance assessment of the structural and functional cardiac adaptations to soccer training in school-aged male children." *Pediatric Cardiology* 39 (5):948–54. doi: 10.1007/s00246-018-1844-5.

Benjamin, E. J., M. J. Blaha, S. E. Chiuve, M. Cushman, S. R. Das, R. Deo, S. D. de Ferranti, J. Floyd, M. Fornage, C. Gillespie, C. R. Isasi, M. C. Jimenez, L. C. Jordan, S. E. Judd, D. Lackland, J. H. Lichtman, L. Lisabeth, S. Liu, C. T. Longenecker, R. H. Mackey, K. Matsushita, D. Mozaffarian, M. E. Mussolino, K. Nasir, R. W. Neumar, L. Palaniappan, D. K. Pandey, R. R. Thiagarajan, M. J. Reeves, M. Ritchey, C. J. Rodriguez, G. A. Roth, W. D. Rosamond, C. Sasson, A. Towfighi, C. W. Tsao, M. B. Turner, S. S. Virani, J. H. Voeks, J. Z. Willey, J. T. Wilkins, J. H. Wu, H. M. Alger, S. S. Wong, and P. Muntner. 2017. "Heart disease and stroke statistics-2017 update: A report from the American Heart Association." *Circulation* 135 (10):e146–e603. doi: 10.1161/cir.0000000000000485.

Bennike, S., J. M. Wikman, and L. S. Ottesen. 2014. "Football fitness: A new version of football? A concept for adult players in Danish football clubs." *Scandinavian Journal of Medicine & Science in Sports* 24 (Suppl 1):138–46. doi: 10.1111/sms.12276.

Boysen, G., and L. H. Krarup. 2009. "Benefits of physical activity for stroke survivors." *Expert Review of Neurotherapeutics* 9 (2):147–9. doi: 10.1586/14737175.9.2.147.

Bradham, W. S., G. Moe, K. A. Wendt, A. A. Scott, A. Konig, M. Romanova, G. Naik, and F. G. Spinale. 2002. "TNF-alpha and myocardial matrix metalloproteinases in heart failure: Relationship to LV remodeling." *American Journal of Physiology: Heart and Circulatory Physiology* 282 (4):H1288–95. doi: 10.1152/ajpheart.00526.2001.

Braunwald, E., and P. Libby. 2008. *Braunwald's heart disease: A textbook of cardiovascular medicine.* Philadelphia: Saunders Elsevier.

Burt, V. L., P. Whelton, E. J. Roccella, C. Brown, J. A. Cutler, M. Higgins, M. J. Horan, and D. Labarthe. 1995. "Prevalence of hypertension in the US adult population: Results from the Third National Health and Nutrition Examination Survey, 1988–1991." *Hypertension (Dallas, Tex.: 1979)* 25 (3):305–13.

Cornelissen, V. A., R. Buys, and N. A. Smart. 2013. "Endurance exercise beneficially affects ambulatory blood pressure: A systematic review and meta-analysis." *Journal of Hypertension* 31 (4):639–48. doi: 10.1097/HJH.0b013e32835ca964.

Cornelissen, V. A., and N. A. Smart. 2013. "Exercise training for blood pressure: A systematic review and meta-analysis." *Journal of the American Heart Association* 2 (1):e004473. doi: 10.1161/jaha.112.004473.

Cvetkovic, N., E. Stojanovic, N. Stojiljkovic, D. Nikolic, A. T. Scanlan, and Z. Milanović. 2018. "Exercise training in overweight and obese children: Recreational football and high-intensity interval training provide similar benefits to physical fitness." *Scandinavian Journal of Medicine and Science in Sports* 1:18–32.

Davies, E. J., T. Moxham, K. Rees, S. Singh, A. J. Coats, S. Ebrahim, F. Lough, and R. S. Taylor. 2010. "Exercise based rehabilitation for heart failure." *The Cochrane Database of Systematic Reviews* (4):Cd003331. doi: 10.1002/14651858.CD003331.pub3.

Fagard, R. H. 2005. "Physical activity, physical fitness and the incidence of hypertension." *Journal of Hypertension* 23 (2):265–7.

Fagard, R. H., and V. A. Cornelissen. 2005. "Physical activity, exercise, fitness and blood pressure." In *Hypertension, principles and practice*, edited by E. J. Battagay, G. Y. H. Lip, and G. L. Bakris. Boca Raton: Taylor adnd Francis Books.

Fagard, R. H., and V. A. Cornelissen. 2007. "Effect of exercise on blood pressure control in hypertensive patients." *European Journal of Cardiovascular Prevention and Rehabilitation: Official Journal of the European Society of Cardiology, Working Groups on Epidemiology & Prevention and Cardiac Rehabilitation and Exercise Physiology* 14 (1):12–7. doi: 10.1097/HJR.0b013e3280128bbb.

Flammer, A. J., Anderson, T., Celermajer, D. S., Creager, M. A., Deanfield, J., Ganz, P. et al. 2012. "The assessment of endothelial function: From research into clinical practice." *Circulation* 126:753–67. doi: 10.1161/CIRCULATIONAHA.112.093245.

Flotum, L. A., L. S. Ottesen, P. Krustrup, and M. Mohr. 2016. "Evaluating a nationwide recreational football intervention: Recruitment, attendance, adherence, exercise intensity, and health effects." *BioMed Research International* 2016:7231545. doi: 10.1155/2016/7231545.

Gopinath, B., Baur, L. A., Wang, J. J., Hardy, L. L., Teber E., Kifley, A. et al. 2011. "Influence of physical activity and screen time on the retinal microvasculature in young children." *Arteriosclerosis Thrombosis and Vascular Biology* 31:1233–39. doi: 10.1161/ATVBAHA.110.219451.

Hansen, P. R., L. J. Andersen, A. N. Rebelo, J. Brito, T. Hornstrup, J. F. Schmidt, S. R. Jackman, J. Mota, C. Rego, J. Oliveira, A. Seabra, and P. Krustrup. 2013. "Cardiovascular effects of 3 months of football training in overweight children examined by comprehensive echocardiography: A pilot study." *Journal of Sports Sciences* 31 (13):1432–40. doi: 10.1080/02640414.2013.792951.

Harrington, D., S. D. Anker, T. P. Chua, K. M. Webb-Peploe, P. P. Ponikowski, P. A. Poole-Wilson, and A. J. Coats. 1997. "Skeletal muscle function and its relation to exercise tolerance in chronic heart failure." *Journal of American College of Cardiology* 30 (7):1758–64.

Hawkins, S. A., and R. A. Wiswell. 2003. "Rate and mechanism of maximal oxygen consumption decline with aging." *Sports Medicine* 33 (12):877–88.

Hu, G., P. Jousilahti, R. Antikainen, and J. Tuomilehto. 2007. "Occupational, commuting, and leisure-time physical activity in relation to cardiovascular mortality among finnish subjects with hypertension." *American Journal of Hypertension* 20 (12):1242–50. doi: 10.1016/j.amjhyper.2007.07.015.

Huang, G., X. Shi, C. A. Gibson, S. C. Huang, N. A. Coudret, and M. C. Ehlman. 2013. "Controlled aerobic exercise training reduces resting blood pressure in sedentary older adults." *Blood Pressure* 22 (6):386–94. doi: 10.3109/08037051.2013.778003.

Hunt, S. A., W. T. Abraham, M. H. Chin, A. M. Feldman, G. S. Francis, T. G. Ganiats, M. Jessup, M. A. Konstam, D. M. Mancini, K. Michl, J. A. Oates, P. S. Rahko, M. A. Silver, L. W. Stevenson, C. W. Yancy, E. M. Antman, S. C. Smith, Jr., C. D. Adams, J. L. Anderson, D. P. Faxon, V. Fuster, J. L. Halperin, L. F. Hiratzka, A. K. Jacobs, R. Nishimura, J. P. Ornato, R. L. Page, and B. Riegel. 2005. "ACC/AHA 2005 guideline update for the diagnosis and management of chronic heart failure in the adult: A report of the American College of Cardiology/American Heart Association task force on practice guidelines (Writing committee to update the 2001 guidelines for the evaluation and management of heart failure): Developed in collaboration with the American College of Chest Physicians and the International Society for Heart and Lung Transplantation: Endorsed by the Heart Rhythm Society." *Circulation* 112 (12):e154–235. doi: 10.1161/circulationaha.105.167586.

Hwang, R., and T. Marwick. 2009. "Efficacy of home-based exercise programmes for people with chronic heart failure: A meta-analysis." *European Journal of Cardiovascular Prevention and Rehabilitation: Official Journal of the European Society of Cardiology, Working Groups on Epidemiology & Prevention and Cardiac Rehabilitation and Exercise Physiology* 16 (5):527–35. doi: 10.1097/HJR.0b013e32832e097f.

Iaia, F. M., E. Rampinini, and J. Bangsbo. 2009. "High-intensity training in football." *International Journal of Sports Physiology and Performance* 4 (3):291–306.

Karlsen, T., I. L. Aamot, M. Haykowsky, and O. Rognmo. 2017. "High intensity interval training for maximizing health outcomes." *Progress in Cardiovascular Diseases* 60 (1):67–77. doi: 10.1016/j.pcad.2017.03.006.

Kearney, P. M., M. Whelton, K. Reynolds, P. Muntner, P. K. Whelton, and J. He. 2005. "Global burden of hypertension: Analysis of worldwide data." *Lancet (London, England)* 365 (9455):217–23. doi: 10.1016/s0140-6736(05)17741-1.

King, M. L., M. Guarracini, L. Lennihan, D. Freeman, B. Gagas, A. Boston, E. Bates, and S. Nori. 1989. "Adaptive exercise testing for patients with hemiparesis." *Journal of Cardiopulmonary Rehabilitation and Prevention* 9 (6):237–42.

Krarup, L. H., T. Truelsen, C. Gluud, G. Andersen, X. Zeng, J. Korv, A. Oskedra, and G. Boysen. 2008. "Prestroke physical activity is associated with severity and long-term outcome from first-ever stroke." *Neurology* 71 (17):1313–8. doi: 10.1212/01.wnl.0000327667.48013.9f.

Krarup, L. H., T. Truelsen, A. Pedersen, H. Lerke, M. Lindahl, L. Hansen, P. Schnohr, and G. Boysen. 2007. "Level of physical activity in the week preceding an ischemic stroke." *Cerebrovascular Diseases (Basel, Switzerland)* 24 (2–3):296–300. doi: 10.1159/000105683.

Krustrup, P., P. Aagaard, L. Nybo, J. Petersen, M. Mohr, and J. Bangsbo. 2010. "Recreational football as a health promoting activity: A topical review." *Scandinavian Journal of Medicine & Science in Sports* 20 (Suppl 1):1–13. doi: 10.1111/j.1600-0838.2010.01108.x.

Krustrup, P., P. R. Hansen, C. M. Nielsen, M. N. Larsen, M. B. Randers, V. Manniche, L. Hansen, J. Dvorak, and J. Bangsbo. 2014. "Structural and functional cardiac adaptations to a 10-week school-based football intervention for 9–10-year-old children." *Scandinavian Journal of Medicine & Science in Sports* 24 (S1):4–9. doi: 10.1111/sms.12277.

Krustrup, P., P. R. Hansen, M. B. Randers, L. Nybo, D. Martone, L. J. Andersen, L. T. Bune, A. Junge, and J. Bangsbo. 2010. "Beneficial effects of recreational football on the cardiovascular risk profile in untrained premenopausal women." *Scandinavian Journal of Medicine & Science in Sports* 20 (Suppl 1):40–9. doi: 10.1111/j.1600-0838.2010.01110.x.

Krustrup, P., E. W. Helge, P. R. Hansen, P. Aagaard, M. Hagman, M. B. Randers, M. de Sousa, and M. Mohr. 2018. "Effects of recreational football on women's fitness and health: Adaptations and mechanisms." *European Journal of Applied Physiology* 118 (1):11–32. doi: 10.1007/s00421-017-3733-7.

Krustrup, P., and B. R. Krustrup. 2018. "Football is medicine: It is time for patients to play!" *British Journal of Sports Medicine.* 52(22):1412–14. doi: 10.1136/bjsports-2018-099377.

Krustrup, P., J. J. Nielsen, B. R. Krustrup, J. F. Christensen, H. Pedersen, M. B. Randers, P. Aagaard, A. M. Petersen, L. Nybo, and J. Bangsbo. 2009. "Recreational soccer is an effective health-promoting activity for untrained men." *British Journal of Sports Medicine* 43 (11):825–31. doi: 10.1136/bjsm.2008.053124.

Krustrup, P., M. B. Randers, L. J. Andersen, S. R. Jackman, J. Bangsbo, and P. R. Hansen. 2013. "Soccer improves fitness and attenuates cardiovascular risk factors in hypertensive men." *Medicine and Science in Sports and Exercise* 45 (3):553–60. doi: 10.1249/MSS.0b013e3182777051.

Lane, R., B. Ellis, L. Watson, and G. C. Leng. 2014. "Exercise for intermittent claudication." *The Cochrane Database of Systematic Reviews* (7):Cd000990. doi: 10.1002/14651858.CD000990.pub3.
Larsen, M. N., C. M. Nielsen, M. Madsen, V. Manniche, L. Hansen, J. Bangsbo, P. Krustrup, and P. R. Hansen. 2018. "Cardiovascular adaptations after 10 months of intense school-based physical training for 8- to 10-year-old children." *Scandinavian Journal of Medicine & Science in Sports* 28 (Suppl 1):33–41. doi: 10.1111/sms.13253.
Laslett, L. J., P. Alagona, Jr., B. A. Clark, 3rd, J. P. Drozda, Jr., F. Saldivar, S. R. Wilson, C. Poe, and M. Hart. 2012. "The worldwide environment of cardiovascular disease: Prevalence, diagnosis, therapy, and policy issues: A report from the American College of Cardiology." *Journal of American College of Cardiology* 60 (25 Suppl):S1–49. doi: 10.1016/j.jacc.2012.11.002.
Law, M. R., J. K. Morris, and N. J. Wald. 2009. "Use of blood pressure lowering drugs in the prevention of cardiovascular disease: Meta-analysis of 147 randomised trials in the context of expectations from prospective epidemiological studies." *BMJ* 338:b1665.
Lewington, S., R. Clarke, N. Qizilbash, R. Peto, and R. Collins. 2002. "Age-specific relevance of usual blood pressure to vascular mortality: A meta-analysis of individual data for one million adults in 61 prospective studies." *Lancet (London, England)* 360 (9349):1903–13.
Mancini, A., D. Vitucci, G. Labruna, E. Imperlini, M. B. Randers, J. F. Schmidt, M. Hagman, T. R. Andersen, R. Russo, S. Orru, P. Krustrup, F. Salvatore, and P. Buono. 2017. "Effect of lifelong football training on the expression of muscle molecular markers involved in healthy longevity." *European Journal of Applied Physiology* 117 (4):721–730. doi: 10.1007/s00421-017-3562-8.
McEwan, G., D. Buchan, D. Cowan, R. Arthur, M. Sanderson, and E. Macrae. 2018. "Recruiting older men to walking football: A pilot feasibility study." *Explore (New York, N.Y.)*. doi: 10.1016/j.explore.2018.12.001.
Midgley, A. W, L. R. McNaughton, and M. Wilkinson. 2006. "Is there an optimal training intensity for enhancing the maximal oxygen uptake of distance runners?" *Sports Medicine* 36 (2):117–32.
Milanović, Z., S. Pantelic, N. Covic, G. Sporis, and P. Krustrup. 2015. "Is recreational soccer effective for improving VO_2 max a systematic review and meta-analysis." *Sports Medicine (Auckland, N.Z.)* 45 (9):1339–53. doi: 10.1007/s40279-015-0361-4.
Milanović, Z., S. Pantelic, N. Covic, G. Sporis, M. Mohr, and P. Krustrup. 2019. "Broad-spectrum physical fitness benefits of recreational football: A systematic review and meta-analysis." *British Journal of Sports Medicine* 53 (15):926–39. doi: 10.1136/bjsports-2017-097885.
Milanović, Z., S. Pantelić, N. Čović, G. Sporiš, and P. Krustrup. 2015. "Is recreational soccer effective for improving VO_2 max? A systematic review and meta-analysis." *Sports Medicine* 45 (9):1339–53.
Mitchell, G. F. 2009. "Arterial stiffness and wave reflection: Biomarkers of cardiovascular risk." *Artery Research* 3 (2):56–64. doi: 10.1016/j.artres.2009.02.002.
Mohr, M., A. Lindenskov, P. M. Holm, H. P. Nielsen, J. Mortensen, P. Weihe, and P. Krustrup. 2014. "Football training improves cardiovascular health profile in sedentary, premenopausal hypertensive women." *Scandinavian Journal of Medicine & Science in Sports* 24 (Suppl 1):36–42. doi: 10.1111/sms.12278.
Myers, J., M. Prakash, V. Froelicher, D. Do, S. Partington, and J. E. Atwood. 2002. "Exercise capacity and mortality among men referred for exercise testing." *The New England Journal of Medicine* 346 (11):793–801. doi: 10.1056/NEJMoa011858.

Nordsborg, N. B., L. Connolly, P. Weihe, E. Iuliano, P. Krustrup, B. Saltin, and M. Mohr. 2015. "Oxidative capacity and glycogen content increase more in arm than leg muscle in sedentary women after intense training." *Journal of Applied Physiology (Bethesda, Md.: 1985)* 119 (2):116–23. doi: 10.1152/japplphysiol.00101.2015.

Pahkala, K., O. J. Heinonen, O. Simell, J. S. Viikari, T. Ronnemaa, H. Niinikoski, and O. T. Raitakari. 2011. "Association of physical activity with vascular endothelial function and intima-media thickness." *Circulation* 124 (18):1956–63. doi: 10.1161/circulationaha.111.043851.

Paolisso, G., S. De Riu, G. Marrazzo, M. Verza, M. Varricchio, and F. D'Onofrio. 1991. "Insulin resistance and hyperinsulinemia in patients with chronic congestive heart failure." *Metabolism: Clinical and Experimental* 40 (9):972–7. doi: 10.1016/0026-0495(91)90075-8.

Paolucci, S., C. Gandolfo, L. Provinciali, R. Torta, and V. Toso. 2006. "The Italian multicenter observational study on post-stroke depression (DESTRO)." *Journal of Neurology* 253 (5):556–62. doi: 10.1007/s00415-006-0058-6.

Pedersen, B. K., and B. Saltin. 2015. "Exercise as medicine: Evidence for prescribing exercise as therapy in 26 different chronic diseases." *Scandinavian Journal of Medicine & Science in Sports* 25 (Suppl 3):1–72. doi: 10.1111/sms.12581.

Price, K. J., B. A. Gordon, S. R. Bird, and A. C. Benson. 2016. "A review of guidelines for cardiac rehabilitation exercise programmes: Is there an international consensus?" *European Journal of Preventive Cardiology* 23 (16):1715–33. doi: 10.1177/2047487316657669.

Radtke, T., K. Khattab, P. Eser, S. Kriemler, H. Saner, and M. Wilhelm. 2012. "Puberty and microvascular function in healthy children and adolescents." *The Journal of Pediatrics* 161 (5):887–91. doi: 10.1016/j.jpeds.2012.04.033.

Rand, D., J. J. Eng, P. F. Tang, J. S. Jeng, and C. Hung. 2009. "How active are people with stroke?: Use of accelerometers to assess physical activity." *Stroke* 40 (1):163–8. doi: 10.1161/strokeaha.108.523621.

Randers, M. B., J. J. Nielsen, J. Bangsbo, and P. Krustrup. 2014. "Physiological response and activity profile in recreational small-sided football: No effect of the number of players." *Scandinavian Journal of Medicine & Science in Sports* 24 (Suppl 1):130–7. doi: 10.1111/sms.12232.

Randers, M. B., L. Nybo, J. Petersen, J. J. Nielsen, L. Christiansen, M. Bendiksen, J. Brito, J. Bangsbo, and P. Krustrup. 2010. "Activity profile and physiological response to football training for untrained males and females, elderly and youngsters: Influence of the number of players." *Scandinavian Journal of Medicine & Science in Sports* 20 (Suppl 1):14–23. doi: 10.1111/j.1600-0838.2010.01069.x.

Rust, P., and C. Ekmekcioglu. 2017. "Impact of salt intake on the pathogenesis and treatment of hypertension." *Advances in Experimental Medicine and Biology* 956:61–84. doi: 10.1007/5584_2016_147.

Schmidt, J. F., T. R. Andersen, L. J. Andersen, M. B. Randers, T. Hornstrup, P. R. Hansen, J. Bangsbo, and P. Krustrup. 2015. "Cardiovascular function is better in veteran football players than age-matched untrained elderly healthy men." *Scandinavian Journal of Medicine & Science in Sports* 25 (1):61–9. doi: 10.1111/sms.12153.

Schmidt, J. F., T. R. Andersen, J. Horton, J. Brix, L. Tarnow, P. Krustrup, L. J. Andersen, J. Bangsbo, and P. R. Hansen. 2013. "Soccer training improves cardiac function in men with type 2 diabetes." *Medicine and Science in Sports and Exercise* 45 (12):2223–33. doi: 10.1249/MSS.0b013e31829ab43c.

Schmidt, J. F., P. R. Hansen, T. R. Andersen, L. J. Andersen, T. Hornstrup, P. Krustrup, and J. Bangsbo. 2014. "Cardiovascular adaptations to 4 and 12 months of football or strength training in 65- to 75-year-old untrained men." *Scandinavian Journal of Medicine & Science in Sports* 24 (Suppl 1):86–97. doi: 10.1111/sms.12217.

Schmidt, J. F., L. J. Andersen, J. Uth, T. Hornstrup, J. Christensen, J. Midtgaard, K. Brasso, P. Krustrup, M. Rørth, and P. R. Hansen. 2017. "Cardiac structure and function in men with prostate cancer receiving androgen-deprivation therapy and the effects of recreational small-sided football training: A randomized controlled trial." *World Journal of Cardiovascular Diseases* 7 (9):308–22. doi: 10.4236/wjcd.2017.79029.

Skoradal, M. B., P. Weihe, P. Patursson, J. Mortensen, L. Connolly, P. Krustrup, and M. Mohr. 2018. "Football training improves metabolic and cardiovascular health status in 55- to 70-year-old women and men with prediabetes." *Scandinavian Journal of Medicine & Science in Sports* 28 (Suppl 1):42–51. doi: 10.1111/sms.13081.

Sui, X., M. J. LaMonte, and S. N. Blair. 2007. "Cardiorespiratory fitness as a predictor of nonfatal cardiovascular events in asymptomatic women and men." *American Journal of Epidemiology* 165 (12):1413–23. doi: 10.1093/aje/kwm031.

Sullivan, M. J., J. D. Knight, M. B. Higginbotham, and F. R. Cobb. 1989. "Relation between central and peripheral hemodynamics during exercise in patients with chronic heart failure: Muscle blood flow is reduced with maintenance of arterial perfusion pressure." *Circulation* 80 (4):769–81.

Swedberg, K., J. Cleland, H. Dargie, H. Drexler, F. Follath, M. Komajda, L. Tavazzi, O. A. Smiseth, A. Gavazzi, A. Haverich, A. Hoes, T. Jaarsma, J. Korewicki, S. Levy, C. Linde, J. L. Lopez-Sendon, M. S. Nieminen, L. Pierard, and W. J. Remme. 2005. "Guidelines for the diagnosis and treatment of chronic heart failure: Executive summary (update 2005): The task force for the diagnosis and treatment of chronic heart failure of the European Society of Cardiology." *European Heart Journal* 26 (11):1115–40. doi: 10.1093/eurheartj/ehi204.

TransAtlantic Inter-Society Consensus (TASC). 2000. " Management of peripheral arterial disease (PAD)" *European Journal of Vascular and Endovascular Surgery: The Official Journal of the European Society for Vascular Surgery* 19 (Suppl A):Si–xxviii, S1–250.

Uth, J., T. Hornstrup, J. F. Christensen, K. B. Christensen, N. R. Jorgensen, J. F. Schmidt, K. Brasso, M. D. Jakobsen, E. Sundstrup, L. L. Andersen, M. Rorth, J. Midtgaard, P. Krustrup, and E. W. Helge. 2016. "Efficacy of recreational football on bone health, body composition, and physical functioning in men with prostate cancer undergoing androgen deprivation therapy: 32-week follow-up of the FC prostate randomised controlled trial." *Osteoporosis International: A Journal Established as Result of Cooperation between the European Foundation for Osteoporosis and the National Osteoporosis Foundation of the USA* 27 (4):1507–18. doi: 10.1007/s00198-015-3399-0.

Weston, K. S., U. Wisloff, and J. S. Coombes. 2014. "High-intensity interval training in patients with lifestyle-induced cardiometabolic disease: A systematic review and meta-analysis." *British Journal of Sports Medicine* 48 (16):1227–34. doi: 10.1136/bjsports-2013-092576.

Chapter 2

Football as Medicine against type 2 diabetes and metabolic syndrome

Maysa Vieira de Sousa, João Brito, Magni Mohr, George P. Nassis, Jørn Wulff Helge, Svein Arne Pettersen, Thomas Rostgaard Andersen and Peter Krustrup

1) Type 2 diabetes and metabolic syndrome: definition, physiopathology and treatment

Metabolic syndrome (MetS) is defined as a cluster of risk factors associated with insulin resistance and an elevated risk of cardiovascular disease and type 2 diabetes mellitus. The prevalence of MetS has increased worldwide in recent years, mainly due to the adoption of a lifestyle characterised by extended sedentarism and increased body adiposity. There have been several definitions of MetS since 1998, when a first definition was published by the World Health Organization (Alberti and Zimmet 1998). According to the WHO, MetS is defined as the presence of insulin resistance plus two of the following risk factors: obesity, hypertension, elevated triglycerides, low high-density lipoprotein (HDL-C) and microalbuminuria. Other MetS definitions, like the one from the National Cholesterol Education Program Adult Treatment Panel III (ATP III), do not include insulin resistance and diagnosis requires three of the following risk factors: abdominal obesity, high blood pressure, high triglycerides (TG) and blood glucose, and reduced HDL-C levels (NCEP 2002). The most recent definition of MetS comes from the joint statement of the International Diabetes Federation and the American Heart Association/National Heart, Lung, and Blood Institute (Alberti et al. 2009). According to this statement, MetS is defined as the presence of any three of five risk factors: elevated waist circumference (population- and country-specific cut-offs), elevated TG (>150 mg/dL), reduced HDL-C (<40 mg/dL), elevated blood pressure (BP) (systolic BP >130 mm Hg, diastolic BP >85 mm Hg) and elevated fasting glucose (>100 mg/dL) (Alberti et al. 2009).

Type 2 diabetes (T2D) is a disease characterised by a defect in both insulin secretion and insulin action on the tissues. For the homeostatic regulation of blood glucose levels, there is cross-talk between pancreatic beta cells and tissues (muscle, liver, fat cells) regarding insulin release. In the presence of high glucose levels in the blood stream, beta cells are stimulated, releasing insulin, which regulates the uptake of excess glucose by the tissues. In turn, these tissues send information to the pancreas regarding the need for insulin. When insulin action at tissue level deteriorates, more insulin is secreted to maintain blood glucose concentration within normal levels. This state, called insulin resistance, is mainly associated with obesity. At some stage, beta cells cannot secrete more insulin and blood glucose levels increase, characterising T2D. The development of T2D is due to an interaction of genetic and environmental factors, mainly obesity. Both abdominal adiposity and ectopic fat (fat accumulated around organs like the heart, liver and skeletal muscle) are considered crucial factors linking adiposity with insulin defects and T2D (Montague and O'Rahilly 2000; Unger 2002). T2D treatment involves lifestyle modification (healthy diet and physical activity), oral medication and, in certain cases, insulin therapy.

2) Why and how to prescribe football training as exercise therapy for T2D and MetS patients

Physical activity is a cornerstone in the treatment and prevention of T2D and MetS, alongside medication and dietary counselling (American Diabetes Association [ADA] 2017). The effects of physical activity on HbA1c levels after aerobic, resistance or combined exercise training have been reported as decreases of −0.7%, −0.6% and −0.5%, respectively (Umpierre et al. 2013). A 1% absolute lowering of HbA1c is associated with a 15–20% reduction in major cardiovascular end-points (Selvin et al. 2004) and, as such, physical activity appears to have a considerable additional effect to the 1.1% reduction in HbA1c levels reported with isolated antidiabetic treatment with metformin alone (Hirst et al. 2012). However, patients with T2D are reluctant to take up regular physical activity regardless of the known therapeutic effects of exercise training (Donahue et al. 2006). Also, dropout rates are high, especially when participants are left to exercise on their own (Williams et al. 2007). Primary perceived barriers to physical activity among people with T2D include lack of time and awareness of where and how to exercise, poor adherence and low self-efficacy in the ability to implement exercise. On the other hand, motivators for physical activity include enjoyment of exercise, mental and physical health benefits, and social interactions (Jepson et al. 2012; Lidegaard et al. 2016).

In recent years, the activity characteristics and health benefits of recreational football have been thoroughly investigated in untrained subjects and in individuals with prediabetes and T2D with no, or only limited, football experience. These studies revealed that recreational football is a high-intensity, intermittent type of training resulting in considerable aerobic load (Randers et al. 2010; Andersen et al. 2014; de Sousa et al. 2014). Moreover, football involves many strength-demanding activities, such as sprints, shots and sudden changes of direction, resulting in a significant anaerobic response (Andersen et al. 2014). The short-term (12–24 weeks) effects of recreational football training in individuals with prediabetes and T2D include marked improvements in physical capacity, body composition and health markers in the blood, including HbA1c and lipid levels. Also, the function and structure of the cardiovascular and musculoskeletal systems are significantly impacted (Schmidt et al. 2013; Andersen et al. 2014; de Sousa et al. 2014, 2017; Skoradal et al. 2018a, 2018b). Collectively, recreational football training in patients with, or at risk of, T2D appears to result in physiological adaptations like those reported after interventions applying a combination of aerobic and strength training (Krustrup et al. 2010). This supports the prescription of recreational football as a multi-purpose exercise treatment for patients with, or at risk of, T2D who do not want to perform other conventional exercise.

It is a remarkable finding that untrained recreational football participants report lower perceived exertion during exercise compared to joggers and interval runners, despite the frequently occurring intense actions and periods of high metabolic loading (Krustrup et al. 2010). This may be linked to the football participants being more focused on psychosocial factors such as enjoyment and team interaction and dynamics (Ottesen et al. 2010). Also, high levels of flow and similar, or even less, experience of worry during football exercise compared to other traditional exercise modalities, such as running or strength training, have been reported (Elbe et al. 2010). All the above may ultimately favour long-term adherence to physical activity (Nielsen et al. 2014). In summary, recreational football provides a non-conventional and joyful group-based training method that offers a unique strategy for increasing adherence, life-long exercise continuation and the promotion of healthy lifestyle behaviours in subjects with T2D and MetS.

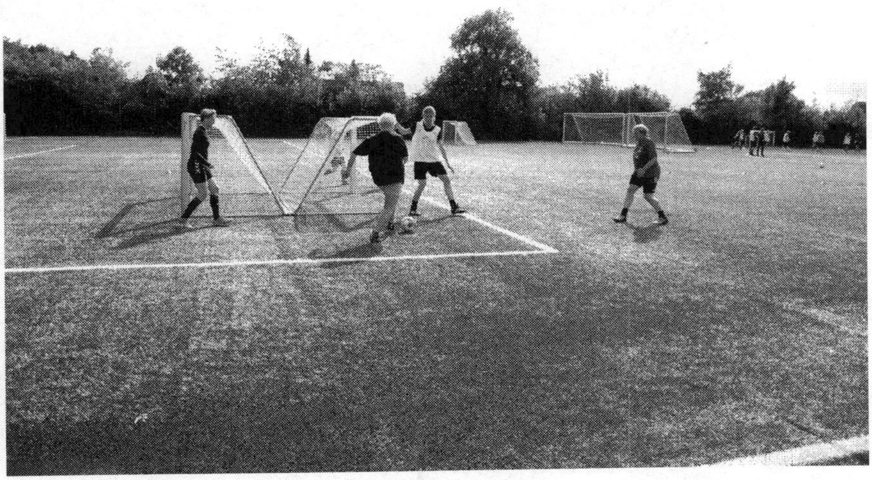

Photo 2.1 Football Fitness training for type 2 diabetes patients.

Source: Photo Credit: Casper Boe Jensen, DBU Zealand.

Recreational football can be played using several formats (e.g., 1v1 to 7v7) and pitch sizes (e.g., 8×11 m to 45×60 m) (Randers et al. 2010), and it can be played outdoors and indoors. As the effect of exercise training on insulin sensitivity appears to be transient, lasting about 24–48 hours (Wojtaszewski et al. 2003), it is recommended engaging in football 2–4 times/week with a total duration of 30–60 min/session. In a recent study by Mohr et al. (2017) GLUT-4 protein expression was upregulated in a group of sedentary middle-aged women after 15 weeks of football training 3 times per week. Thus, skeletal muscle glucose uptake capacity can by upregulated with recreational football training over a 3–4 month treatment period. In relation to organization, a training session can comprise game periods lasting 6–12 min interspersed with short rest periods to allow for sufficient recovery, rehydration and refuelling. Especially at the beginning of a training period, it is important to carefully match the above factors to the fitness and skill levels of the players to favour ball involvement and enjoyment (Williams and Hodges 2005). With minor adjustments in rules, risk of injury during recreational football training is considered low (Krustrup et al. 2010) and, as such, heterogeneous groups across age, gender, skill and fitness levels can easily and safely engage in the same training session. It is advised that players undergo appropriate medical screening prior to exercise. Specifically, subjects suffering from uncontrolled T2D and progressed diabetic complications, as well as cardiovascular disease and musculoskeletal complaints, have not been included in the previous studies on football in T2D and pre-diabetic subjects. As such, at this stage it cannot be concluded that these subjects are able to adhere to recreational football training.

3) Football training improves physical fitness and body composition in patients with T2D and MetS

There is strong evidence of the positive effects of regular exercise training on body composition and physical fitness in patients with T2D and MetS. Overall, the value and appropriateness of routine exercise training are measured by the extent to which the positive adaptive effects of regular exercise outweigh the risks associated with physical inactivity. In this regard, regular recreational football training has great potential for enhancing aerobic fitness. Moreover, recreational football is a practically sound strategy for tackling the lack of motivation to exercise, which is a key component of treatment guidelines for T2D and MetS.

Patients with T2D and MetS tend to have hampered physical fitness. VO_2peak and VO_2 kinetics might be impaired early in patients with T2D, and might lead to subclinical cardiac dysfunctions such as decreased perfusion during exercise. Impaired nutritive blood flow limits exercise kinetics and decreases exercise capacity. Moreover, several endothelial-specific impairments are active mediators of exercise dysfunction in patients with T2D, including insulin resistance, endothelial dysfunction, decreased myocardial perfusion, slowed tissue haemoglobin oxygen saturation and impairment in mitochondrial function (Reusch et al. 2013).

Recreational football can potentially reverse these complications. Overall, significant improvements in VO_2max have been observed in patients with T2D and hypertension engaging in regular recreational football training (Milanović et al. 2015). Interestingly, 48- to 68-year-old patients with T2D engaging in a 12-week recreational football training programme (40 min, 3 times per week) combined with a calorie-restricted diet improved their VO_2max by 10 ± 4%, which has not been observed with calorie-restricted diet alone (−3 ± 4%) (de Sousa et al. 2014). Similarly, football training combined with dietary advice had broad-spectrum effects on metabolic and cardiovascular health profile, with greater overall effects than dietary advice alone for 55- to 70-year-old women and men with prediabetes (Skoradal et al. 2018a, 2018b). In the study by Skoradal and colleagues (2018a, 2018b) VO_2max increased by 14% for football training combined with dietary advice, with a higher change score than for dietary advice alone (2%).

Individuals with T2D and MetS can also engage in regular recreational football training to improve body composition. There is an inverse association between physical activity and risk of T2D, which may partly be mediated by reduced adiposity (Aune et al. 2015). Thus, T2D can be associated with obesity and low levels of muscle mass (Pedersen and Saltin 2015). Moderate to vigorous physical activity is recommended for patients with T2D. However, patients with T2D can be physically weak, making it difficult for them to engage in the recommended levels of physical activity (Hamasaki 2016). It is thus noteworthy that recreational football training combined with a calorie-restricted diet reduced fat mass to the same extent as a calorie-restricted diet alone (3.4 ± 0.4 kg vs 3.7 ± 0.4 kg, respectively) (de Sousa et al. 2014). Similarly, football training combined with dietary advice resulted in greater fat loss (−3.4 ± 2.8 vs −1.2 ± 2.0 kg) and increases in lean body mass than professional dietary advice *per se* (0.7 ± 1.5 vs −0.3 ± 1.6 kg).

4) Football training improves biomarkers of bone health and metabolic parameters, and reduces cardiovascular risk in T2D and MetS patients

T2D constitutes a global health challenge associated with considerable morbidity and mortality, and is also imposing a great economic burden on the healthcare system (Yang et al. 2013). Patients with T2D usually suffer from multiple pathological conditions, since they are not only struggling with deteriorated blood glucose control. For example, they have higher prevalence of other health complications including poor physical fitness and cardiovascular deficiencies (Flores-Le Roux et al. 2011), as well as impaired muscle mitochondrial function (Wojtaszewski 2009) and poor bone health (Kulkarni et al. 2017), compared to age-matched healthy individuals. Thus, the treatment of patients with T2D, as well as individuals with prediabetes (impaired fasting glycaemia or impaired glucose tolerance), should consist of a broad-spectrum approach while focusing on normalisation of blood glucose levels. Exercise training has been shown to improve blood glucose regulation and is proposed for inclusion in the treatment of patients with prediabetes and T2D (Pedersen and Saltin 2015). However, it is extremely important that this patient group receives exercise treatment that is potent enough to induce a broad-spectrum impact. Football training may therefore be suitable as a treatment for these pathological conditions, as it targets both metabolic and cardiovascular components.

In a study by de Sousa et al. (2014), improved blood glucose control has been demonstrated in male and female patients with T2D. Moreover, a combination of 12 weeks of football training and diet alterations markedly improved blood glucose regulation as well as muscle catabolism, with greater changes than for dietary changes alone (de Sousa et al. 2017). In support of these findings, it was recently shown in a group of 55- to 70-year-old individuals with prediabetes that football training in combination with dietary advice appeared superior for blood glucose control than dietary advice alone (Skoradal et al. 2018a). Indeed, fasting blood glucose concentrations declined from 6.2 to 5.8 mmol $\cdot l^{-1}$ in both intervention groups in the latter study, and this blood glucose level is below the clinical threshold related to impaired blood glucose control. It is noteworthy that the football intervention group displayed lower post-intervention blood glucose concentrations at 60 and 120 min of the oral glucose tolerance test (OGTT) and had a lower total area under the curve in comparison with the diet group. Finally, the football group, in contrast to the diet group, was able to normalise the glucose concentration to baseline values at the end of the OGTT, which indicates a decreased risk of progression of diabetes (de Sousa et al. 2017).

An independent risk factor for insulin resistance and T2D is obesity, and especially abdominal fat accumulation, which is also detrimental to cardiovascular health. In the study by Skoradal et al. (2018a), the football intervention induced a markedly greater fat loss (~3.5 kg) compared to dietary advice alone. The effect of football training in reducing body fat content is well-documented in a new meta-analysis (Milanović et al. 2019). Moreover, cross-sectional studies in elderly football players showed markedly lower body fat content than age-matched sedentary controls (Randers et al. 2014). Recently, it was demonstrated that 15 weeks of football training in sedentary hypertensive women upregulated skeletal muscle mitochondrial function and β-oxidative capacity in both lower and upperbody muscle groups (Nordsborg et al. 2015), which is also supported by increased whole-body fat oxidation during exercise after a football training intervention (Krustrup et al. 2010). Thus, increased muscle fat oxidative capacity after football training may contribute to the decrease in body fat content observed in patients with T2D by de Sousa et al. (2014) and of prediabetic individuals by Skoradal et al. (2018a). Part of the pathology of T2D is low skeletal muscle mitochondrial function (Wojtaszewski 2009), which seems to be upregulated after football training (Bangsbo et al. 2009; Nordsborg et al. 2015).

T2D is associated with a decline in muscle mass (Pedersen and Saltin 2015), and our studies of patients with prediabetes (Skoradal et al. 2018a, 2018b) and T2D show a ~1 kg increase in lean body mass after 12–16 weeks of treatment. The higher muscle mass provides a larger total muscle glycogen storage capacity, which is likely to improve clearance of glucose from the bloodstream. It seems, therefore, that football can improve blood glucose control by exerting a beneficial effect on mechanisms associated with pre- and post-insulin receptor binding events. Briefly, football can improve muscle mass (Skoradal et al. 2018a, 2018b) and the capillary network, adaptations that will increase insulin and blood glucose delivery to the targeted tissues (muscle, liver and fat cells). At post-receptor locations, it has been shown that football can improve mitochondria metabolism (Bangsbo et al. 2009; Nordsborg et al. 2015), which is beneficial to blood glucose regulation.

Patients with T2D, prediabetes or MetS have a higher prevalence of cardiovascular deficiencies compared to healthy individuals (Flores-Le Roux et al. 2011). In the study by Skoradal et al. (2018a), the prediabetic prediabetic were moderately hypertensive prior to the football treatment. The treatment resulted in an 8 mmHg drop in mean arterial pressure, which is comparable to conventional pharmacological agents used for blood pressure management. Indeed, the patients were actually able to normalise systolic and diastolic blood pressure (127 and 77 mmHg) in just 16 weeks of football training. Small-sided football games have been shown to induce high cardiovascular loading (Randers et al. 2010), confirmed by mean and peak heart rates of 80 and 95% HRmax, respectively (Skoradal et al. 2018a). Finally, the studies by de Sousa et al. (2014) and Skoradal et al. (2018a) both showed a markedly improved blood lipid profile after only 12 and 16 weeks of combined football and diet treatment. Thus, football treatment improves cardiovascular health in patients with T2D and individuals with prediabetes.

A meta-analysis review has shown that football training 2–3 times weekly increases VO_2max by about 25% in only 12 weeks (Milanović et al. 2015). Nearly similar and clinically significant increases in maximal oxygen uptake (Milanović et al. 2015) are observed after 12 and 16 weeks of football training in patients with T2D (de Sousa et al. 2014) and prediabetes (Skoradal et al. 2018a). Low cardiorespiratory fitness is a common characteristic in patients with T2D (Regensteiner et al. 1995; de Sousa et al. 2014). Physiological aging causes a decline in VO_2max of 5–10% per decade (Hawkins and Wiswell 2003). Thus, patients with prediabetes or T2D at a relatively high age are likely to display very low aerobic fitness, which impacts on their cardiorespiratory health. Indeed, patients with T2D who increase their cardiorespiratory fitness by ~5 mL/kg/min presented a significant reduction in overall cardiovascular mortality of 39–70% (Church et al. 2005). Thus, football training appears to be a highly efficient and important treatment method for increasing the cardiorespiratory health status of patients with T2D and prediabetes.

Patients with T2D have relatively poor bone health (Kulkarni et al. 2017). Since poor glycaemic control negatively affects several aspects of bone structure, density, skeletal integrity and biochemical markers of bone turnover, it remains a frequently overlooked complication of prediabetes and T2D (Starup-Linde 2013). Patients with deteriorated glycaemic control are at higher risk of fractures than healthy controls (Sharifi et al. 2006), which is associated with impaired or poor glycaemic control, longer disease duration and complications of diabetes (Kulkarni et al. 2017). In a recently published study, 16 weeks of football training markedly improved bone mineral density at clinically critical sites, such as the femur shaft, and upregulated blood markers of elevated bone turnover (Skoradal et al. 2018b). Thus, treating T2D and MetS patients with football training also facilitates bone health in these patient groups.

In conclusion, there is strong evidence that regular recreational football training can improve blood glucose regulation and blood lipids in patients with T2D. Moreover, football training can ameliorate the T2D-associated decline in cardiorespiratory and bone health in patients with T2D. Accordingly, it is expected that regular football training will improve overall health status and wellbeing for these patients.

5) Football training and nutritional advice prevent decline in muscle mass in patients with T2D

Football training and diet have been shown to be a good strategy as a lifestyle intervention, alongside glucose-lowering medication, for improving metabolic control and reducing cardiovascular events (de Sousa et al. 2017; de Sousa et al. 2014).

Inappropriate lifestyle and aging, starting in the fourth decade of life, are associated with a decline in pancreatic function and growth hormone production, resulting in central adiposity, sarcopenia and a higher prevalence of metabolic diseases. It is also known that a decrease in pancreatic islet function is also an important factor in the development of hyperglycaemia (Nguyen et al. 2011; Karakelides and Nair 2005).

The aging process induces changes in body composition, such as increased visceral fat and reduced muscle mass. Thus, a new concept called sarcopenic obesity has emerged (Kemmler et al. 2017). Sarcopenic obesity was first defined by Baumgartner (2000) as the coexistence of sarcopenia and obesity in one individual, i.e. a low amount of muscle tissue (sarcopenia) and an excess of adipose tissue (Lee et al. 2016). It has been more common in older adults than in young adults due to natural changes in body composition predicted in aging (Lee et al. 2016). Besides muscle tissue reduction, low muscle strength (hand-grip strength) and low physical capacity (slow walking) has been predicted as a modern definition of sarcopenia (Leong et al. 2015).

However, gains or losses in body mass, mainly measured as a reduction in lean body mass, are due to acute and chronic imbalances in protein turnover (Morton et al. 2015). The synthesis and degradation of proteins in the human body is affected by a number of variables, including age, activity level, gender, hormones, diseases and diet (Rennie et al. 2004). The body's proteins are constantly being transferred. This constant synthesis and degradation of proteins provides a mechanism for maintaining protein in the event of damage related to oxidative stress, protein malformation or other processes (Phillips 2017).

Regarding nutritional assessment, healthy meals with reduced portion sizes and low energy density generally favour weight loss and diabetes control. In addition, we know that the population with T2D consists particularly of elderly and sedentary people, and loss of lean mass is a natural part of the aging process and can lead to sarcopenic obesity. However, adherence to these better lifestyle actions in the long term is uncommon in this population, impairing the maintenance of weight loss in the short term after a period of energy restriction. Thus, interventions that lead to weight loss as well as its maintenance are strategies that result in more robust changes in long-term control of diabetes, impacting on better quality of life in the elderly population as well as lower public-health expenditure. In this context, the use of different types of protein supplementation has been less mentioned in the nutrition guidelines applied in the treatment of T2D as a strategy for preserving the loss of lean mass, improving the functional capacity of the muscle and ultimately controlling the glycaemia and the prevention of sarcopenic obesity, a common phenomenon in the elderly population with diabetes (de Sousa et al. 2019).

It has been shown that a minimum safe protein intake would be 1.0–1.2 g/kg/day for normal healthy people and at least 1.2 g/kg/day to 1.4 g/kg/day for the elderly (Rafii et al. 2016; Elango et al. 2010). However, according to Phillips (2017) it is important to emphasise that even these estimates may not be optimal and should be tested in long-term trials to establish the ramifications of this consumption and recommendation.

According to the Standards of Medical Care in Diabetes (ADA 2018), there is no evidence that adjusting daily protein intake (typically 1–1.5 g/kg body weight/day or 15–20% total calories) will improve health in individuals without diabetic kidney disease, and research is inconclusive regarding the ideal amount of dietary protein to optimise either glycaemic control or cardiovascular disease risk. Protein intake goals should therefore be individualised based on current eating patterns.

It has been shown that slightly higher levels of protein (20–30%) may contribute to increased satiety, which might favour the management and reduction of weight. However, the long-term effects of protein intake greater than 20% of calories on diabetes management and its complications are unknown (ADA 2018; Hamdy and Horton 2011). Although such diets may produce short-term weight loss and improved glycaemia, it has not been established that these benefits are maintained long term, and long-term effects on kidney function for persons with diabetes are unknown.

Reducing the amount of dietary protein below the recommended daily allowance (0.8 g/kg body weight/day) is not advised because it does not alter glycaemic measures, cardiovascular risk measures or the rate at which the glomerular filtration rate declines (ADA 2018). In individuals with T2D, protein intake may increase the insulin response to dietary carbohydrates. Carbohydrate sources high in protein should not therefore be used to treat or prevent hypoglycaemia due to the potential concurrent rise in endogenous insulin (ADA 2018).

The long-term health outcome in older people is impacted by the consumption of protein at levels of at least 1.2 g/kg/day in relation to maintenance of the muscular tissue of these individuals. This point is even more relevant if we consider that 25% of older men and up to 50% of elderly women are not consuming even the 0.8 g/kg/day recommended by the RDA (Fulgoni et al. 2008). Protein supplementation may therefore be considered in the event that this requirement is not met by food protein sources.

The best protein supplement studied so far is whey protein (milk serum). It contains high levels of branched-chain amino acids compared to other sources of protein and especially high concentrations of leucine, an amino acid responsible for activating protein synthesis (Jonker et al. 2017).

Whey protein is rapidly digested and therefore results in a rapid increase in blood amino acid concentrations. Another milk protein, casein, has a slower digestion profile than whey protein. As a result, casein prolongs higher hyperaminoacidaemia than milk serum. Although the increase in blood amino acids after ingestion of casein does not reach the magnitude observed with whey intake, protein synthesis is still activated post-exercise (Reitelseder et al. 2011). Milk is not the only source of protein for post-exercise supplementation. In addition, soy, which contains many antioxidants, is a good alternative source of protein for those on a vegetarian diet (Wang et al. 2013).

In the studies by de Sousa et al. (2014, 2017), 3 months of recreational football combined with dietary advice that consisted of 45–60% carbohydrate, 20–30% fat, and 15–20% of total energy intake from protein (0.8–1.0 g/kg/ body weight) distributed in five to six meals a day, favoured weight loss of ~3 kg and preserved lean body mass in type 2 diabetes mellitus patients. Moreover, this treatment was efficient at improving physical capacity, dyslipidaemic status and insulin sensitivity, and decreased markers of muscle catabolism in elderly patients with T2D (de Sousa et al. 2017; de Sousa et al. 2014). See Figure 2.1.

This intervention increased the use of glucose and fat as substrate during football sessions, evidenced by lower FFA and glucose blood levels, as well as improved

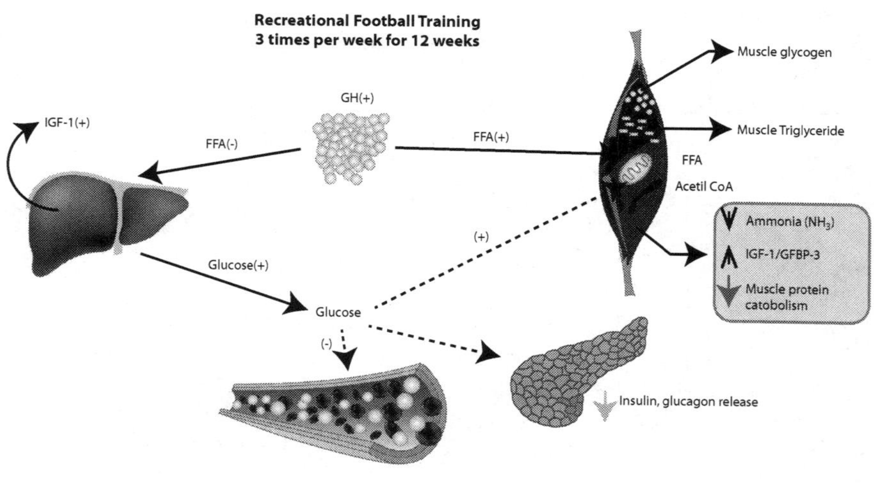

Figure 2.1 Recreational football training and nutritional intervention increase substrate utilisation and reduce markers of protein catabolism (de Sousa et al. 2017).

lipid profile and glucoregulatory markers (de Sousa et al. 2014). Football training resulted in a higher IGF-1/IGFBP-3 ratio and lower ammonia concentration, suggestive of attenuated muscle protein catabolism. Also, the intervention decreased insulin resistance through lower IGFBP-3 and glucose levels, increased lipolytic activity and prevented loss of lean body mass, improving health outcomes in patients with T2D (de Sousa et al. 2017).

6) Future study directions for recreational football and T2D

Based on the current chapter, we have reached the following conclusions and considerations for future research. Metabolic syndrome and T2D mainly occur in the middle-aged and elderly population. Aging induces changes in body composition, such as increased visceral fat and progressive loss of muscle mass, strength and functional capacity, leading to the phenomenon of sarcopenic obesity, decreasing the degree of activity with advancing age and predisposing subjects to the development of chronic diseases such as obesity and T2D and its complications. Evidence shows that the prevalence of T2D is higher in obese, overweight and physically inactive individuals, and physical inactivity is independently related to an increased risk of each of these. Thus, avoiding a sedentary lifestyle is important in T2D prevention and treatment. In this chapter, we have demonstrated that recreational football improves physical capacity, body composition and glucose tolerance parameters as well as decreasing the risks of cardiovascular outcome in the T2D population.

Football training contributes to decreases in the deleterious effects of T2D such as muscle frailty and sarcopenia. In addition to this, daily protein intake should be adjusted based on current eating patterns. Both strategies are aimed at increasing and/or preserving muscle mass loss as the main pillars of anabolism. As a guide for future research, investigating the impact of football training in improving metabolic outcomes and decreasing frailty with aging becomes necessary in T2D. From the molecular point of view, the study of the football training-induced mechanisms that improve insulin sensitivity and protect against premature mortality is of vital importance.

Regarding nutrition, one future challenge is to investigate the optimal daily therapeutic dosage of protein that, in combination with football training, will ameliorate aging-induced muscle mass loss.

Acknowledgements: Chapter revised by Maria Elizabeth Rossi da Silva, MD, PhD Endocrinology Division, School of Medicine, University of Sao Paulo, Brazil.

References

Alberti, K. G., R. H. Eckel, S. M. Grundy, P. Z. Zimmet, J. I. Cleeman, K. A. Donato, J. C. Fruchart, et al. 2009. "Harmonizing the metabolic syndrome: A joint interim statement of the International Diabetes Federation Task Force on Epidemiology and

Prevention; National Heart, Lung, and Blood Institute; American Heart Association; World Heart Federation; International Atherosclerosis Society; and International Association for the Study of Obesity." *Circulation* 120 (16):1640–1645. doi: 10.1161/CIRCULATIONAHA.109.192644.

Alberti, K. G., and P. Z. Zimmet. 1998. "Definition, diagnosis and classification of diabetes mellitus and its complications, part 1: Diagnosis and classification of diabetes mellitus provisional report of a WHO consultation." *Diabetic Medicine* 15 (7):539–553. doi: 10.1002/(SICI)1096-9136(199807)15:7<539::AID-DIA668>3.0.CO;2-S.

Andersen, T. R., J. F. Schmidt, M. Thomassen, T. Hornstrup, U. Frandsen, M. B. Randers, P. R. Hansen, P. Krustrup, and J. Bangsbo. 2014. "A preliminary study: Effects of football training on glucose control, body composition, and performance in men with type 2 diabetes." *Scandinavian Journal of Medicine & Science in Sports* 24 (1):43–56. doi: 10.1111/sms.12259.

American Diabetes Association (ADA). 2017. "4: Lifestyle management." *Diabetes Care* 40 (1):S33–S43.

American Diabetes Association (ADA). 2018. "4: Lifestyle management: Standards of medical care in diabetes-2018." *Diabetes Care* 41 (1):S38–S50.

Aune, D., T. Norat, M. Leitzmann, S. Tonstad, and L. J. Vatten. 2015. "Physical activity and the risk of type 2 diabetes: A systematic review and dose-response meta-analysis." *European Journal of epidemiology* 30 (7):529–542. doi: 10.1007/s10654-015-0056-z.

Bangsbo, J., T. P. Gunnarsson, J. Wendell, L. Nybo, and M. Thomassen. 2009. "Reduced volume and increased training intensity elevate muscle Na+-K+ pump α2-subunit expression as well as short-and long-term work capacity in humans." *Journal of Applied Physiology* 107 (6):1771–1780.

Baumgartner, R. N. 2000. "Body composition in healthy aging." *Annals of the New York Academy of Sciences* 904 (1):437–448.

Church, T. S., M. J. LaMonte, C. E. Barlow, and S. N. Blair. 2005. "Cardiorespiratory fitness and body mass index as predictors of cardiovascular disease mortality among men with diabetes." *Archives of Internal Medicine* 165 (18):2114–2120. doi: 10.1001/archinte.165.18.2114.

de Sousa, M. V., R. Fukui, P. Krustrup, S. Dagogo-Jack, and M. E. Rossi da Silva. 2017. "Combination of recreational soccer and caloric restricted diet reduces markers of protein catabolism and cardiovascular risk in patients with type 2 diabetes." *The Journal of Nutrition, Health & Aging* 21 (2):180–186.

de Sousa, M. V., R. Fukui, P. Krustrup, R. M. R. Pereira, P. R. S. Silva, A. C. Rodrigues, J. L. de Andrade, A. J. Hernandez, and M. E. Rossi da Silva. 2014. "Positive effects of football on fitness, lipid profile, and insulin resistance in Brazilian patients with type 2 diabetes." *Scandinavian Journal of Medicine & Science in Sports* 24:57–65.

de Sousa M.V.R., da Silva Soares D.B., Caraça E.R., Cardoso R. 2019. "Dietary protein and exercise for preservation of lean mass and perspectives on type 2 diabetes prevention." *Experimental Biology and Medicine* (Maywood) 244 (12):992–1004. doi.org/10.1177/1535370219861910.

Donahue, K. E., T. J. Mielenz, P. D. Sloane, L. F. Callahan, and R. F. Devellis. 2006. "Identifying supports and barriers to physical activity in patients at risk for diabetes." *Preventing Chronic Disease* 3 (4):A119.

Elango, R., M. A. Humayun, R. O. Ball, and P. B. Pencharz. 2010. "Evidence that protein requirements have been significantly underestimated." *Current Opinion in Clinical Nutrition and Metabolic Care* 13 (1):52–57. doi: 10.1097/MCO.0b013e328332f9b7.

Elbe, A. M., K. Strahler, P. Krustrup, J. Wikman, and R. Stelter. 2010. "Experiencing flow in different types of physical activity intervention programs: Three randomized studies." *Scandinavian Journal of Medicine & Science in Sports* 20 (1):111–117. doi: 10.1111/j.1600-0838.2010.01112.x.

Flores-Le Roux, J. A., J. Comin, J. Pedro-Botet, D. Benaiges, J. Puig-de Dou, J. J. Chillaron, A. Goday, J. Bruguera, and J. F. Cano-Perez. 2011. "Seven-year mortality in heart failure patients with undiagnosed diabetes: An observational study." *Cardiovascular Diabetology* 10 (1):39. doi: 10.1186/1475-2840-10-39.

Fulgoni III, V. L. 2008. "Current protein intake in America: Analysis of the National Health and Nutrition Examination Survey, 2003–2004." *The American Journal of Clinical Nutrition* 87 (5):1554S–1557S.

Hamasaki, H. 2016. "Daily physical activity and type 2 diabetes: A review." *World Journal of Diabetes* 7 (12):243–251. doi: 10.4239/wjd.v7.i12.243.

Hamdy, O., and E. S. Horton. 2011. "Protein content in diabetes nutrition plan." *Current Diabetes Reports* 11 (2):111–119. doi: 10.1007/s11892-010-0171-x.

Hawkins, S., and R. Wiswell. 2003. "Rate and mechanism of maximal oxygen consumption decline with aging: Implications for exercise training." *Sports Medicine* 33 (12):877–888. doi: 10.2165/00007256-200333120-00002.

Hirst, J. A., A. J. Farmer, R. Ali, N. W. Roberts, and R. J. Stevens. 2012. "Quantifying the effect of metformin treatment and dose on glycemic control." *Diabetes Care* 35 (2):446–454. doi: 10.2337/dc11-1465.

Jepson, R., F. M. Harris, A. Bowes, R. Robertson, G. Avan, and A. Sheikh. 2012. "Physical activity in South Asians: An in-depth qualitative study to explore motivations and facilitators." *PLoS One* 7 (10):e45333. doi: 10.1371/journal.pone.0045333.

Jonker, R., N. E. Deutz, M. L. Erbland, P. J. Anderson, and M. P. Engelen. 2017. "Effectiveness of essential amino acid supplementation in stimulating whole body net protein anabolism is comparable between COPD patients and healthy older adults." *Metabolism-Clinical and Experimental* 69:120–129. doi: 10.1016/j.metabol.2016.12.010.

Karakelides, H., and K. S. Nair. 2005. "Sarcopenia of aging and its metabolic impact." *Current Topics in Developmental Biology* 68:123–148. doi: 10.1016/S0070-2153(05)68005-2.

Kemmler, W., M. Teschler, A. Weissenfels, C. Sieber, E. Freiberger, and S. von Stengel. 2017. "Prevalence of sarcopenia and sarcopenic obesity in older German men using recognized definitions: High accordance but low overlap!" *Osteoporosis International* 28 (6):1881–1891. doi: 10.1007/s00198-017-3964-9.

Krustrup, P., P. Aagaard, L. Nybo, J. Petersen, M. Mohr, and J. Bangsbo. 2010. "Recreational football as a health promoting activity: A topical review." *Scandinavian Journal of Medicine & Science in Sports* 20 (1):1–13. doi: 10.1111/j.1600-0838.2010.01108.x.

Kulkarni, S. V., S. Meenatchi, R. Reeta, R. Ramesh, A. R. Srinivasan, and C. Lenin. 2017. "Association of glycemic status with bone turnover markers in type 2 diabetes mellitus." *International Journal of Applied & Basic Medical Research* 7 (4):247–251. doi: 10.4103/ijabmr.IJABMR_35_17.

Lee, D. C., R. P. Shook, C. Drenowatz, and S. N. Blair. 2016. "Physical activity and sarcopenic obesity: Definition, assessment, prevalence and mechanism." *Future science OA* 2 (3):FSO127. doi: 10.4155/fsoa-2016-0028.

Leong, D. P., K. K. Teo, S. Rangarajan, P. Lopez-Jaramillo, A. Avezum, Jr., A. Orlandini, P. Seron, S. H. Ahmed, et al. 2015. "Prognostic value of grip strength: Findings from the Prospective Urban Rural Epidemiology (PURE) study." *Lancet* 386 (9990):266–273. doi: 10.1016/S0140-6736(14)62000-6.

Lidegaard, L. P., N. Schwennesen, I. Willaing, and K. Faerch. 2016. "Barriers to and motivators for physical activity among people with type 2 diabetes: Patients' perspectives." *Diabetic Medicine* 33 (12):1677–1685. doi: 10.1111/dme.13167.

Milanović, Z., S. Pantelic, N. Covic, G. Sporis, and P. Krustrup. 2015. "Is recreational soccer effective for improving VO2max a systematic review and meta-analysis." *Sports Medicine* 45 (9):1339–1353. doi: 10.1007/s40279-015-0361-4.

Milanović, Z., S. Pantelic, N. Covic, G. Sporis, M. Mohr, and P. Krustrup. 2019. "Broad-spectrum physical fitness benefits of recreational football: A systematic review and meta-analysis." *British Journal of Sports Medicine* 53(15): 926–939. doi: 10.1136/bjsports-2017-097885.

Mohr, M., T. S. Nielsen, P. Weihe, J. A. Thomsen, G. Aquino, P. Krustrup, and N. B. Nordsborg. 2017. "Muscle ion transporters and antioxidative proteins have different adaptive potential in arm than in leg skeletal muscle with exercise training." *Physiological Reports* 5 (19):e13470. https://www.ncbi.nlm.nih.gov/pubmed/29038365. doi: 10.14814/phy2.13470.

Montague, C. T., and S. O'Rahilly. 2000. "The perils of portliness: Causes and consequences of visceral adiposity." *Diabetes* 49 (6):883–888.

Morton, R. W., C. McGlory, and S. M. Phillips. 2015. "Nutritional interventions to augment resistance training-induced skeletal muscle hypertrophy." *Frontiers in Physiology* 6:245. doi: 10.3389/fphys.2015.00245.

National Cholesterol Education Program Expert Panel on Detection, Evaluation, and Adults Treatment of High Blood Cholesterol in. 2002. "Third Report of the National Cholesterol Education Program (NCEP) expert panel on detection, evaluation, and treatment of high blood cholesterol in adults (adult treatment panel III) final report." *Circulation* 106 (25):3143–3421.

Nguyen, K. H., X. H. Yao, S. Moulik, S. Mishra, and B. L. Nyomba. 2011. "Human IGF binding protein-3 overexpression impairs glucose regulation in mice via an inhibition of insulin secretion." *Endocrinology* 152 (6):2184–2196. doi: 10.1210/en.2010-1324.

Nielsen, G., J. M. Wikman, C. J. Jensen, J. F. Schmidt, L. Gliemann, and T. R. Andersen. 2014. "Health promotion: The impact of beliefs of health benefits, social relations and enjoyment on exercise continuation." *Scandinavian Journal of Medicine & Science in Sports* 24 (1):66–75. doi: 10.1111/sms.12275.

Nordsborg, N. B., L. Connolly, P. Weihe, E. Iuliano, P. Krustrup, B. Saltin, and M. Mohr. 2015. "Oxidative capacity and glycogen content increase more in arm than leg muscle in sedentary women after intense training." *Journal of Applied Physiology* 119 (2):116–123. doi: 10.1152/japplphysiol.00101.2015.

Ottesen, L., R. S. Jeppesen, and B. R. Krustrup. 2010. "The development of social capital through football and running: Studying an intervention program for inactive women." *Scandinavian Journal of Medicine & Science in Sports* 20:118–131. doi: 10.1111/j.1600-0838.2010.01123.x.

Pedersen, B. K., and B. Saltin. 2015. "Exercise as medicine: Evidence for prescribing exercise as therapy in 26 different chronic diseases." *Scandinavian Journal of Medicine & Science in Sports* 25:1–72.

Phillips, S. M. 2017. "Current Concepts and Unresolved Questions in Dietary Protein Requirements and Supplements in Adults." *Frontiers in Nutrition* 4:13. doi: 10.3389/fnut.2017.00013.

Rafii, M., K. Chapman, R. Elango, W. W. Campbell, R. O. Ball, P. B. Pencharz, and G. Courtney-Martin. 2016. "Dietary protein requirement of men >65 years old determined by the indicator amino acid oxidation technique is higher than the current estimated average requirement." *The Journal of Nutrition.* doi: 10.3945/jn.115.225631.

Randers, M. B., J. L. Andersen, J. Petersen, E. Sundstrup, M. D. Jakobsen, J. Bangsbo, B. Saltin, and P. Krustrup. 2014. "Exercise performance and cardiovascular health variables in 70-year-old male soccer players compared to endurance-trained, strength-trained and untrained age-matched men." *Journal of Sports Sciences* 32 (13):1300–1308. doi: 10.1080/02640414.2014.898857.

Randers, M. B., L. Nybo, J. Petersen, J. J. Nielsen, L. Christiansen, M. Bendiksen, J. Brito, J. Bangsbo, and P. Krustrup. 2010. "Activity profile and physiological response to football training for untrained males and females, elderly and youngsters: Influence of the number of players." *Scandinavian Journal of Medicine & Science in Sports* 20 (1):14–23. doi: 10.1111/j.1600-0838.2010.01069.x.

Regensteiner, J. G., J. Sippel, E. T. McFarling, E. E. Wolfel, and W. R. Hiatt. 1995. "Effects of non-insulin-dependent diabetes on oxygen consumption during treadmill exercise." *Medicine and Science in Sports and Exercise* 27 (6):875–881.

Reitelseder, S., J. Agergaard, S. Doessing, I. C. Helmark, P. Lund, N. B. Kristensen, J. Frystyk, et al. 2011. "Whey and casein labeled with L-[1-13C]leucine and muscle protein synthesis: Effect of resistance exercise and protein ingestion." *American Journal of Physiology-Endocrinology and Metabolism* 300 (1):E231–E242. doi: 10.1152/ajpendo.00513.2010.

Rennie, M. J., H. Wackerhage, E. E. Spangenburg, and F. W. Booth. 2004. "Control of the size of the human muscle mass." *Annual Review of Physiology* 66:799–828. doi: 10.1146/annurev.physiol.66.052102.134444.

Reusch, J. E., M. Bridenstine, and J. G. Regensteiner. 2013. "Type 2 diabetes mellitus and exercise impairment." *Reviews in Endocrine and Metabolic Disorders* 14 (1):77–86. doi: 10.1007/s11154-012-9234-4.

Schmidt, J. F., T. R. Andersen, J. Horton, J. Brix, L. Tarnow, P. Krustrup, L. J. Andersen, J. Bangsbo, and P. R. Hansen. 2013. "Soccer training improves cardiac function in men with type 2 diabetes." *Medicine & Science in Sports & Exercise* 45 (12):2223–2233. doi: 10.1249/MSS.0b013e31829ab43c.

Selvin, E., S. Marinopoulos, G. Berkenblit, T. Rami, F. L. Brancati, N. R. Powe, and S. H. Golden. 2004. "Meta-analysis: Glycosylated hemoglobin and cardiovascular disease in diabetes mellitus." *Annals of Internal Medicine* 141 (6):421–431.

Sharifi, S., H. Mirzadeh, M. Imani, M. Atai, R. Bakhshi, and F. Ziaee. 2006. "Synthesis and characterization of novel injectable, biodegradable and in situ crosslinkable poly (hexamethylene-carbonate-fumarate), poly (hexamethylene carbonate) diacrylate and poly (ethylene glycol fumarate-co-hexamethylene carbonate-fumarate) scaffolds for bone tissue engineering." International Conference of the IEEE Engineering in Medicine and Biology Society.

Skoradal, M. B., P. Weihe, P. Patursson, J. Mortensen, L. Connolly, P. Krustrup, and M. Mohr. 2018a. "Football training improves metabolic and cardiovascular health status in 55- to 70-year-old women and men with prediabetes." *Scandinavian Journal of Medicine & Science in Sports* 28 (1):42–51. doi: 10.1111/sms.13081.

Skoradal, M. B., E. W. Helge, N. R. Jørgensen, J. Mortensen, P. Weihe, P. Krustrup, and M. Mohr. 2018b. "Osteogenic impact of football training in 55- to 70-year-old women and men with prediabetes." *Scandinavian Journal of Medicine & Science in Sports* 28 (1):52–60. doi: 10.1111/sms.13252.

Starup-Linde, J. 2013. "Diabetes, biochemical markers of bone turnover, diabetes control, and bone." *Frontiers in Endocrinology* 4:21. doi: 10.3389/fendo.2013.00021.

Umpierre, D., P. A. Ribeiro, B. D. Schaan, and J. P. Ribeiro. 2013. "Volume of supervised exercise training impacts glycaemic control in patients with type 2 diabetes: A systematic review with meta-regression analysis." *Diabetologia* 56 (2):242–251. doi: 10.1007/s00125-012-2774-z.

Unger, R. H. 2002. "Lipotoxic diseases." *Annual Review of Medicine* 53 (1):319–336. doi: 10.1146/annurev.med.53.082901.104057.

Wang, Q., X. Ge, X. Tian, Y. Zhang, J. Zhang, and P. Zhang. 2013. "Soy isoflavone: The multipurpose phytochemical (review)." *Biomedical Reports* 1 (5):697–701. doi: 10.3892/br.2013.129.

Williams, A. M., and N. J. Hodges. 2005. "Practice, instruction and skill acquisition in soccer: Challenging tradition." *Journal of Sports Sciences* 23 (6):637–650. doi: 10.1080/02640410400021328.

Williams, N. H., M. Hendry, B. France, R. Lewis, and C. Wilkinson. 2007. "Effectiveness of exercise-referral schemes to promote physical activity in adults: Systematic review." *The British Journal of General Practice: The Journal of the Royal College of General Practitioners* 57 (545):979–986. doi: 10.3399/096016407782604866.

Wojtaszewski, J. F. 2009. "AMP-activated protein kinase in sickness and health: From molecule to man." *Acta Physiologica (Oxford, England)* 196 (1):1. doi: 10.1111/j.1748-1716.2009.01966.x.

Wojtaszewski, J. F., S. B. Jørgensen, C. Frøsig, C. MacDonald, J. B. Birk, and E. A. Richter. 2003. "Insulin signalling: Effects of prior exercise." *Acta Physiologica Scandinavica* 178 (4):321–328. doi: 10.1046/j.1365-201X.2003.01151.x.

Yang, W., T. M. Dall, P. Halder, P. Gallo, S. L. Kowal, P. F. Hogan, and M. Petersen. 2013. "Economic costs of diabetes in the U.S. in 2012." *Diabetes Care* 36 (4):1033–1046. doi: 10.2337/dc12-2625.

Chapter 3

Football for promotion of bone health across the lifespan

Dimitris Vlachopoulos, Craig A. Williams, Eva Wulff Helge, Per Aagaard, Niklas Rye Jørgensen and Peter Krustrup

3.1 Introduction

Osteoporosis is characterised by compromised bone strength predisposing a person to an increased risk of fracture (NIH Consensus Development Panel on Osteoporosis Prevention and Therapy 2001). Approximately 200 million people are affected by osteoporosis worldwide, and in the European Union, 22 million women (Melton et al. 1992) and 5.5 million men are estimated to have osteoporosis (Hernlund et al. 2013). The prevalence of osteoporosis is expected to increase due to an aging population (Reginster and Burlet 2006) and the world population ≥65 years of age is predicted to double from about 506 million in 2008 to 1.3 billion by 2040, at which time it will account for 14% of the world's total population (Kinsella and Wan 2008). The economic burden of osteoporosis in Europe is higher than most types of cancer (except lung cancer) or chronic cardiorespiratory diseases (Kanis et al. 2008; Johnell and Kanis 2006), and represents a direct annual cost of ~ €31.7 billion to health care and social services (Kanis and Johnell 2005). Approximately 30% of all postmenopausal women have osteoporosis in the United States and Europe, and at least 40% of these women and 15–30% of men will sustain one or more fragility fractures in their remaining lifetime. The economic burden of incident and prior fragility fractures are estimated at €37 billion, and due to the aging of the population, the costs are expected to increase by 25% in 2025 (Hernlund et al. 2013; Randell et al. 1995). Approximately 20% of all patients with a hip fracture do not survive for more than 1 year from diagnosis, and more than 50% never completely regain their previous functional status (Boonen et al. 2005). The increased mortality and morbidity, physical disabilities and chronic pain after fractures can lead to loss of independence, hence primary prevention remains the most important policy action in public health to reduce the prevalence of osteoporosis and fractures.

Determinants of osteoporosis include a high genetic component with epidemiological studies indicating that heritable factors account for 60–80% of the variability in bone mineral density (BMD) and bone mineral content (BMC) (Mitchell et al. 2015; Stewart and Ralston 2000; Bachrach 2001), while environmental and modifiable factors (e.g., calcium, vitamin D and exercise) (Courteix et al. 2005; Ward et al. 2007; Lappe et al. 2014; Mouratidou et al. 2013; Valtuena et al. 2012;

Vlachopoulos et al. 2016) account for the remaining BMD variance. Peak bone mass (PBM) attainment typically occurs between the second and third decade of life, with 80–90% acquired by late adolescence, although this is dependent on the specific skeletal site (Baxter-Jones et al. 2011; Henry, Fatayerji, and Eastell 2004). During the years of puberty, girls acquire approximately 40% of their PBM, meaning they had achieved approximately 90% of PBM by the age of 18 (Theintz et al. 1992). The PBM is relatively stable until the onset of bone loss with aging. In addition to age-related bone loss for both men and women, women experience an accelerated loss for 3–6 years at menopause (Faulkner and Bailey 2007). Moderate to vigorous physical activity (MVPA) contributes to achieving the full potential of PBM (Gordon et al. 2017), which is an important predictor for BMD in elderly and hence, maximising the PBM should be an essential prevention strategy for reducing the incidence and prevalence of osteoporosis (Bonjour and Chevalley 2007).

Exercise is well known to play an important role in bone development and maintenance of bone mass due to the mechanical loads produced and the forces applied on the skeleton that subsequently trigger bone modeling and remodeling (Wolff et al. 1999). It has been suggested that short-duration and high-intensity loading movements of a sufficient magnitude stimulate bone cell activity and induce bone adaptations that lead to increased bone strength (Turner 1998). The relationship between muscle and bone led to the functional 'bone-muscle unit' theory, suggesting that long-term changes in muscle strength (either increased or decreased) affects bone strength linearly (Schoenau and Frost 2002). According to the potential to augment bone mass and geometry during growth, exercises can be categorised as osteogenic (weight-bearing and high-intense exercise) or non-osteogenic (non-weight-bearing and low-intense exercise) (Courteix et al. 1998; Bass et al. 2002; Duncan et al. 2002; Faulkner et al. 2003; Ward et al. 2005; Tournis et al. 2010; Dowthwaite, Rosenbaum, and Scerpella 2012; Ferry et al. 2013; Maimoun et al. 2013). Training including weight-bearing activities may elicit greater improvements in BMC and BMD than non-weight bearing activities, while non-weight bearing activities may have no osteogenic effect or even inflict a negative effect on bone development in children and adolescents (Hind and Burrows 2007). Considering that the majority of children and adults in developed countries are participating in sports during growth and adulthood, it is important to understand how participation in different loading sports can promote bone health and reduce the prevalence of osteoporosis and the incidence of fractures.

Football is the most popular sport worldwide, with around 300 million registered football players, accounting for approximately 4% of the world's total population (Dvorak and Junge 2015). Football includes intermittent high-intensity movements involving various types of runs, multiple and rapid changes of directions, accelerations and decelerations, jumps and kicks, which produce large ground reaction forces that can stimulate bone formation and skeletal adaptations during childhood and adolescence (Ara et al. 2006; Vicente-Rodriguez et al. 2004; Krustrup et al. 2010; Calbet et al. 2001). Additionally, football training can improve bone health outcomes during adulthood, including untrained populations (Helge et al. 2010), clinical populations (Uth et al. 2018), women (Krustrup et al. 2010; Jackman et al. 2013) and men (Helge, Andersen, et al. 2014; Hagman et al. 2018). Cross-sectional and longitudinal studies investigating the effect of football participation on bone health during growth and in adulthood have mainly used dual-energy X-ray absorptiometry (DXA) (Hagman et al. 2018; Vicente-Rodriguez et al. 2004; Jackman et al. 2013) and geometry estimates, such as hip structural analysis (HSA) (Nikander et al. 2005; El Hage 2013) and trabecular bone score (TBS) (Vlachopoulos, Barker, Ubago-Guisado, et al. 2017; Heinio, Nikander, and Sievanen 2015). But there are also studies that have included peripheral quantitative computed tomography (pQCT) (Helge et al. 2010), Quantitative Ultrasound (QUS) (Torres-Costoso et al. 2018; Falk et al. 2010) and bone turnover markers (Mohr et al. 2015; Weiler, Keen, and Wolman 2012; Helge, Randers, et al. 2014). This chapter will comprehensively outline the role of football participation to promote bone health across the lifespan and reduce the prevalence of osteoporosis and non-traumatic fractures.

3.2 Football participation for promotion of bone health during growth

3.2.1 Cross-sectional studies on football and bone health during growth

During developmental growth, participation in football positively affects bone mass in both sexes in children and adolescents according to a recent systematic review and meta-analysis (Lozano-Berges et al. 2018). The meta-analysis indicated that the mean differences in total body BMD between football players and sedentary controls were 0.061 (95% CI, 0.042–0.079) in males and 0.063 (95% CI, 0.026–0.099) in females (Lozano-Berges et al. 2018). Additionally, the effects of football practice on BMD were greater during pubertal years compared to pre-pubertal years (Lozano-Berges et al. 2018). Cross-sectional data in prepubescent male footballers demonstrate that long-term football participation for at least 3 hours per week leads to greater BMC at the lumbar spine, femoral neck and trochanter skeletal sites compared to that observed in non-athletic controls (Vicente-Rodriguez et al. 2003) (Figure 3.1), which indicates that the effects of football practice on skeletal bone health may be evident when training at least 3 hours per week. However, it should be noted that the optimal volume of football training for osteogenic stimulus has not yet been established. A recent cross-sectional study found that adolescent male footballers had significantly higher BMD (8.8% to 25.1 %) and BMC (7.9 % to 29.5 %) than active controls at all sites of the skeleton except for the lumbar spine and arms after adjusting for age, height, region-specific lean mass, calcium intake and MVPA (Vlachopoulos, Barker, Williams, et al. 2017). A comparison between adolescent female swimmers and footballers found that swimmers had significantly lower BMD at all body sites compared to footballers, while also showing lower values compared with untrained age-matched controls (Ferry et al. 2011). Site-specific adaptations from football practice were investigated by Seabra et al. that found total body BMD and lower limb BMD at dominant and non-dominant site were substantially higher in footballers compared to controls after controlling for maturity offset. However, no significant differences were found for BMC (Seabra et al. 2013). Nebigh and colleagues showed similar results in pubertal but not in pre-pubertal male football players compared to controls (Nebigh et al. 2009). Moreover, Silva et al. showed that male adolescent footballers had significantly higher hip BMD than controls at the end of puberty (16–18 years), and that footballers at the end of puberty had higher total body, lumbar spine and proximal femur BMD than footballers at the initial age of puberty (10–12 years) (Silva et al. 2011). These findings can be explained by the greater muscle strength of young footballers, which was found to be the strongest predictor of bone mass and structure (Vlachopoulos, Ubago-Guisado, et al. 2017; Vicente-Rodriguez et al. 2005). Notably, the magnitude of the differences reported among various studies appears to stem from the use of different confounders (e.g., height, lean mass, hours of training and nutritional intakes) and highly differing characteristics of study participants (e.g., sexual maturation status).

3.2.2 *Longitudinal studies on football and bone health during growth*

Longitudinal studies evaluating the effect of football participation on bone health during childhood and adolescence are limited, and a study performed by Agostinete et al. found no BMD accrual differences between young football players and controls after 9 months of football training (Agostinete et al. 2016). In support of this observation, following 1 year of football training, no differences in BMD and BMC could be noted between a football group and the active controls after adjusting for baseline bone status, age, height, lean mass, MVPA and maturity (Vlachopoulos et al. 2018). A study conducted by Zouch et al. also found no differences between footballers and controls at baseline, but after 10 months of football training there were significant improvements in BMC at whole body, lumbar spine, total hip and lower limbs compared to controls, with amplified increases observed in those who trained for 4 hours per week compared with individuals who trained for 2 hours per week (Zouch et al. 2008). After 1 year of football training, the pubertal football players have demonstrated higher BMC compared to controls. After 1 year, greater increases in BMC at whole body, total hip and lower limbs were observed for pre-pubertal football players compared to controls, whereas pubertal players also showed greater increases at lumbar spine BMC. When both groups of football players were compared, greater BMC increases were reported in pubertal players than in pre-pubertal players (Zouch et al. 2014). Also, it was noted that the bone gains were greater when evaluated for the total body and weight-bearing bones (the lumbar spine, total hip and supporting leg) compared to non-weight-bearing bones (dominant arm and non-dominant arm) in boys who became pubescent during the 1-year study period. No differential gains were observed in boys who remained prepubescent (Zouch et al. 2014). After 3 years of football training, football players showed larger BMC and BMD gains for whole body, lumbar spine, total hip and lower limbs compared to non-exercising controls (Zouch et al. 2015). Another study followed 9-year-old male footballers for 3 years and compared selected bone health parameters with that of controls (Figure 3.1). The data revealed that footballers gained twice as much femoral neck and intertrochanteric BMC than the control group, and their mean hip BMD increased 33% more than the control group (Vicente-Rodriguez et al. 2004). Likewise, muscle-skeletal structures were found to respond positively to the weight-bearing and impact-loading imposed by football practice (Seabra et al. 2013) and enhancement of lean mass was found to be the best predictor of this bone mass accumulation during growth (Vicente-Rodriguez et al. 2005).

Randomised controlled trials allocating only football to improve musculo-skeletal outcomes during growth have not been conducted, however a recent 10-month school-based intervention in children aged 8–10 years compared the musculoskeletal effects of small-sided ball games and circuit strength training for 40 minutes 3 times per week. The small-sided ball game training consisted of 75% 3x3 football training and 25% of 3v3 basketball and floorball games. The study showed that the small-sided ball game group significantly improved total body BMD and leg BMC compared to age-matched controls, and had significantly

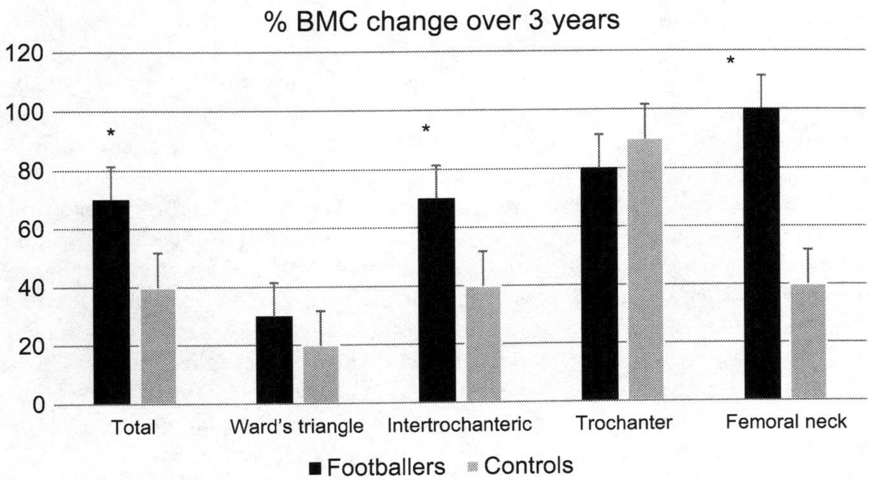

Figure 3.1 Changes in BMC with 3 years of football training in young footballers (9 to 12 years) for the whole femur and femoral regions after adjustment for the concurrent increase in age, height and body mass.

Source: Adapted from (Vicente-Rodriguez et al. 2004).

higher change in leg BMD compared with controls and the circuit strength training group. These findings indicate that small-sided ball games, mainly football, can improve bone mineralisation and can be implemented in the school system (Larsen et al. 2018).

3.2.3 Football and structural bone adaptations during growth

In addition to BMD and BMC gains, exercise can also influence the structural bone outcomes (Hind et al. 2012). A combination of bone quantity, quality and microarchitecture outcomes can provide important information regarding bone adaptations during growth. In addition, bone turnover markers can provide further information on cellular bone responses (Jurimae, Maestu, and Jurimae 2010). In parallel with the findings for BMD and BMC, the geometrical adaptations examined by HSA at the narrow neck of the femoral neck also supported a superior bone geometry in footballers (Vlachopoulos, Barker, Williams, et al. 2017). The study used HSA software analysis at the narrow neck of the femur and reported that male adolescent footballers had a significantly larger cross-sectional moment of inertia (CSMI) (17%), cross-sectional area (CSA) (19%), section modulus (21%) and hip strength index (39%) than controls. Additionally, using QUS analysis, footballers demonstrated higher bone stiffness than controls in the dominant foot (20.1%), as well as in the non-dominant foot (12.9%), while non-footballers showed no significant differences between the dominant vs. non-dominant foot (Vlachopoulos, Barker, Williams, et al. 2017). A study in oligomenorrheic female athletes reported that engagement in weight-bearing sports for 4 hours per week resulted in significantly higher HSA outcomes compared to non-athletes (Ackerman et al. 2013), which is consistent with the improved structural rigidity previously found in footballers. In a study of adolescent female athletes, greater increase in subperiosteal width was observed in footballers compared to swimmers, while the endocortical diameter was significantly reduced in swimmers after 8 months of training (Ferry et al. 2013). The differences observed in bone mass between osteogenic and non-osteogenic sports (i.e. football vs. swimming) are likely to be explained by differences in the specific mechanical loading pattern on the skeleton (Greene and Naughton 2006). Using QUS analysis, Falk et al. found that child and adolescent male football players had higher values of speed of sound (SOS) than controls (Falk et al. 2010). Madic et al. also compared QUS between footballers and controls and found that footballers had significantly higher SOS values at right and left calcaneus sites than the control (Madic et al. 2010). The only cross-sectional study using pQCT to compare dominant and non-dominant leg bone geometry in adolescent male footballers found that footballers had higher bone mass and improved geometry at 4% of the distal tibia, 14% and 38% of diaphyseal tibia in the non-dominant leg than the dominant leg (Anliker, Sonderegger, and Toigo 2013). These differences between dominant and non-dominant legs might be explained by the higher ground reaction forces experienced by the non-dominant leg when kicks and tackles are performed by the dominant leg (Seabra et al. 2013).

3.3 Football participation for promotion of bone health in adulthood

3.2.1 *Cross-sectional studies on football and bone health in adulthood*

Football participation can be beneficial for bone health across the ages of adulthood and evidence suggests that the football participation can improve or maintain bone outcomes (Helge, Andersen, et al. 2014; Hagman et al. 2018; Jackman et al. 2013; Krustrup et al. 2010; Helge et al. 2010). A recent systematic review examined the health benefits of recreational football in middle-aged and older adults and concluded that recreational football can be considered an alternative exercise modality for untrained, healthy or unhealthy middle-aged and older adults of both sexes to maintain an active lifestyle and mitigate a wide array of physical and physiological age-related changes (Luo et al. 2018). A cross-sectional study compared BMD of footballers and long-distance runners aged 20–30 years old and showed that leg and calcaneal BMD was significantly higher in football players than controls. Additionally, footballers had significantly higher right hip and spine BMD than runners, and runners had higher calcaneal BMD than controls (Fredericson et al. 2007). A previous study of 22 year old footballers who had been playing football for the last 12 years found a 13–24% higher BMC than in non-active controls (Calbet et al. 2001), indicating the long-term potential benefits of football participation on bone health. A cross-sectional evaluation in adults showed that participation in repeated moderate-impact loading sports may result in lower TBS at the lumbar spine and

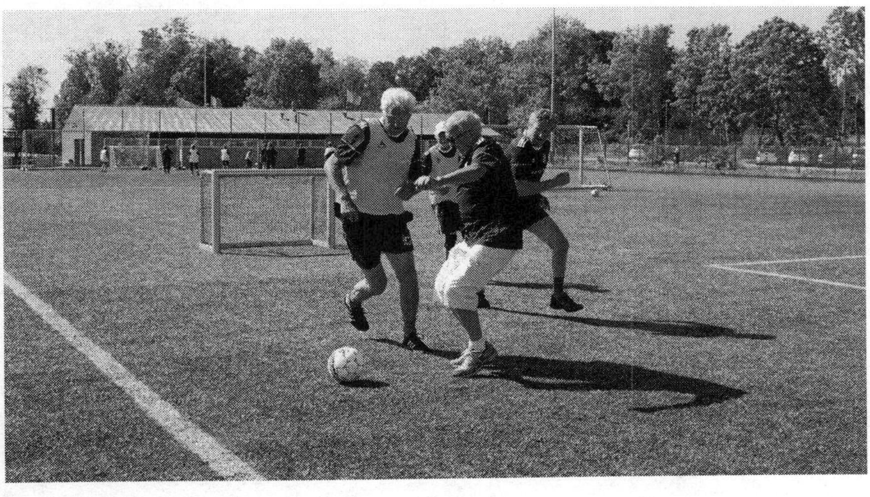

Photo 3.1 Small-sided football training for elderly.

Source: Photo Credit: Bo Kousgaard, University of Southern Denmark.

increased fracture risk compared to high-impact loading sports (Heinio, Nikander, and Sievanen 2015). Another cross-sectional study comparing bone geometry estimates using hip structural analysis in 22-year-old female football players and sedentary controls found that total hip BMD, femoral neck BMD and HSA parameters (7–17%) were significantly higher in football players compared to controls after adjusting for body mass (El Hage 2013). Exercises that involve maximal muscle contractions and rapid accelerations and decelerations can place substantial loads on bones and stimulate an increase in bone strength even during adulthood (Schoenau and Frost 2002), which might explain the findings of the previous studies. A recent study by Hagman et al. has shown that BMD of the proximal femur and total body BMD were significantly higher in lifelong trained male football players aged 65–80 years and young elite football players aged 18–30 years compared to age-matched untrained men. Interestingly, elderly football players even had significantly higher BMD in femoral trochanter and leg BMD than untrained young males despite an age difference of 47 years. It should be noted that adjustments for lean mass and height have been conducted as part of the study (Hagman et al. 2018).

3.3.2 *Acute and long-term skeletal adaptations from football in adulthood*

The effect of football participation on BMD during adulthood and in elderly populations was investigated by randomised controlled trials that reported small site-specific skeletal benefits (Helge et al. 2010; Krustrup et al. 2009; Randers et al. 2010). The effect of 14 weeks of recreational football and endurance running on volumetric BMD and muscle power was investigated in untrained premenopausal women aged 36.5 years and compared with a control group. The findings showed that volumetric BMD in left and right tibia increased significantly by 2.6% and 2.1% respectively in footballers and by 0.7% and 1.1% respectively in runners (Figure 3.2), without any significant changes in controls (Helge et al. 2010). However, no significant improvements were observed in areal BMD at any skeletal sites of the groups, possibly due to the short duration of the programme. Additionally, significant improvements were observed in the football group in peak jump power by 3%, hamstring strength during fast (240°·s^{-1}) and slow (30°·s^{-1}) contractions by 11% and 9% respectively, but there were no significant improvements in the endurance running and control groups (Helge et al. 2010). These findings highlight the potential of a 14-week football training programme (1.8 hours per week) to significantly improve peak jump power, maximal hamstring strength and volumetric BMD in premenopausal women that could potentially decrease the risk of falling and fracture. Similarly, a 16-week football training study in elite and untrained young women aged 24 years showed that at baseline total and leg BMD and BMC were 13–24% and 23–28%, significantly higher in the elite group compared to the untrained group. After 16 weeks of football training for the untrained group, lean body mass was significantly increased by 1.4 kg and the number of falls was decreased by 29%, but no significant changes occurred in

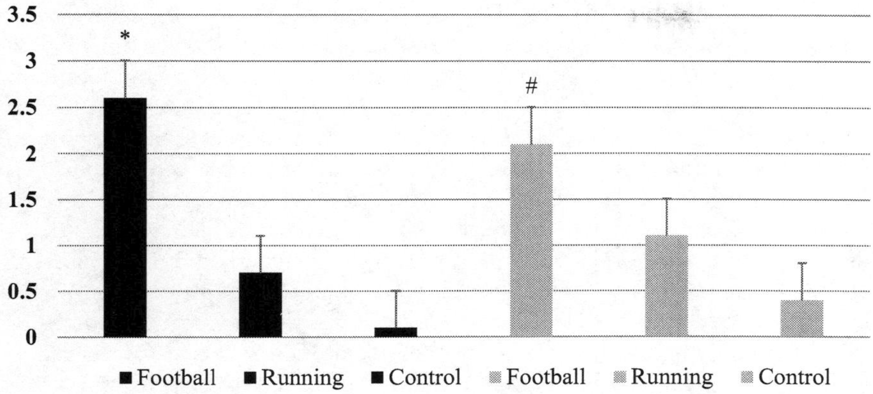

Figure 3.2 Percentage change in total volumetric BMD in distal tibia for untrained premenopausal women after 14 weeks of training football (n=12), running (n=16) and an inactive lifestyle (n=9). Results from the left leg are shown in black and results from the right leg in grey. Means ± standard deviation. * denotes significant difference from running and control groups (P<0.05); # denotes significant difference from control group (P<0.05).

Source: Adapted from (Helge et al. 2010).

BMD or BMC (Jackman et al. 2013). A study compared the effect of recreational football and running for 12 weeks on BMD in 20- to 43-year-old sedentary men. The results showed that total body BMD was not significantly increased in any group, while lower-extremity BMD was increased by 2% following the 12-week short-term soccer training, but unaltered in the running group. The increase in lean body mass and lower-extremity bone mass over 12 weeks were greater in the football group than in runners and controls, with no significant difference between runners and controls (Krustrup et al. 2009). A different study in untrained adult males that measured at baseline, at 12 weeks and at 52 weeks showed that the BMD and the BMC at the legs was significantly higher (2.0 and 3.5%, respectively) at 52 weeks, but it was not different at baseline and at 12 weeks (Randers et al. 2010). It is likely that the movement characteristics in the football group include many changes of direction and jumps, which can augment BMD after a period of training, since the osteogenic stimulus from exercise depends on the strain rate and magnitude induced by muscle contraction and ground reaction forces (Kohrt, Barry, and Schwartz 2009).

3.3.3 Football participation and cellular bone adaptations in adulthood

The positive effects of football participation can also be observed at the cellular level of bones by using bone turnover markers, such as osteocalcin and

N-terminal propeptide of type 1 procollagen (P1NP) as bone formation markers, and C-terminal telopeptide of type 1 collagen (CTX) as a bone resorption marker. A 15-week study in sedentary women aged 45 years showed that football training can improve the bone turnover marker profile, while swimming training did not have similar effects (Mohr et al. 2015). Specifically, it was found that osteocalcin and P1NP significantly increased by 37% and 42%, respectively, in the football training group, whereas no increases were observed in the high-intensity intermittent, moderate-intensity swimming and the control group. Additionally, in the football group, leg BMC significantly increased by 3.1% and BMD in the femoral shaft and trochanter significantly increased by 1.7% and 2.4%, respectively. There were no increases observed in the other groups over 15 weeks. A longer-duration study investigated the effects of 12 months of recreational football and resistance training on BMD and bone turnover markers in elderly men, aged 68.2 years. In footballers, BMD in proximal femur significantly increased by 1.8% from 0 to 4 months, and by 5.4% from 0 to 12 months, while total body BMD remained unchanged. After 4 and 12 months of football, osteocalcin was increased by 45% and 46% from baseline, and P1NP was 41% and 40% higher from baseline. CTX only increased after 12 months, by 43% from baseline. In resistance training and controls, BMD and bone turnover markers remained unchanged. These findings indicate that an osteogenic adaptation was initiated after 4 months of recreational football for elderly men, which was further increased after 12 months, while the resistance training group did not have similar improvements (Helge, Andersen, et al. 2014). These findings show that the osteogenic BMD response in elderly men is not lower, but rather slower, compared to their younger counterparts. Measurements of biochemical bone turnover markers in the elderly also showed that the anabolic response might be due to the improvements in P1NP with no change in CTX. The changes in the elderly population are higher than previously observed in other intervention studies examining the skeletal effect of physical activity (Vincent and Braith 2002; Bolam, van Uffelen, and Taaffe 2013). The effects of football participation on bone metabolism were also investigated by a case-control study in homeless men who were monitored over 12 weeks, and the findings showed that osteocalcin increased by 27% along with minor improvements (1.0%) in trunk BMD (Helge, Randers, et al. 2014). Another mechanistic study in females compared the acute effects of a short-duration vibration exercise session and two football sessions of 15 minutes and 1 hour duration, respectively, on bone turnover markers. These findings revealed that 48 hours after a single bout of exercise, plasma osteocalcin concentration increased by 10% in all groups, whereas P1NP increased by 15% after 15 minutes of small-sided football training, but in contrast to P1NP, that failed to increase in the short-duration vibration group (Bowtell et al. 2016). These findings indicate that the observed beneficial effects of football participation may to some extent be attributable to the repeated stimulation of osteoblast activity within each single training session.

3.4 Conclusions

Football is the most popular sport practised worldwide and there is conclusive evidence that football participation has site-specific positive effects on skeletal bone mass during growth and in adulthood. The positive effects of football participation during the pubertal years might be greater compared to pre- or post-pubertal years, partially due to the rapid increases of sex and growth hormones that have an independent effect on bone accretion in these periods. Additionally, participation in football for many years starting from childhood might induce greater adaptations due to the greater exposure to weight-bearing loads, which then leads to more pronounced bone development. The benefits of football practise are observed in both male and female athletes during growth and in adulthood with evidence indicating structural, cellular and clinically relevant bone adaptations. During adulthood, football can be considered an effective exercise modality to not only maintain but also improve bone health in untrained middle-aged and older men and women inclusive of clinical patient groups. The skeletal benefits are site-specific with lower limbs skeletal regions, such as hip, femoral neck, trochanter, and intertrochanteric, being particularly stimulated by the mechanical loads elicited by football-specific movements such as jumps, changes of direction, and vigorous accelerations and decelerations. Due to the paucity and variation in quality of available studies, future research should comprise high-quality randomised controlled trials and longitudinal studies to establish more comprehensive evidence on the positive effects of football practise in childhood, adolescence and adulthood. Considerations about research focusing on football and bone health should include the use of important covariates, i.e. lean body mass and size, and the justification of covariates selected in the statistical models. Future applied research should focus on providing evidence on the dose-response relationship for inducing positive bone adaptations during developmental growth and in adulthood to allow global policy stakeholders to incorporate football as an effective and feasible sports medicine strategy across the lifespan.

References

Ackerman, K. E., L. Pierce, G. Guereca, M. Slattery, H. Lee, M. Goldstein, and M. Misra. 2013. "Hip structural analysis in adolescent and young adult oligoamenorrheic and eumenorrheic athletes and nonathletes." *The Journal of Clinical Endocrinology & Metabolism* 98 (4):1742–1749. doi: 10.1210/jc.2013-1006.

Agostinete, R. R., K. R. Lynch, L. A. Gobbo, M. C. Lima, I. H. Ito, R. Luiz-de-Marco, M. A. Rodrigues-Junior, and R. A. Fernandes. 2016. "Basketball affects bone mineral density accrual in boys more than swimming and other impact sports: 9-mo Follow-Up." *Journal of Clinical Densitometry* 19(3): 375–81. doi: 10.1016/j.jocd.2016.04.006.

Anliker, E., A. Sonderegger, and M. Toigo. 2013. "Side-to-side differences in the lower leg muscle-bone unit in male soccer players." *Medicine and Science in Sports and Exercise* 45 (8):1545–1552. doi: 10.1249/MSS.0b013e31828cb712.

Ara, I., G. Vicente-Rodriguez, J. Perez-Gomez, J. Jimenez-Ramirez, J. A. Serrano-Sanchez, C. Dorado, and J. A. Calbet. 2006. "Influence of extracurricular sport activities on body composition and physical fitness in boys: A 3-year Longitudinal Study." *International Journal of Obesity (Lond)* 30 (7):1062–1071. doi: 10.1038/sj.ijo.0803303.

Bachrach, L. K. 2001. "Acquisition of optimal bone mass in childhood and adolescence." *Trends in Endocrinology and Metabolism* 12 (1):22–28.

Bass, S. L., L. Saxon, R. M. Daly, C. H. Turner, A. G. Robling, E. Seeman, and S. Stuckey. 2002. "The effect of mechanical loading on the size and shape of bone in pre-, peri-, and postpubertal girls: A study in tennis players." *J Bone Miner Res* 17 (12):2274–2280. doi: 10.1359/jbmr.2002.17.12.2274.

Baxter-Jones, A. D., R. A. Faulkner, M. R. Forwood, R. L. Mirwald, and D. A. Bailey. 2011. "Bone mineral accrual from 8 to 30 years of age: An estimation of peak bone mass." *Journal of Bone and Mineral Research* 26 (8):1729–1739. doi: 10.1002/jbmr.412.

Bolam, K. A., J. G. van Uffelen, and D. R. Taaffe. 2013. "The effect of physical exercise on bone density in middle-aged and older men: A systematic review." *Osteoporosis International* 24 (11):2749–2462. doi: 10.1007/s00198-013-2346-1.

Bonjour, J.-P., and T. Chevalley. 2007. "Pubertal timing, peak bone mass and fragility fracture risk." *BoneKEy-Osteovision* 4 (2):30–48. doi: 10.1138/20060247.

Boonen, S., R. F. Laan, I. P. Barton, and N. B. Watts. 2005. "Effect of osteoporosis treatments on risk of non-vertebral fractures: Review and meta-analysis of intention-to-treat studies." *Osteoporosis International* 16 (10):1291–1298. doi: 10.1007/s00198-005-1945-x.

Bowtell, J. L., S. R. Jackman, S. Scott, L. J. Connolly, M. Mohr, G. Ermidis, R. Julian, F. Yousefian, E. W. Helge, N. R. Jorgensen, J. Fulford, K. M. Knapp, and P. Krustrup. 2016. "Short duration small sided football and to a lesser extent whole body vibration exercise induce acute changes in markers of bone turnover." *Biomed Research International* 2016:3574258. doi: 10.1155/2016/3574258.

Calbet, J. A., C. Dorado, P. Diaz-Herrera, and L. P. Rodriguez-Rodriguez. 2001. "High femoral bone mineral content and density in male football (soccer) players." *Medicine and Science in Sports and Exercise* 33 (10):1682–1687.

Courteix, D., C. Jaffre, E. Lespessailles, and L. Benhamou. 2005. "Cumulative effects of calcium supplementation and physical activity on bone accretion in premenarchal children: A double-blind randomised placebo-controlled trial." *International Journal of Sports Medicine* 26 (5):332–338. doi: 10.1055/s-2004-821040.

Courteix, D., E. Lespessailles, S. L. Peres, P. Obert, P. Germain, and C. L. Benhamou. 1998. "Effect of physical training on bone mineral density in prepubertal girls: A comparative study between impact-loading and non-impact-loading sports." *Osteoporosis International* 8 (2):152–158. doi: Doi 10.1007/Bf02672512.

Dowthwaite, J. N., P. F. Rosenbaum, and T. A. Scerpella. 2012. "Site-specific advantages in skeletal geometry and strength at the proximal femur and forearm in young female gymnasts." *Bone* 50 (5):1173–1183. doi: 10.1016/j.bone.2012.01.022.

Duncan, C. S., C. J. Blimkie, C. T. Cowell, S. T. Burke, J. N. Briody, and R. Howman-Giles. 2002. "Bone mineral density in adolescent female athletes: Relationship to exercise type and muscle strength." *Medicine and Science in Sports and Exercise* 34 (2):286–294.

Dvorak, J., and A. Junge. 2015. "Twenty years of the FIFA medical assessment and research centre: From 'medicine for football' to 'football for health'." *British Journal of Sports Medicine* 49 (9):561–563. doi: 10.1136/bjsports-2015-094805.

El Hage, R. 2013. "Geometric indices of hip bone strength in young female football players." *Journal of Musculoskeletal and Neuronal Interactions* 13 (2):206–212.

Falk, B., S. Braid, M. Moore, M. Yao, P. Sullivan, and N. Klentrou. 2010. "Bone properties in child and adolescent male hockey and soccer players." *Journal of Science and Medicine in Sport* 13 (4):387–391. doi: 10.1016/j.jsams.2009.03.011.

Faulkner, R. A., and D. A. Bailey. 2007. "Osteoporosis: A pediatric concern?" *Medicine and Sports Science* 51:1–12. doi: 10.1159/0000102993.

Faulkner, R. A., M. R. Forwood, T. J. Beck, J. C. Mafukidze, K. Russell, and W. Wallace. 2003. "Strength indices of the proximal femur and shaft in prepubertal female gymnasts." *Medicine and Science in Sports and Exercise* 35 (3):513–518. doi: 10.1249/01.MSS.0000053724.33480.8B.

Ferry, B., M. Duclos, L. Burt, P. Therre, F. Le Gall, C. Jaffre, and D. Courteix. 2011. "Bone geometry and strength adaptations to physical constraints inherent in different sports: Comparison between elite female soccer players and swimmers." *Journal of Bone and Mineral Research* 29 (3):342–351. doi: 10.1007/s00774-010-0226-8.

Ferry, B., E. Lespessailles, P. Rochcongar, M. Duclos, and D. Courteix. 2013. "Bone health during late adolescence: Effects of an 8-month training program on bone geometry in female athletes." *Joint Bone Spine* 80 (1):57–63. doi: 10.1016/j.jbspin.2012.01.006.

Fredericson, M., K. Chew, J. Ngo, T. Cleek, J. Kiratli, and K. Cobb. 2007. "Regional bone mineral density in male athletes: A comparison of soccer players, runners and controls." *British Journal of Sports Medicine* 41 (10):664–668; discussion 668. doi: 10.1136/bjsm.2006.030783.

Gordon, C. M., B. S. Zemel, T. A. Wren, M. B. Leonard, L. K. Bachrach, F. Rauch, V. Gilsanz, C. J. Rosen, and K. K. Winer. 2017. "The determinants of peak bone mass." *The Journal of Pediatrics* 180:261–269. doi: 10.1016/j.jpeds.2016.09.056.

Greene, D. A., and G. A. Naughton. 2006. "Adaptive skeletal responses to mechanical loading during adolescence." *Sports Medicine* 36 (9):723–732.

Hagman, M., E. W. Helge, T. Hornstrup, B. Fristrup, J. J. Nielsen, N. R. Jorgensen, J. L. Andersen, J. W. Helge, and P. Krustrup. 2018. "Bone mineral density in lifelong trained male football players compared with young and elderly untrained men." *Journal of Sport and Health Science* 7 (2):159–168. doi: 10.1016/j.jshs.2017.09.009.

Heinio, L., R. Nikander, and H. Sievanen. 2015. "Association between long-term exercise loading and lumbar spine trabecular bone score (TBS) in different exercise loading groups." *Journal of Musculoskeletal and Neuronal Interactions* 15 (3):279–285.

Helge, E. W., P. Aagaard, M. D. Jakobsen, E. Sundstrup, M. B. Randers, M. K. Karlsson, and P. Krustrup. 2010. "Recreational football training decreases risk factors for bone fractures in untrained premenopausal women." *Scandinavian Journal of Medicine & Science in Sports* 20 (1):31–39. doi: 10.1111/j.1600-0838.2010.01107.x.

Helge, E. W., T. R. Andersen, J. F. Schmidt, N. R. Jorgensen, T. Hornstrup, P. Krustrup, and J. Bangsbo. 2014. "Recreational football improves bone mineral density and bone turnover marker profile in elderly men." *Scandinavian Journal of Medicine & Science in Sports* 24:98–104. doi: 10.1111/sms.12239.

Helge, E. W., M. B. Randers, T. Hornstrup, J. J. Nielsen, J. Blackwell, S. R. Jackman, and P. Krustrup. 2014. "Street football is a feasible health-enhancing activity for homeless men: Biochemical bone marker profile and balance improved." *Scandinavian Journal of Medicine & Science in Sports* 24:122–129. doi: 10.1111/sms.12244.

Henry, Y. M., D. Fatayerji, and R. Eastell. 2004. "Attainment of peak bone mass at the lumbar spine, femoral neck and radius in men and women: Relative contributions of bone size and volumetric bone mineral density." *Osteoporosis International* 15 (4):263–273. doi: 10.1007/s00198-003-1542-9.

Hernlund, E., A. Svedbom, M. Ivergard, J. Compston, C. Cooper, J. Stenmark, E. V. McCloskey, B. Jonsson, and J. A. Kanis. 2013. "Osteoporosis in the European Union: Medical management, epidemiology and economic burden: A report prepared in collaboration with the International Osteoporosis Foundation (IOF) and the European Federation of Pharmaceutical Industry Associations (EFPIA)." *Archives of Osteoporosis* 8:136. doi: 10.1007/s11657-013-0136-1.

Hind, K., and M. Burrows. 2007. "Weight-bearing exercise and bone mineral accrual in children and adolescents: A review of controlled trials." *Bone* 40 (1):14–27. doi: 10.1016/j.bone.2006.07.006.

Hind, K., L. Gannon, E. Whatley, C. Cooke, and J. Truscott. 2012. "Bone cross-sectional geometry in male runners, gymnasts, swimmers and non-athletic controls: A hip-structural analysis study." *European Journal of Applied Physiology* 112 (2):535–541. doi: 10.1007/s00421-011-2008-y.

Jackman, S. R., S. Scott, M. B. Randers, C. Orntoft, J. Blackwell, A. Zar, E. W. Helge, M. Mohr, and P. Krustrup. 2013. "Musculoskeletal health profile for elite female footballers versus untrained young women before and after 16 weeks of football training." *Scandinavian Journal of Medicine & Science in Sports* 31 (13):1468–1474. doi: 10.1080/02640414.2013.796066.

Johnell, O., and J. A. Kanis. 2006. "An estimate of the worldwide prevalence and disability associated with osteoporotic fractures." *Osteoporosis International* 17 (12):1726–1733. doi: 10.1007/s00198-006-0172-4.

Jurimae, J., J. Maestu, and T. Jurimae. 2010. "Bone turnover markers during pubertal development: Relationships with growth factors and adipocytokines." *Medicine and Sport Science* 55:114–127. doi: 10.1159/000321976.

Kanis, J. A., N. Burlet, C. Cooper, P. D. Delmas, J. Y. Reginster, F. Borgstrom, and R. Rizzoli. 2008. "European guidance for the diagnosis and management of osteoporosis in postmenopausal women." *Osteoporosis International* 19 (4):399–428.

Kanis, J. A., and O. Johnell. 2005. "Requirements for DXA for the management of osteoporosis in Europe." *Osteoporosis International* 16 (3):229–238.

Kinsella, K., and H. Wan. 2008. "International population reports, P95/09-1, an aging world: 2008." US Census Bureau, US Government Printing Office, Washington, DC (2009).

Kohrt, W. M., D. W. Barry, and R. S. Schwartz. 2009. "Muscle forces or gravity: What predominates mechanical loading on bone?" *Medicine and Science in Sports and Exercise* 41 (11):2050–2055. doi: 10.1249/MSS.0b013e3181a8c717.

Krustrup, P., P. R. Hansen, L. J. Andersen, M. D. Jakobsen, E. Sundstrup, M. B. Randers, L. Christiansen, E. W. Helge, M. T. Pedersen, P. Sogaard, A. Junge, J. Dvorak, P. Aagaard, and J. Bangsbo. 2010. "Long-term musculoskeletal and cardiac health effects of recreational football and running for premenopausal women." *Scandinavian Journal of Medicine & Science in Sports* 20 (1):58–71. doi: 10.1111/j.1600-0838.2010.01111.x.

Krustrup, P., J. J. Nielsen, B. R. Krustrup, J. F. Christensen, H. Pedersen, M. B. Randers, P. Aagaard, A. M. Petersen, L. Nybo, and J. Bangsbo. 2009. "Recreational soccer is an effective health-promoting activity for untrained men." *British Journal of Sports Medicine* 43 (11):825–831. doi: 10.1136/bjsm.2008.053124.

Lappe, J. M., P. Watson, V. Gilsanz, T. Hangartner, H. J. Kalkwarf, S. Oberfield, J. Shepherd, K. K. Winer, and B. Zemel. 2015. "The longitudinal effects of physical activity and dietary calcium on bone mass accrual across stages of pubertal development." *Journal of Bone and Mineral Research* 30 (1): 156–64. doi: 10.1002/jbmr.2319.

Larsen, M. N., C. M. Nielsen, E. W. Helge, M. Madsen, V. Manniche, L. Hansen, P. R. Hansen, J. Bangsbo, and P. Krustrup. 2018. "Positive effects on bone mineralisation and muscular fitness after 10 months of intense school-based physical training for children aged 8–10 years: The FIT FIRST randomised controlled trial." *British Journal of Sports Medicine* 52 (4):254. doi: 10.1136/bjsports-2016-096219.

Lozano-Berges, G., A. Matute-Llorente, A. Gonzalez-Aguero, A. Gomez-Bruton, A. Gomez-Cabello, G. Vicente-Rodriguez, and J. A. Casajus. 2018. "Soccer helps build strong bones during growth: A systematic review and meta-analysis." *European Journal of Pediatrics* 177 (3):295–310. doi: 10.1007/s00431-017-3060-3.

Luo, H., R. U. Newton, F. Ma'ayah, D. A. Galvão, and D. R. Taaffe. 2018. "Recreational soccer as sport medicine for middle-aged and older adults: A systematic review." *BMJ Open Sport & Exercise Medicine* 4 (1): e000336. doi: 10.1136/bmjsem-2017-000336.

Madic, D., B. Obradovic, M. Smajic, J. Obradovic, D. Maric, and K. Boskovic. 2010. "Status of bone mineral content and body composition in boys engaged in intensive physical activity." *Vojnosanitetski Pregled* 67 (5):386–390.

Maimoun, L., O. Coste, T. Mura, P. Philibert, F. Galtier, D. Mariano-Goulart, F. Paris, and C. Sultan. 2013. "Specific bone mass acquisition in elite female athletes." *The Journal of Clinical Endocrinology & Metabolism* 98 (7):2844–2853. doi: 10.1210/jc.2013-1070.

Melton, L. J., E. A. Chrischilles, C. Cooper, A. W. Lane, and B. L. Riggs. 1992. "How many women have osteoporosis." *The Journal of Bone and Mineral Research* 7 (9):1005–1010.

Mitchell, J. A., A. Chesi, O. Elci, S. E. McCormack, H. J. Kalkwarf, J. M. Lappe, V. Gilsanz, S. E. Oberfield, J. A. Shepherd, A. Kelly, B. S. Zemel, and S. F. Grant. 2015. "Genetics of bone mass in childhood and adolescence: Effects of sex and maturation interactions." *The Journal of Bone and Mineral Research* 30 (9):1676–1683. doi: 10.1002/jbmr.2508.

Mohr, M., E. W. Helge, L. F. Petersen, A. Lindenskov, P. Weihe, J. Mortensen, N. R. Jorgensen, and P. Krustrup. 2015. "Effects of soccer vs swim training on bone formation in sedentary middle-aged women." *European Journal of Applied Physiology* 115 (12):2671–2679. doi: 10.1007/s00421-015-3231-8.

Mouratidou, T., G. Vicente-Rodriguez, L. Gracia-Marco, I. Huybrechts, I. Sioen, K. Widhalm, J. Valtuena, M. Gonzalez-Gross, L. A. Moreno, and Helena Study Group. 2013. "Associations of dietary calcium, vitamin D, milk intakes, and 25-hydroxyvitamin D with bone mass in Spanish adolescents: The Helena study." *Journal of Clinical Densitometry* 16 (1):110–117. doi: 10.1016/j.jocd.2012.07.008.

Nebigh, A., H. Rebai, M. Elloumi, A. Bahlous, M. Zouch, M. Zaouali, C. Alexandre, S. Sellami, and Z. Tabka. 2009. "Bone mineral density of young boy soccer players at different pubertal stages: Relationships with hormonal concentration." *Joint Bone Spine* 76 (1):63–69. doi: 10.1016/j.jbspin.2008.03.002.

NIH Consensus Development Panel on Osteoporosis Prevention, Diagnosis, and Therapy. 2001. "Osteoporosis prevention, diagnosis, and therapy." *JAMA* 285 (6):785–795.

Nikander, R., H. Sievanen, A. Heinonen, and P. Kannus. 2005. "Femoral neck structure in adult female athletes subjected to different loading modalities." *Journal of Bone and Mineral Research* 20 (3):520–8. doi: 10.1359/JBMR.041119.

Randell, A., P. N. Sambrook, T. V. Nguyen, H. Lapsley, G. Jones, P. J. Kelly, and J. A. Eisman. 1995. "Direct clinical and welfare costs of osteoporotic fractures in elderly men and women." *Osteoporosis International* 5 (6):427–432. doi: 10.1007/Bf01626603.

Randers, M. B., J. J. Nielsen, B. R. Krustrup, E. Sundstrup, M. D. Jakobsen, L. Nybo, J. Dvorak, J. Bangsbo, and P. Krustrup. 2010. "Positive performance and health effects of a football training program over 12 weeks can be maintained over a 1-year period with reduced training frequency." *Scandinavian Journal of Medicine & Science in Sports* 20:80–89. doi: 10.1111/j.1600-0838.2010.01091.x.

Reginster, J. Y., and N. Burlet. 2006. "Osteoporosis: A still increasing prevalence." *Bone* 38 (2):4–9. doi: 10.1016/j.bone.2005.11.024.
Schoenau, E., and H. M. Frost. 2002. "The 'muscle-bone unit' in children and adolescents." *Calcif Tissue International* 70 (5):405–407. doi: 10.1007/s00223-001-0048-8.
Seabra, A. F., J. Brito, E. Marques, S. Abreu, J. Oliveira, J. Mota, P. Krustrup, C. Rego, and A. Rebelo. 2012. "Muscle strength and soccer practice as major determinants of bone mineral density in adolescents." *Joint Bone Spine* 79 (4):403–408.
Silva, C. C., T. B. Goldberg, A. S. Teixeira, and J. C. Dalmas. 2011. "The impact of different types of physical activity on total and regional bone mineral density in young Brazilian athletes." *Journal of Sports Sciences* 29 (3):227–234. doi: 10.1080/02640414.2010.529456.
Stewart, T. L., and S. H. Ralston. 2000. "Role of genetic factors in the pathogenesis of osteoporosis." *Journal of Endocrinology* 166 (2):235–245.
Theintz, G., B. Buchs, R. Rizzoli, D. Slosman, H. Clavien, P. C. Sizonenko, and J. P. Bonjour. 1992. "Longitudinal monitoring of bone mass accumulation in healthy adolescents: Evidence for a marked reduction after 16 years of age at the levels of lumbar spine and femoral neck in female subjects." *The Journal of Clinical Endocrinology & Metabolism* 75 (4):1060–1065. doi: 10.1210/jcem.75.4.1400871.
Torres-Costoso, A., D. Vlachopoulos, E. Ubago-Guisado, A. Ferri-Morales, I. Cavero-Redondo, V. Martinez-Vizcaino, and L. Gracia-Marco. 2018. "Agreement between dual-energy X-ray absorptiometry and quantitative ultrasound to evaluate bone health in adolescents: The PRO-BONE study." *Pediatric Exercise Science*:1–8. doi: 10.1123/pes.2017-0217.
Tournis, S., E. Michopoulou, I. G. Fatouros, I. Paspati, M. Michalopoulou, P. Raptou, D. Leontsini, A. Avloniti, M. Krekoukia, V. Zouvelou, A. Galanos, N. Aggelousis, A. Kambas, I. Douroudos, G. P. Lyritis, K. Taxildaris, and N. Pappaioannou. 2010. "Effect of rhythmic gymnastics on volumetric bone mineral density and bone geometry in premenarcheal female athletes and controls." *Journal of Clinical Endocrinology & Metabolism* 95 (6):2755–2762. doi: 10.1210/jc.2009-2382.
Turner, C. H. 1998. "Three rules for bone adaptation to mechanical stimuli." *Bone* 23 (5):399–407.
Uth, J., B. Fristrup, R. D. Haahr, K. Brasso, J. W. Helge, M. Rorth, J. Midtgaard, E. W. Helge, and P. Krustrup. 2018. "Football training over 5 years is associated with preserved femoral bone mineral density in men with prostate cancer." *Scandinavian Journal of Medicine & Science in Sports* 28:61–73. doi: 10.1111/sms.13242.
Valtuena, J., L. Gracia-Marco, G. Vicente-Rodriguez, M. Gonzalez-Gross, I. Huybrechts, J. P. Rey-Lopez, T. Mouratidou, I. Sioen, M. I. Mesana, A. E. Martinez, K. Widhalm, L. A. Moreno, and Helena Study Group. 2012. "Vitamin D status and physical activity interact to improve bone mass in adolescents. The Helena study." *Osteoporosis International* 23 (8):2227–2237. doi: 10.1007/s00198-011-1884-7.
Vicente-Rodriguez, G., I. Ara, J. Perez-Gomez, C. Dorado, and J. A. Calbet. 2005. "Muscular development and physical activity as major determinants of femoral bone mass acquisition during growth." *British Journal of Sports Medicine* 39 (9):611–666. doi: 10.1136/bjsm.2004.014431.
Vicente-Rodriguez, G., I. Ara, J. Perez-Gomez, J. A. Serrano-Sanchez, C. Dorado, and J. A. Calbet. 2004. "High femoral bone mineral density accretion in prepubertal soccer players." *Medicine and Science in Sports and Exercise* 36 (10):1789–1795.
Vicente-Rodriguez, G., J. Jimenez-Ramirez, I. Ara, J. A. Serrano-Sanchez, C. Dorado, and J. A. Calbet. 2003. "Enhanced bone mass and physical fitness in prepubescent footballers." *Bone* 33 (5):853–859.

Vincent, K. R., and R. W. Braith. 2002. "Resistance exercise and bone turnover in elderly men and women." *Medicine and Science in Sports and Exercise* 34 (1):17–23.

Vlachopoulos, D., A. R. Barker, E. Ubago-Guisado, I. G. Fatouros, K. M. Knapp, C. A. Williams, and L. Gracia-Marco. 2017. "Longitudinal adaptations of bone mass, geometry, and metabolism in adolescent male athletes: The PRO-BONE study." *Journal of Bone and Mineral Research* 32 (11):2269–2277. doi: 10.1002/jbmr.3206.

Vlachopoulos, D., A. R. Barker, E. Ubago-Guisado, F. B. Ortega, P. Krustrup, B. Metcalf, J. C. Pinero, J. R. Ruiz, K. M. Knapp, C. A. Williams, L. A. Moreno, and L. Gracia-Marco. 2018. "The effect of 12-month participation in osteogenic and non-osteogenic sports on bone development in adolescent male athletes. The PRO-BONE study." *The Journal of Science and Medicine in Sport* 21 (4):404–409. doi: 10.1018/j.jsams.2017.08.018.

Vlachopoulos, D., A. R. Barker, C. A. Williams, A. RNGRiMSSON SA, K. M. Knapp, B. S. Metcalf, I. G. Fatouros, L. A. Moreno, and L. Gracia-Marco. 2017. "The impact of sport participation on bone mass and geometry in male adolescents." *Medicine and Science in Sports and Exercise* 49 (2):317–326. doi: 10.1249/MSS.0000000000001091.

Vlachopoulos, D., L. Gracia-Marco, A. R. Barker, I. Huybrechts, L. A. Moreno, and T. Mouratidou. 2016. "Bone health: The independent and combined effects of calcium, vitamin D and exercise in children and adolescents." In *Calcium: Chemistry, Analysis, Function and Effects*, edited by V. R. Preedy, 530–546. London, UK: The Royal Society of Chemistry.

Vlachopoulos, D., E. Ubago-Guisado, A. R. Barker, B. S. Metcalf, I. G. Fatouros, A. Avloniti, K. M. Knapp, L. A. Moreno, C. A. Williams, and L. Gracia-Marco. 2017. "Determinants of bone outcomes in adolescent athletes at baseline: The PRO-BONE study." *Medicine and Science in Sports and Exercise* 49 (7):1389–1396. doi: 10.1249/MSS.0000000000001233.

Ward, K. A., S. A. Roberts, J. E. Adams, S. Lanham-New, and M. Z. Mughal. 2007. "Calcium supplementation and weight bearing physical activity: Do they have a combined effect on the bone density of pre-pubertal children?" *Bone* 41 (4):496–504. doi: 10.1016/j.bone.2007.06.007.

Ward, K. A., S. A. Roberts, J. E. Adams, and M. Z. Mughal. 2005. "Bone geometry and density in the skeleton of pre-pubertal gymnasts and school children." *Bone* 36 (6):1012–1018. doi: 10.1016/j.bone.2005.03.001.

Weiler, R., R. Keen, and R. Wolman. 2012. "Changes in bone turnover markers during the close season in elite football (soccer) players." *The Journal of Science and Medicine in Sport* 15 (3):255–258. doi: 10.1016/j.jsams.2011.09.004.

Wolff, I., J. J. van Croonenborg, H. C. Kemper, P. J. Kostense, and J. W. Twisk. 1999. "The effect of exercise training programs on bone mass: A meta-analysis of published controlled trials in pre- and postmenopausal women." *Osteoporosis International* 9 (1):1–12.

Zouch, M., C. Jaffre, T. Thomas, D. Frere, D. Courteix, L. Vico, and C. Alexandre. 2008. "Long-term soccer practice increases bone mineral content gain in prepubescent boys." *Joint Bone Spine* 75 (1):41–49. doi: 10.1016/j.jbspin.2006.12.008.

Zouch, M., L. Vico, D. Frere, Z. Tabka, and C. Alexandre. 2014. "Young male soccer players exhibit additional bone mineral acquisition during the peripubertal period: 1-year longitudinal study." *European Journal of Pediatrics* 173 (1):53–61. doi: 10.1007/s00431-013-2115-3.

Zouch, M., A. Zribi, C. Alexandre, H. Chaari, D. Frere, Z. Tabka, and L. Vico. 2015. "Soccer increases bone mass in prepubescent boys during growth: A 3-yr longitudinal study." *Journal of Clinical Densitometry* 18 (2):179–186. doi: 10.1016/j.jocd.2014.10.004.

Chapter 4

Football as rehabilitation for cancer patients

Jacob Uth, Mikael Rørth, Klaus Brasso, Therese Hornstrup and Peter Krustrup

Background

In 2015, there were 17.5 million cancer cases and 8.7 million deaths worldwide (Global Burden of Disease Cancer Collaboration et al., 2018). The number of cancer survivors, i.e. people living with and beyond cancer, is increasing due to earlier detection of cancer and improvements in treatment options (Hashim et al., 2016; Garcia and Thomson, 2014). While improvements in survival for cancer patients is inherently good, survivors often face long-term debilitating health problems that are attributable to the cancer treatment, whether curative or not, although patients managed with surgery alone for small non-metastatic tumours, i.e. stage I cancer, often only have minor sequelae. Late effects include increased risk of recurrent cancer (Low et al., 2014), diabetes, cardiovascular disease, osteoporosis, chronic fatigue (Low et al., 2014), self-reported poor health (Elliott et al., 2011) and poor health-related quality of life (Corner et al., 2013). An extensive body of literature has established that physical exercise is beneficial for cancer patients and cancer survivors, and may improve both physical function and quality of life (Stout et al., 2017).

On this basis, the American College of Sports Medicine (ACSM) recommends that cancer patients should adhere to national guidelines for physical activity: 150 min of moderate-intensity or 75 min of vigorous-intensity aerobic activity (or an equivalent combination of moderate- and vigorous-intensity activity) and 2–3 weekly bouts of resistance exercise and stretching. If achieving these goals is not realistic, it is recommended that patients should be as active as possible and, first and foremost, avoid inactivity (Schmitz et al., 2010).

Prostate cancer

The most common non-cutaneous malignancy in men in developed countries is prostate cancer (PCa). The disease often develops slowly, and this, combined with successful treatment strategies, results in 5- and 10-year survival rates in the United States of 99.7% and 98.8% (DeSantis et al., 2014). Androgen deprivation therapy (ADT) is a cornerstone in the management of the disease, with approximately 50% of men diagnosed with PCa receiving ADT (Gillessen et al., 2015; Meng et al., 2002). The treatment reduces circulating testosterone to castrate levels, which in turn reduces tumour growth and may thus improve the curative potential of radiotherapy or provide palliation for patients with disseminated disease. ADT is associated with significant side effects, including loss of lean and bone mass, gains in fat mass, deteriorating physical functioning and increased bone fracture rates. Aerobic and resistance exercise may ameliorate some of the side effects, but most men with PCa are predominantly sedentary and rarely make healthy lifestyle changes spontaneously after the point of diagnosis (Karlsen et al., 2012). Novel approaches to lifestyle interventions have therefore been warranted.

The FC Prostate RCT

In 2012, a research group from Copenhagen, Denmark, initiated the FC Prostate RCT (randomised controlled trial) to test the feasibility and effects of football training in relation to health outcomes in men with PCa (Uth et al., 2013). Fifty-seven men with locally advanced or metastatic PCa undergoing ADT for a minimum of 6 months were randomly assigned to a football training group (FTG) or a usual care control group (CON) (Uth et al., 2014). Before randomisation, participants were assessed for body composition, bone turnover markers, bone mineral content (BMC) and bone mineral density (BMD), muscle strength, peak oxygen uptake (VO_2max) and parameters of physical functioning, with repeat assessments after 12 and 32 weeks. The participants in FTG were offered football training for 45–60 minutes, 2–3 times per week for 32 weeks. Activity profile and intensity during training were monitored with GPS units and heart-rate monitors.

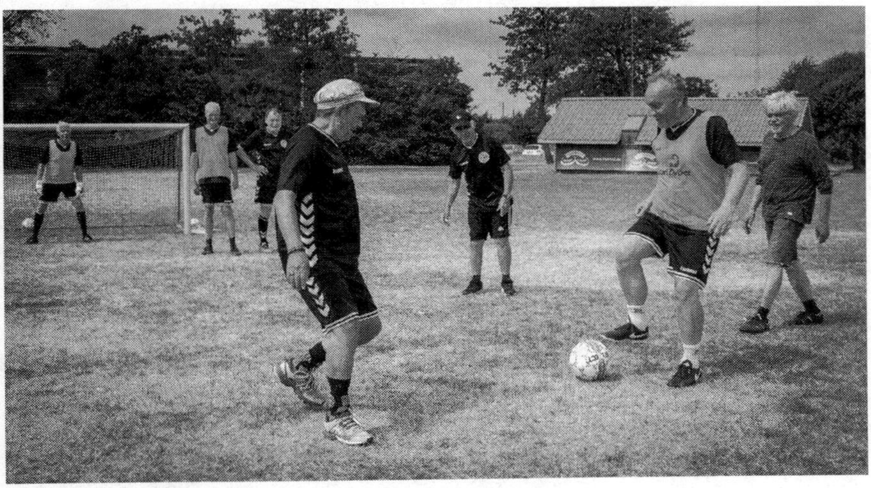

Photo 4.1 The FC Prostate 2012 team.

Source: Photo Credit: Bo Kousgaard, University of Southern Denmark.

The participants allocated to CON were offered football training after the final follow-up assessments.

Attendance, intensity and physiological adaptations

The participants in FTG attended 76.5 ± 24.2% (means±SD) and 46.2 ± 24.3% of the training sessions in the first 12 and next 20 weeks, respectively. Mean heart rate during training was 84.6 ± 3.9% of maximal heart rate, with 26.8 ± 22.2% of training time at heart rates above 90% of maximal heart rate (Uth et al., 2014). During a regular football training session, the participants in FTG performed 194 ± 41 accelerations and 296 ± 65 decelerations >0.6 m/s/s, and covered 905 ± 297 m at speeds >6 km/h and 2646 ± 705 m in total (Uth et al., 2016). Compared to usual care, 12 weeks of football training significantly improved LBM by 0.7 kg, one-repetition maximum for knee extension by 6.7 kg (Uth et al., 2014), leg BMC by 13.8 g and whole-body BMC by 26.4 g (Uth et al., 2016). Additionally, between-group differences in change scores for markers of bone formation, i.e. P1NP (36.6 μg/L) and osteocalcin (8.6 μg/L), were observed after 12 weeks in favour of FTG (Uth et al., 2016). After 32 weeks, the researchers observed between-group differences in mean changes for BMD in right and left femoral shaft and in right and left total hip in favour of FTG, ranging from 0.015 g/mm^2 (total hip right) to 0.024 g/mm^2 (femoral shaft left) (Uth et al., 2016). Additionally, after 32 weeks, between-group differences in changes favouring FTG were observed for jump height (1.7 cm) and stair-climbing time (-0.21 s). VO_2max did not improve in FTG compared to CON after 12 or 32 weeks.

Cancer patients' experiences of football training

In the FC Prostate RCT, the experiences of the men participating in football training were investigated through focus group interviews (Bruun et al., 2014). The men stressed how the social component embodied in football was essential for their perception of exercise as meaningful and relevant to them and described how they felt obligated to show up for training and that team spirit was crucial for their motivation and adherence to the training. They expressed that playing together and relying on each other as teammates contributed to a feeling of positive mutual interdependency and unity. The men explained how the feeling of being secure and close to each other gave rise to frank discussions about PCa and treatment, which they perceived as their 'common destiny', without them feeling forced to bare their souls. The changing room was described as a place that provided an intimate environment for these discussions (Bruun et al., 2014).

With regard to the physical aspects of the training, the men stated that playing football was much harder physically than they expected, but at the same time they expressed an appreciation of the feeling of being naturally exhausted and in good health. The patients emphasised that the team coach played an important role, both as a respectful authority pushing them to try harder and challenge themselves, and as a thoughtful teammate contributing to the social bonding of the team, resulting in everyone feeling included and well cared for (Bruun et al., 2014).

Injury risk prevention

Men with PCa are often elderly and may be undergoing ADT, which increases the risk of osteoporosis. This, combined with the nature of the game with its unforeseen movements and actions from opponents, potentially increases the risk of injury compared to, e.g., closed-chain movements on resistance exercise machines. Patients were therefore screened for comorbidity, including osteoporosis, before participating in the FC Prostate RCT (Uth et al., 2013). During football training, the participants were instructed to avoid hard tackles and other actions that carried a risk of injury. Despite these precautions, 5 participants in the FC Prostate RCT sustained musculoskeletal injuries, of which 3 were characterised as serious. After conservative management, 3 of the 5 injured participants rejoined the football training programme (Uth et al., 2014).

Summary of the FC Prostate RCT

The results of the FC Prostate RCT provide early evidence that football training offered 2–3 times weekly improves lean body mass, muscle strength, leg- and whole-body BMC, and bone formation markers after 12 weeks, and femoral shaft and total-hip BMD and jump and stair-climbing performance after 32 weeks. Evaluation of the physiological demands during training demonstrated that football involves high-intensity running and numerous accelerations and decelerations, and that most of the training is performed at heart rates above 80% of individual maximal heart rate. Injuries related to the football training emphasise the importance of injury prevention regimes for this population. The risk of injury may to some extent be outweighed by the observed improvements in lean body mass, BMD and physical functioning, which may decrease the risk of falls and fractures in the long term. A qualitative investigation of the patients' experiences of participation in football training revealed that, in general, the training was regarded as a welcome opportunity to regain control and acquire a sense of responsibility for their own health without assuming the patient role (Bruun et al., 2014).

Effects of long-term adherence to football training in men with prostate cancer

A study from 2018 in our group evaluated the association of long-term adherence to football training with changes in BMD, VO_2max, body composition, muscle strength, sit-to-stand performance, postural balance and blood lipid profile (Uth et al., 2018). The study involved 22 patients from the FC Prostate RCT, of whom 11 had continued football training for 4.5 years after the original study intervention terminated and 11 of whom had not been playing football after their participation in the original study. The results indicated that the men who had continued self-organised football training had maintained their BMD of the right femoral neck, whereas the men not participating in football training in the 4.5-year follow-up period had decreased levels of right femoral neck BMD. The difference in changes over 5 years between the two groups was almost 5 percentage points. Right femur shaft, right total hip and L2-L4 BMD exhibited similar differences between the two groups, though not reaching statistical significance. The researchers noted that body composition and physical capacity deteriorated over 5 years irrespective of football participation.

Since osteoporosis and bone fractures are associated with aging and ADT, the researchers conclude that the observed association between long-term adherence to unsupervised recreational football training and BMD may be of clinical importance for men with advanced-stage PCa and their carers. Importantly, the long-term adherence to training, which is rarely seen in exercise intervention studies (Mutrie et al., 2012), suggests that participation in football for this group of patients was very motivating and associated with meaningfulness, joy and peer support.

Recommendations for future research and applied practices

The early available data from an RCT, including 5-year follow-up data, suggest that football training is a high-intensity interval training modality that may improve important clinical outcomes in men with PCa and that football is regarded as relevant and meaningful by patients. The positive results of the FC Prostate RCT raise the question of whether football training may be feasible and effective for managing negative side effects of treatment in other cancer populations such as women with breast cancer. Future studies seeking an answer to this question would be a welcome addition to the existing evidence on football as medicine for cancer patients. A key feature of the FC Prostate RCT was a close collaboration between clinicians responsible for managing cancer treatment and experts within exercise and sports physiology and psychology. Future applied practice may include prescription or recommendation of football training in local football clubs by the treating physician or specialist nurse. Before large-scale implementation of football training as an adjuvant to cancer treatment is realistic, it is essential that future studies investigate the effectiveness and safety of football training provided by local football clubs and collect data on those who screen out, thereby providing information about the generalisability of football training for men with PCa. Regarding prevention of injuries, it is worth noting that a Norwegian study by Soligard and colleagues found that a comprehensive warm-up programme aimed at improving strength, awareness and neuromuscular control during static and dynamic movements reduced the risk of injury in female youth players (Soligard et al., 2008). A similar approach to injury prevention in patient groups appears to be rational, although no empirical data are currently available to support this notion. The outline for a study evaluating some of these outcomes has been suggested by Bjerre and colleagues (Bjerre et al., 2016). To reach the next level towards mainstream adaptation of football for PCa patients, the researchers plan to include 200 patients from multiple centres and evaluate the effects of football training on health-related quality of life, body composition and safety for men with PCa where training is provided through local football clubs. In addition to the proposed trial, it is essential that future studies evaluate the cost-to-benefit ratio of football training for cancer patients to inform local, regional and national policymakers.

References

Bjerre, E., D. M. Bruun, A. Tolver, K. Brasso, P. Krustrup, C. Johansen, R. Christensen, M. Rørth, and J. Midtgaard. 2016. "Effectiveness of Community-Based Football Compared to Usual Care in Men with Prostate Cancer: Protocol for a Randomised, Controlled, Parallel Group, Multicenter Superiority Trial (The FC Prostate Community Trial)." *BMC Cancer* 16 (October). https://doi.org/10.1186/s12885-016-2805-0.

Bruun, D. M., P. Krustrup, T. Hornstrup, J. Uth, K. Brasso, M. Rørth, J. F. Christensen, and J. Midtgaard. 2014. "'All Boys and Men Can Play Football': A Qualitative Investigation of Recreational Football in Prostate Cancer Patients." *Scandinavian Journal of Medicine & Science in Sports* 24 (1, August): 113–121. https://doi.org/10.1111/sms.12193.

Corner, J., R. Wagland, A. Glaser, and Sir M. Richards. 2013. "Qualitative Analysis of Patients' Feedback from a PROMs Survey of Cancer Patients in England." *BMJ Open* 3 (4). https://doi.org/10.1136/bmjopen-2012-002316.

DeSantis, C. E., C. C. Lin, A. B. Mariotto, R. L. Siegel, K. D. Stein, J. L. Kramer, R. Alteri, A. S. Robbins, and A. Jemal. 2014. "Cancer Treatment and Survivorship Statistics, 2014." *CA: A Cancer Journal for Clinicians* 64 (4): 252–271. https://doi.org/10.3322/caac.21235.

Elliott, J., A. Fallows, L. Staetsky, P. W. F. Smith, C. L. Foster, E. J. Maher, and J. Corner. 2011. "The Health and Well-Being of Cancer Survivors in the UK: Findings from a Population-Based Survey." *British Journal of Cancer* 105 (1, November): S11–S20. https://doi.org/10.1038/bjc.2011.418.

Garcia, D. O., and C. A. Thomson. 2014. "Physical Activity and Cancer Survivorship." *Nutrition in Clinical Practice: Official Publication of the American Society for Parenteral and Enteral Nutrition* 29 (6): 768–779. https://doi.org/10.1177/0884533614551969.

Gillessen, S., A. Omlin, G. Attard, J. S. de Bono, E. Efstathiou, K. Fizazi, S. Halabi, et al. 2015. "Management of Patients with Advanced Prostate Cancer: Recommendations of the St. Gallen Advanced Prostate Cancer Consensus Conference (APCCC) 2015." *Annals of Oncology* (June): mdv257. https://doi.org/10.1093/annonc/mdv257.

Global Burden of Disease Cancer Collaboration, C. Fitzmaurice, T. F. Akinyemiju, F. H. Al Lami, T. Alam, R. Alizadeh-Navaei, C. Allen, et al. 2018. "Global, Regional, and National Cancer Incidence, Mortality, Years of Life Lost, Years Lived with Disability, and Disability-Adjusted Life-Years for 29 Cancer Groups, 1990 to 2016: A Systematic Analysis for the Global Burden of Disease Study." *JAMA Oncology* (June). https://doi.org/10.1001/jamaoncol.2018.2706.

Hashim, D., P. Boffetta, C. La Vecchia, M. Rota, P. Bertuccio, M. Malvezzi, and E. Negri. 2016. "The Global Decrease in Cancer Mortality: Trends and Disparities." *Annals of*

Oncology: Official Journal of the European Society for Medical Oncology 27 (5): 926–933. https://doi.org/10.1093/annonc/mdw027.

Karlsen, R. V., P. E. Bidstrup, J. Christensen, S. B. Larsen, A. Tjønneland, S. O. Dalton, and C. Johansen. 2012. "Men with Cancer Change Their Health Behaviour: A Prospective Study from the Danish Diet, Cancer and Health Study." *British Journal of Cancer* 107 (1): 201–206. https://doi.org/10.1038/bjc.2012.238.

Low, C. A., E. Beckjord, D. H. Bovbjerg, M. Amanda Dew, D. M. Posluszny, J. E. Schmidt, A. E. Lowery, S. A. Nutt, S. R. Arvey, and R. Rechis. 2014. "Correlates of Positive Health Behaviors in Cancer Survivors: Results from the 2010 LIVESTRONG Survey." *Journal of Psychosocial Oncology* 32 (6): 678–695. https://doi.org/10.1080/07347332.2014.955243.

Meng, M. V., G. D. Grossfeld, N. Sadetsky, S. S. Mehta, D. P. Lubeck, and P. R. Carroll. 2002. "Contemporary Patterns of Androgen Deprivation Therapy Use for Newly Diagnosed Prostate Cancer." *Urology* 60 (3 Suppl 1): 7–11, discussion 11–12.

Mutrie, N., A. Campbell, S. Barry, K. Hefferon, A. McConnachie, D. Ritchie, and S. Tovey. 2012. "Five-Year Follow-Up of Participants in a Randomised Controlled Trial Showing Benefits from Exercise for Breast Cancer Survivors during Adjuvant Treatment: Are There Lasting Effects?" *Journal of Cancer Survivorship* 6 (4): 420–430. https://doi.org/10.1007/s11764-012-0233-y.

Schmitz, K. H., K. S. Courneya, C. Matthews, W. Demark-Wahnefried, D. A. Galvão, B. M. Pinto, M. L. Irwin, et al. 2010. "American College of Sports Medicine Roundtable on Exercise Guidelines for Cancer Survivors." *Medicine and Science in Sports and Exercise* 42 (7): 1409–1426. https://doi.org/10.1249/MSS.0b013e3181e0c112.

Soligard, T., G. Myklebust, K. Steffen, I. Holme, H. Silvers, M. Bizzini, A. Junge, J. Dvorak, R. Bahr, and T. E. Andersen. 2008. "Comprehensive Warm-Up Programme to Prevent Injuries in Young Female Footballers: Cluster Randomised Controlled Trial." *BMJ (Clinical Research Ed.)* 337: a2469.

Stout, N. L., J. Baima, A. K. Swisher, K. M. Winters-Stone, and J. Welsh. 2017. "A Systematic Review of Exercise Systematic Reviews in the Cancer Literature (2005–2017)." *PM & R: The Journal of Injury, Function, and Rehabilitation* 9 (9S2): S347–S384. https://doi.org/10.1016/j.pmrj.2017.07.074.

Uth, J., B. Fristrup, R. D. Haahr, K. Brasso, J. W. Helge, M. Rørth, J. Midtgaard, E. W. Helge, and P. Krustrup. 2018. "Football Training over 5 Years Is Associated with Preserved Femoral Bone Mineral Density in Men with Prostate Cancer." *Scandinavian Journal of Medicine & Science in Sports* 28 (1, August): 61–73. https://doi.org/10.1111/sms.13242.

Uth, J., T. Hornstrup, J. F. Christensen, K. B. Christensen, N. R. Jørgensen, J. F. Schmidt, K. Brasso, et al. 2016. "Efficacy of Recreational Football on Bone Health, Body Composition, and Physical Functioning in Men with Prostate Cancer Undergoing Androgen Deprivation Therapy: 32-Week Follow-Up of the FC Prostate Randomised Controlled Trial." *Osteoporosis International: A Journal Established as Result of Cooperation between the European Foundation for Osteoporosis and the National Osteoporosis Foundation of the USA* 27 (4): 1507–1518. https://doi.org/10.1007/s00198-015-3399-0.

Uth, J., T. Hornstrup, J. F. Christensen, K. B. Christensen, N. R. Jørgensen, E. W. Helge, J. F. Schmidt, et al. 2016. "Football Training in Men with Prostate Cancer Undergoing Androgen Deprivation Therapy: Activity Profile and Short-Term Skeletal and Postural Balance Adaptations." *European Journal of Applied Physiology* 116 (3): 471–480. https://doi.org/10.1007/s00421-015-3301-y.

Uth, J., T. Hornstrup, J. F. Schmidt, J. F. Christensen, C. Frandsen, K. B. Christensen, E. W. Helge, et al. 2014. "Football Training Improves Lean Body Mass in Men with Prostate

Cancer Undergoing Androgen Deprivation Therapy." *Scandinavian Journal of Medicine & Science in Sports* 24 (1, August): 105–112. https://doi.org/10.1111/sms.12260.

Uth, J., J. F. Schmidt, J. F. Christensen, T. Hornstrup, L. J. Andersen, P. R. Hansen, K. B. Christensen, et al. 2013. "Effects of Recreational Soccer in Men with Prostate Cancer Undergoing Androgen Deprivation Therapy: Study Protocol for the 'FC Prostate' Randomized Controlled Trial." *BMC Cancer* 13: 595. https://doi.org/10.1186/1471-2407-13-595.

Chapter 5

Football as broad-spectrum prevention for children and youth – in club and school settings

André Seabra, Malte Nejst Larsen, Peter Riis Hansen, Amri Hammami, Jiri Dvorak, Anne-Marie Elbe, Laila Ottesen and Peter Krustrup

Introduction

The expansion of industrialisation, technological advances, urbanism and economic development have profoundly changed lifestyles and collectively mark an unprecedented turning point in human life. Examples of such transformations are easily observed in the urban planning of modern cities (e.g., high residential density, reduced living space and decreased availability of sports facilities), means of transport (e.g., increased mobility via motorised private transport ['passive mobility']), work activities (e.g., increased focus on intellectual work), academic activities and facilities (e.g., lack of access to sports facilities due to budgetary constraints and increased academic requirements) and patterns of leisure activities (e.g., increased time spent watching television, playing computer games and surfing the web) (Shields and Tremblay, 2008; Tremblay et al., 2011). This multivariate set of transformations has consequently contributed to the emergence of physical inactivity and sedentary lifestyles, which, along with the acquisition of inappropriate behaviours and eating habits (e.g., increased consumption of processed and high-calorie foods), has spurred the development of a wide range of chronic diseases, including cardiovascular disease, cancer, diabetes and obesity (Lee et al., 2012; Pearson and Biddle, 2011).

Physical activity, defined as any bodily movement performed by the skeletal muscles that increases energy expenditure relative to the resting metabolic rate (Caspersen et al., 1985), when performed daily at moderate to vigorous intensity and associated with reduced time dedicated to sedentary activities, plays a vital role in promoting active, healthy lifestyles. Physical activity can entail numerous benefits for children, including improvements in growth and development, bone health, metabolic health, psychological wellbeing, physical fitness and academic performance (Janssen and LeBlanc, 2010; Strong et al., 2005), as well as the lowering of risk factors of cardiometabolic disease. Although there are conflicting data, evidence also suggests that regular participation in physical activity during childhood increases the likelihood of continued physical activity into adolescence and adulthood (Telama et al., 2014). Given the accumulation of systematic and rigorous findings about the benefits of participation in physical activity, several guidelines have been presented. The most recent proposals recommend that children and adolescents should accumulate at least 60 min or more of moderate-to-vigorous aerobic physical activity per day and perform muscle- and bone-strengthening activities at least three days per week (World Health Organization, 2010). The activities should be age appropriate, enjoyable and offer variety.

Despite the recognised benefits of physical activity, the prevalence of children's and adolescents' engagement in inactive lifestyles continues to increase. Epidemiological studies conducted in various regions worldwide have shown that 60–85% of people living in developed or developing countries lead inactive lifestyles, and that more than 80% of children do not achieve daily levels of physical activity considered to benefit health (World Health Organization, 2015). In view of these results, several international medical and scientific organisations (including the World Health Organization, the American College of Sports Medicine, the Centers for Disease Control and Prevention, and the American Academy of Pediatrics) have declared physical inactivity a major problem for public health in modern societies and have emphasised the urgent need to develop and implement effective programmes that promote physical activity among children and adolescents in different contexts (e.g., communities, sports clubs and schools). However, for such programmes to effectively achieve their results, it is first important to describe the levels and patterns of physical activity among children and to identify variables that can explain such behaviour.

Epidemiology of physical activity

In epidemiology, researchers have described the levels and patterns of physical activity among children and adolescents in terms of demographic and biological factors, as well as longitudinally assessing changes in those values (Katzmarzyk et al., 2017; Van Hecke et al., 2016). Despite some conceptual and methodological divergence, most of these studies have suggested that girls are less physically active than boys. Overweight and obese children are overrepresented in families with low socioeconomic status, whereas normal-weight children are overrepresented in families with high socioeconomic status. Results have also shown that older children are often less physically active than younger children, indicating that adolescence is a critical period during which physical inactivity tends to increase (Katzmarzyk et al., 2017; Van Hecke et al., 2016).

Such descriptive information is particularly useful in identifying and characterising populations or groups at risk of inactivity, thus enabling the development and implementation of more effective physical activity intervention programmes. Although some demographic and biological factors can influence levels and patterns of physical activity among children and adolescents, most factors cannot be modified. Accordingly, researchers have conducted various studies to identify modifiable factors that can influence levels and patterns of physical activity among children and adolescents (Ferreira et al., 2007; Sallis et al., 2000; Uijtdewilligen et al., 2011; Van Der Horst et al., 2007). In addition to demographic and biological factors, some psychological, social and environmental factors have also been considered. For example, Sallis et al. (2000) found that male gender, access to infrastructure and athletic equipment, barriers to participating in physical activity, and preference for a specific physical activity or sport consistently related to children's levels of physical activity, while Van der Horst et al. (2007) showed that self-efficacy, parental physical activity and parental support were equally important factors. Somewhat similarly, Seabra et al. (2008) observed that higher socioeconomic status and family and peer participation in physical activity were correlates that most influenced children's physical activity habits, with age correlating negatively. In Ferreira et al.'s (2007) literature review addressing environmental factors of physical activity, parental physical activity, time spent in outdoors activities and school policies related to physical activity best explained interindividual variation in physical activity. More recently, Uijtdewilligen et al. (2011) reported that the intention to be active positively associated with physical activity among children.

Physical activity programmes to promote active, healthy lifestyles

Considering these findings, several intervention programmes to promote active, healthy lifestyles among children and adolescents have been implemented in different settings (communities, sports clubs and schools) (Dobbins et al., 2013; Geidne et al., 2013; Parrish et al., 2013; Salmon et al., 2007; van Sluijs et al., 2007). Three approaches have been tested in the community setting (Salmon et al., 2007; van Sluijs et al., 2007). Firstly, in informational approaches, the transmission of information that motivates children and adolescents to change their behaviour and maintain such changes over time has been pursued in community-based campaigns and strategic decision-making. Presenting information about the possible benefits for health and wellbeing of practising physical activity, about opportunities and facilities available in the community and at sports clubs, and about strategies to overcome barriers and negative attitudes towards physical activity seems to promote children's acquisition of active lifestyles. Secondly, behavioural and social approaches have involved teaching behaviour management skills and structuring social environments to support children in initiating and maintaining their participation in physical activity, reducing or eliminating barriers to participation (e.g., lack of safety and lack of motivation) and creating or strengthening social networks and social environments outside the family that facilitate collaborative behavioural change. Thirdly, environmental and political approaches have advocated increased access to programmes that create and improve built environments that enable children's greater involvement in physical activity. Recommended examples of the third approach are developing and enhancing public recreational spaces, implementing policies that promote active transportation, and designing communities capable of encouraging children's and adolescents' participation in physical activity.

Sports clubs, a primary setting for children's and adolescents' leisure-time physical activities, can also promote the acquisition of active, healthy lifestyles (Geidne et al., 2013). Strategies tested with promising results include having motivating coaches with positive attitudes and enthusiasm for sport, ensuring quality athletic activity with motivating, enjoyable instructional and training content, and organising sports events (e.g., sport tournaments and sport-focused days, seminars and workshops) (Duda and Appleton, 2016). However, difficulties have arisen in implementing these strategies given that most sports clubs focus on developing athletic, technical and tactical skills and promoting the competitive performance of children and adolescents (Geidne et al., 2013).

Schools are considered an ideal setting for implementing strategies and programmes that can promote physical activity (Dobbins et al., 2013). Children and adolescents spend a large proportion of their daily lives in school, which underscores the importance of schools in their acquisition and continuance of active lifestyles. Several interventions to promote children's and adolescents' physical activity have been implemented in curricular and extracurricular activities, and evidence strongly suggests that creating new policies for physical education can contribute to children's and adolescents' increased participation in physical activity. To that end, three proposed policies stand out: adding and lengthening classes; altering the teaching-learning process to allow students to remain more active during lessons; and introducing diverse, motivating and challenging athletic activities into curricula. Another proposal has been scheduling time for physical activity between classes and after school. Above all, multicomponent interventions encompassing various strategies (e.g., diversifying the availability of sports facilities and equipment) seem to effectively increase physical activity among children and adolescents at school (Dobbins et al., 2013; Parrish et al., 2013).

Despite the demonstrated positive benefits of such programmes and strategies, more than 80% of children and adolescents worldwide do not meet recommended international guidelines for physical activity (World Health Organization, 2015). Although factors accounting for such low adherence remain poorly understood, a plausible explanation relates to limited possibilities of facilitating recommended types of physical activity, as well as barriers to increasing the duration, frequency and intensity of physical activity in schools, athletic clubs and other community settings. Another possible explanation is that children and adolescents perceive prescribed physical activity, inasmuch as it is imposed by others, to be less enjoyable than physical activity in which they choose to participate. Although most proposed physical activity programmes for children and adolescents have incorporated various aerobic and resistance activities that accommodate individual differences in interest (e.g., running, walking and circuit training), these programmes have rarely incorporated team games and sports activities of specific interest to children (Lavelle et al., 2012). Another problem is that most programmes do not accommodate natural patterns of spontaneous physical activity among children, who tend to participate in relatively short (<5 min) bouts of physical activity and seldom participate in sustained (>20 min) activities, as results of continuous heart rate (HR) monitoring studies have shown (Armstrong and

Bray, 1991). Children and adolescents in several cultures have indicated that having fun, improving self-perceived competence, making friends and being part of a team are major motivations for participating in physical activity (Deci, 2000). It is therefore crucial to identify forms of physical activity that satisfy basic psychological needs (Deci, 2000).

Recreational football programmes to promote active, healthy lifestyles

There are four reasons why recreational football could be one such activity. Firstly, as the most commonly played sport worldwide, football is universally known, easily accessible, and socially and culturally meaningful to children and adolescents at different levels of training, regardless of their gender, socioeconomic status and nutritional status. Secondly, football is a team-based activity with the potential to promote teamwork and social interactions that provide opportunities to enhance children's and adolescents' psychological state and, in turn, their levels of physical activity. After all, children and adolescents enjoy participating in team sports significantly more than in individual sports (Elbe et al., 2017; McCarthy, Jones, & Clark-Carter, 2008). Thirdly, football has clear, simple rules that can be easily followed in nearly any setting, as well as minimal requirements in terms of equipment (e.g., ball and goals). Fourthly, the physical and physiological demands of recreational football practice fulfil the international physical activity guidelines for children and adolescents. Randers et al. (2010) demonstrated that recreational small-team football practice for 9- to 12-year-old boys and girls was associated with relatively high energy expenditure, an exceptional aerobic component and a mean greater than 80% of maximum HR for the entire training session. Along this line, Bendiksen et al. (2014) reported that mean HR and time spent in the so-called 'aerobic high-intensity zone' were significantly greater for 8- to 9-year-old schoolchildren who participated in matches with small teams than those who engage in circuit training, walking or Nintendo Wii games. Interestingly, those authors also observed high HRs during football matches with small teams for schoolchildren with the greatest need for physical training (i.e. children with no sports club participation, poor fitness and/or a high body mass index). Being a relatively high-impact sport, football is a muscle- and bone-strengthening activity in which forces generated while rapidly changing direction, stopping and landing, jumping and kicking can confer excellent osteogenic benefits for weight-bearing bone sites. In cross-sectional studies, researchers have also shown that prepubertal and pubertal male football players showed significantly greater bone mineral density and content in their lower limbs and throughout their bodies than their physically inactive age-, weight- and height-matched control counterparts. According to Vicente-Rodríguez (2006), physical exercise during football promotes bone resistance in two ways: due to the high-impact loads characteristic of sport in general and as a result of indirect, osteogenic mechanisms due to the development of muscles in specific areas that increase tension on the bones attached to them. In light of these findings,

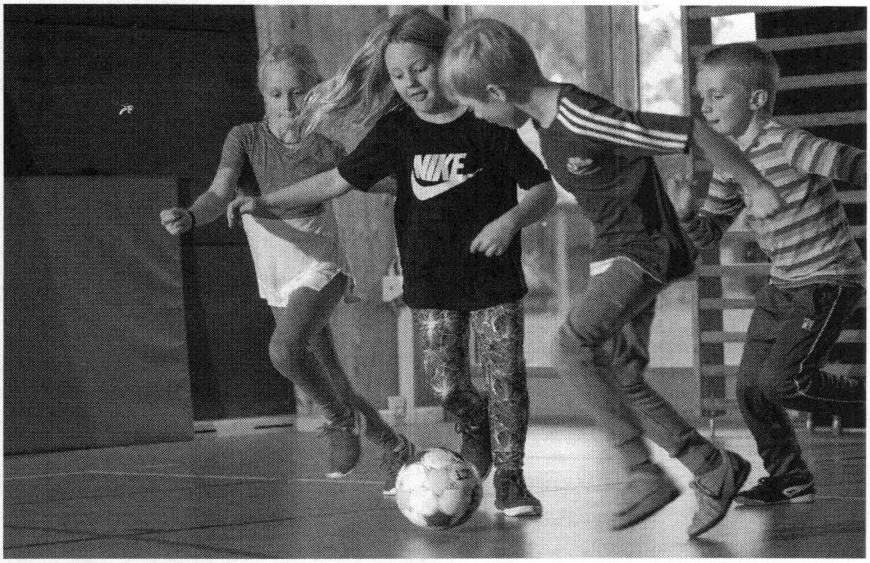

(a)

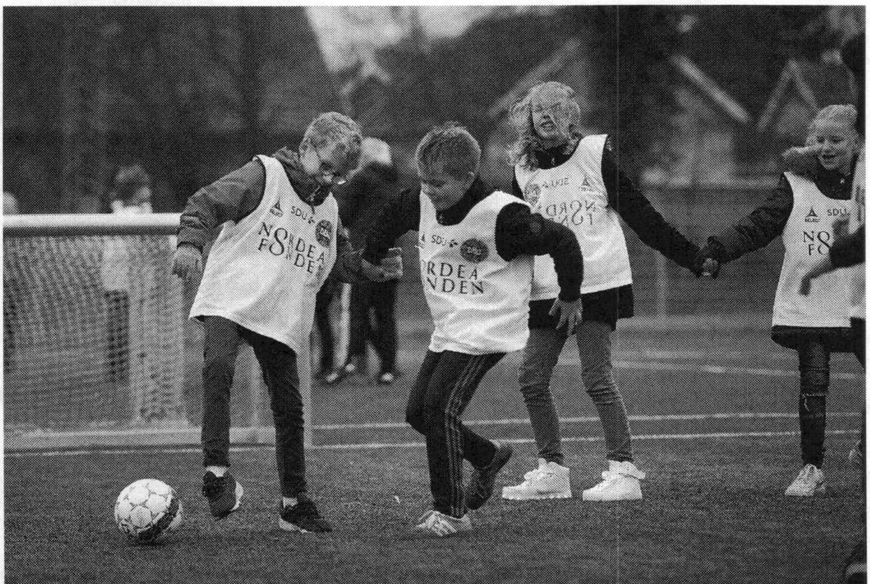

(b)

Photo 5.1 Two large-scale school football projects are currently running in Denmark, i.e. the FIT FIRST (a) and the 11 for Health project (b).

Source: Photo Credit: Mikal Schlosser, University of Copenhagen (a) and Bo Kousgaard, University of Southern Denmark (b).

football should be regarded as a sport with the potential to improve bone mass density and content during childhood and adolescence, since fulfilling the physical demands of the game requires the activation of a wide range of body muscles.

Of thirteen recent studies (Cvetkovic et al., 2018; Faude et al., 2010; Hammami et al., 2016; Hammami et al., 2018; Hansen et al., 2013; Krustrup et al., 2014; Madsen et al., 2013; Orntoft et al., 2016; Seabra et al., 20142016; Skoradal et al., 2018; Vasconcellos et al., 2015; Weintraub et al., 2008) conducted to examine the effects of recreational football programmes on the health status of children: six had samples of overweight or obese participants only; ten addressed recreational football-only programmes, whereas the other three also included another kind of physical activity intervention; twelve took place in schools, whereas the other took place in communities as well; eight included both genders, whereas the other five included males only; and eight had follow-up periods of no more than twelve weeks, whereas the other five had longer follow-up periods. Table 5.1 summarises the effects of the studied programmes on participants' body composition, cardiovascular parameters, biochemical variables, physical fitness and psychological wellbeing.

Although the researchers in all thirteen studies analysed the effects of recreational football on participants' body mass index, only two programmes effectively reduced those scores. Of the seven studies in which the researchers measured body fat percentage, they only observed a decrease in four. In one study, the researchers assessed the participants' bone mass, which ultimately increased subsequent to their engagement in the programmes, whereas in three studies the researchers reported significant decreases in the participants' C-reactive protein, insulin resistance, total cholesterol, low-density lipoprotein cholesterol and triglyceride levels, as well as increases in high-density lipoprotein cholesterol, following their participation in the programmes. Regarding the inflammatory variables of leptin, researchers analysed the participants' resistin and adiponectin levels in only two studies, which ultimately had improved significantly after the programmes. In five studies, the results regarding cardiovascular variables (e.g., arterial pressure, cardiac structure and cardiac function) indicated decreased blood pressure and a positive effect on the cardiovascular system, including in the modulation of cardiac structure and function, due to participation in recreational football programmes. In one study, the researchers showed an improvement in autonomic function measured through heart-rate variability in untrained adolescents. In three studies, the researchers measured physical activity levels, which increased significantly in two of the studies. By contrast, in nine studies the researchers assessed changes in cardiorespiratory fitness, which improved in seven of them. Finally, with regard to variables related to psychological wellbeing, improvements in self-esteem emerged in three studies. It is also noteworthy that three other studies showed significant improvements in quality of life, self-perception of physical competence, body image and attraction to physical activity among the participants.

These results highlight the need for further studies. Nevertheless, the available evidence clearly suggests that recreational football can represent a promising broad-spectrum intervention for promoting physical activity, physical fitness and

Table 5.1 Recreational football intervention studies among children and adolescents

Study	Sample	Design/Setting	Intervention	Outcomes	Results
Weintraub et al. (2008)	G–B; 9–11 years; BMI ≥85 RFG:9; CG:12	RCT/S	3–4x/wk – 75min 24 weeks	BMI, PA, DS, SE	↑ PA
Faude et al. (2010)	G–B; 8–12 years; BMI≥95 RFG: 11; SAG:11	RCT/S	3x/wk – 60min 24 weeks	BMI, CRF, CMJ, AGL, FL, QL, SE	↑ BMI, CMJ, AGL, OLS, FL, QL, SE
Hansen et al. (2013)	G–B; 8–12 years; BMI≥85 RFG:20; CG:11	QE/S	4x/wk – 60–90min 12 weeks	BMI, SBP, DBP, LVDD, LVSD, LVPWD, LV, LVEF, IVSD, LA, E/A, IVRT, RVDD, TAPSE	↓ SBP ↑ LVPWD, IVRT, TAPSE
Madsen et al. (2013)	G–B; 9–11 years RFG:79; CG:71	RCT/S-C	2–3x/wk – 120min 40 weeks	BMI, PA, CRF	↑ PA
Krustrup et al. (2014)	G–B; 9–10 years RFG:46; CG:51	RCT/S	3x/wk – 40min 10 weeks	BMI, SBP, DBP, LVDD, LVSD, LVPWD, LV, LVEF, IVSD, LA, IVT, IVRT, RVDD, TAPSE	↑ IVT, LVPWD, IVRT
Seabra et al. (2014)	B; 8–12 years; BMI≥85 RFG:12; CG:8	QE/S	4x/wk – 60–90min 20 weeks	BMI, %FAT, LBM, SE, BI, PC, AP	↑ LBM, SE, BI, PC, AP
Vasconcellos et al. (2015)	G–B; 12–17 years; BMI≥85 RFG:10; CG:10	RCT/S	3x/wk – 60min 12 weeks	BMI, %FAT, LBM WC, SBP, DBP, HDLC, LDLC, TRG, TC, FG, INS, HOMA-IR, CRP, TNF-α, LEP, IL-6, ADP, RES, CRF	↓ BMI, %FAT, WC, SBP, TRG, TC, CRP, TNF-α ↑ HDLC, CRF
Hammami et al. (2016)	B; 14–16 years RFG: 10; CG: 10	RCT/S	2x/wk – 45–60min 8 weeks	HRV, SBP, DBP, CRF, SP, PB	↓ SP ↑ HRV, CRF
Orntoft et al. (2016)	G–B; 10–12 years RFG: 402; CG: 144	RCT/S	2x/wk – 45min 11 weeks	BMI, %FAT, LBM, SBP, DBP, PB, SP, HJ, CRF,	↓ %FAT, SBP, DBP, SP ↑ LBM, PB, CRF
Seabra et al. (2016)	B; 8–12 years; BMI≥85 RFG:29; SAG:29; CG:30	QE/S	3x/wk – 60–90min 24 weeks	BMI, %FAT, LBM, BM, WC, SBP, DBP, HDLC, LDLC, TRG, TC, FG, CRP, LEP, ADP, RES, CRF, QL, SE, BI, PC, APA	↓ %FAT, WC, LDLC, TRG, TC, CRP ↑ LBM, BM, HDLC, ADP, LEP, RES, CRF, QL, SE, BI, PC, APA
Hammami et al. (2018)	B; 14–16 years RFG: 10; CG: 10	RCT/S	2x/wk – 45–60min 8 weeks	BMI, %FAT, LBM; CMJ, CRF, FL, SP, PB	↓ SP ↑ LBM, CRF, CMJ, PB

(Continued)

Table 5.1 (Continued)

Study	*Sample*	*Design/Setting*	*Intervention*	*Outcomes*	*Results*
Cvetkovic et al. (2018)	B; 11–13 years; BMI≥85 RFG: 14; HIG:11; CG: 14	RCT/S	3x/wk – 60min 12 weeks	BMI, %FAT, LBM, SBP, DBP, CMJ, AGL, FL, CRF	↑ CMJ, AGL, CRF
Skoradal et al. (2018)	G–B; 10–12 years RFG: 292; CG: 100	RCT/S	2x/wk – 45min 11 weeks	BMI, %FAT, LBM, SBP, DBP, PB, HJ, CRF,	↓ BMI, %FAT, SBP ↑ LBM, PB, CRF

A: peak transmitral flow velocity during atrial contraction; ADP: adiponectin; AGL: agility; APA: attraction to physical activity; BI: body image; BM: bone mass; BMI: body mass index; B: boys; CG: control group; CMJ: counter movement jump; CRF: cardiorespiratory fitness; DBP: diastolic blood pressure; CRP: C-reactive protein; DS: depressive symptoms; E: peak transmitral flow velocity in early diastole; FG: fasting glucose; FL: flexibility; G/B: girls and boys; HDLC: high-density lipoprotein cholesterol; HIG: high-intensity group; HJ: horizontal jump; HRV: heart rate variability; IL-6: interleukin-6; INS: insulin; IVT: interventricular septum thickness; IVRTglobal: global isovolumetric relaxation time; IVSD: interventricular septum diameter; LA: left atrial volume; LBM: lean body mass; LDL: low-density lipoprotein cholesterol; LEP: leptin; LVDD: left ventricular diastolic diameter; LVEF: left ventricular ejection fraction; LVPWD: left ventricular posterior wall diameter; LVSD: left ventricular systolic diameter; OLS: one-leg standing; PA: physical activity; PB: postural balance; PC: perceived physical competence; QL: quality of life; QE: quasi-experimental; RCT: randomised controlled trial; RES: resistin; RFG: recreational football group; RVDD: right ventricular diastolic diameter; S: school; SAG: standard activity group; SBP: systolic blood pressure; SC: school and community; SE: self-esteem; SP: sprint; TAPSE: tricuspid annular plane systolic excursion; TC: total cholesterol; TRG: triglycerides; WC: waist circumference; %FAT: body fat percentage; ↓: significant decrease in the mean value; ↑: significant increase of the mean value.

health status among children and adolescents, regardless of gender, age, socioeconomic status and nutritional status. Considering these benefits and that football is a highly popular sport that is accessible to all, relatively inexpensive and easy to implement in different settings, recreational football should be incorporated in public-health programmes to promote active, healthy lifestyles among children and adolescents.

References

Armstrong, N., and S. Bray. 1991. "Physical activity patterns defined by continuous heart rate monitoring." *Archives of Disease in Childhood, 66*(2): 245–247.

Bendiksen, M., C. A. Williams, T. Hornstrup, H. Clausen, J. Kloppenborg, D. Shumikhin, J. Brito, et al. 2014. "Heart rate response and fitness effects of various types of physical education for 8- to 9-year-old schoolchildren." *European Journal of Sport Science*. doi:10.1080/17461391.2014.884168

Caspersen, C. J., K. E. Powell, and G. M. Christenson. 1985. "Physical activity, exercise, and physical fitness: Definitions and distinctions for health-related research." *Public Health Reports, 100*(2): 126–131.

Cvetkovic, N., E. Stojanovic, N. Stojiljkovic, D. Nikolic, A. T. Scanlan, and Z. Milanović. 2018. "Exercise training in overweight and obese children: Recreational football and high-intensity interval training provide similar benefits to physical fitness." *Scandinavian Journal of Medicine and Science in Sports 28*(1): 18–32. doi:10.1111/sms.13241

Deci, E. L., & R. M. Ryan. 2000. "The 'what' and 'why' of goal pursuits: Human needs and the self-determination of behavior." *Psychological Inquiry, 11*(4): 227.

Dobbins, M., H. Husson, K. Decorby, and R. L. Larocca. 2013. "School-based physical activity programs for promoting physical activity and fitness in children and adolescents aged 6 to 18." *Cochrane Database Syst Rev, 2*: CD007651. doi:10.1002/14651858.CD007651.pub2

Duda, J. L., and P. Appleton (2016). "Empowering and disempowering coaching behaviors: Conceptualization, measurement considerations, and intervention implications." In Raab, M., Wylleman, P., Seiler, R., Elbe, A.-M., and Hatzigeorgiadis, A. (Ed.), *Sport and Exercise Psychology Research: From Theory to Practice*: 373–388. London: Elsevier.

Elbe, A. M., J. M. Wikman, M. Zheng, M. N. Larsen, G. Nielsen, and P. Krustrup. 2017. "The importance of cohesion and enjoyment for the fitness improvement of 8–10-year-old children participating in a team and individual sport school-based physical activity intervention." *European Journal of Sport Science, 17*(3): 343–350. doi:10.1080/17461391.2016.1260641

Faude, O., O. Kerper, M. Multhaupt, C. Winter, K. Beziel, A. Junge, and T. Meyer. 2010. "Football to tackle overweight in children." *Scandinavian Journal of Medicine & Science in Sports, 20*(s1): 103–110.

Ferreira, I., K. Horst, S. Wendel-Vos Kremers, F. J. Van Lenthe, and J. Brug. 2007. "Environmental correlates of physical activity in youth: A review and update." *Obesity Reviews, 8*: 129–154.

Geidne, S., M. Quennerstedt, and C. Eriksson. 2013. "The youth sports club as a health-promoting setting: An integrative review of research." *Scandinavian Journal of Public Health, 41*(3): 269–283. doi:10.1177/1403494812473204

Hammami, A., S. Kasmi, M. Razgallah, Z. Tabka, R. Shephard, and E. Bouhlel. 2016. "Recreational soccer training improves heart-rate variability indices and physical performance in untrained healthy adolescent." *Sport Sciences for Health, 13*(3): 507–514.

Hammami, A., M. B. Randers, S. Kasmi, M. Razgallah, Z. Tabka, K. Chamari, and E. Bouhlel. 2018. "Effects of soccer training on health-related physical fitness measures in male adolescents." *Journal of Sport and Health Sciences, 7*(2): 169–175. doi:10.1016/j.jshs.2017.10.009

Hansen, P. R., L. J. Andersen, A. N. Rebelo, J. Brito, T. Hornstrup, J. F. Schmidt, S. R. Jackman, et al. 2013. "Cardiovascular effects of 3 months of football training in overweight children examined by comprehensive echocardiography: A pilot study." *Journal of Sports Science, 31*(13): 1432–1440. doi:10.1080/02640414.2013.792951

Janssen, I., and A. Leblanc. 2010. "Systematic review of the health benefits of physical activity and fitness in school-aged children and youth." *International Journal of Behavioral Nutrition and Physical Activity, 7*(1): 40.

Katzmarzyk, P. T., I. M. Lee, C. K. Martin, and S. N. Blair. 2017. "Epidemiology of physical activity and exercise training in the United States." *Progress in Cardiovascular Diseases, 60*(1): 3–10. doi:10.1016/j.pcad.2017.01.004

Krustrup, P., P. R. Hansen, C. M. Nielsen, M. N. Larsen, M. B. Randers, V. Manniche, L. Hansen, J. Dvorak, and J. Bangsbo. 2014. "Structural and functional cardiac adaptations to a 10-week school-based football intervention for 9–10-year-old children." *Scandinavian Journal of Medicine and Science in Sports, 24*(1): 4–9. doi:10.1111/sms.12277

Lavelle, H. V., D. F. Mackay, and J. P. Pell. 2012. "Systematic review and meta-analysis of school-based interventions to reduce body mass index." *Journal of Public Health, 34*(3): 360–369.

Lee, I. M., E. J. Shiroma, F. Lobelo, P. Puska, S. N. Blair, P. T. Katzmarzyk, and Group "Lancet Physical Activity Series Working". 2012. "Effect of physical inactivity on major non-communicable diseases worldwide: An analysis of burden of disease and life expectancy." *Lancet, 380*(9838): 219–229. doi:10.1016/S0140-6736(12)61031-9

Madsen, K., H. Thompson, A. Adkins, and Y. Crawford. 2013. "School-community partnerships: A cluster-randomized trial of an after-school soccer program." *JAMA Pediatrics, 167*(4): 321–326. doi:10.1001/jamapediatrics.2013.1071

McCarthy, P. J., Jones, M. V., & Clark-Carter, D. 2008. "Understanding enjoyment in youth sport: A developmental perspective." *Psychology of Sport and Exercise, 9*(2): 142–156.

Orntoft, C., C. W. Fuller, M. N. Larsen, J. Bangsbo, J. Dvorak, and P. Krustrup. 2016. "'FIFA 11 for Health' for Europe II: Effect on health markers and physical fitness in Danish schoolchildren aged 10–12 years." *British Journal of Sports Medicine, 50*(22): 1394–1399. doi:10.1136/bjsports-2016-096124

Parrish, A. M., A. D. Okely, R. M. Stanley, and N. D. Ridgers. 2013. "The effect of school recess interventions on physical activity: A systematic review." *Sports Medicine, 43*(4): 287–299. doi:10.1007/s40279-013-0024-2

Pearson, N., and S. J. Biddle. 2011. "Sedentary behavior and dietary intake in children, adolescents, and adults: A systematic review." *American Journal of Preventive Medicine, 41*(2): 178–188.

Randers, M. B., L. Nybo, J. Petersen, J. J. Nielsen, L. Christiansen, M. Bendiksen, J. Brito, J. Bangsbo, and P. Krustrup. 2010. "Activity profile and physiological response to football training for untrained males and females, elderly and youngsters: Influence of the number of players." *Scandinavian Journal of Medicine & Science in Sports, 20*(S1): 14–23.

Sallis, J. F., J. J. Prochaska, and W. C. Taylor. 2000. "A review of correlates of physical activity of children and adolescents." *Medicine & Science in Sports & Exercise, 32*(5): 963–975.

Salmon, J., M. L. Booth, P. Phongsavan, N. Murphy, and A. Timperio. 2007. "Promoting physical activity participation among children and adolescents." *Epidemiologic Reviews, 29*: 144–159.

Seabra, A. C., A. F. Seabra, J. Brito, P. Krustrup, P. R. Hansen, J. Mota, A. Rebelo, C. Rego, and R. M. Malina. 2014. "Effects of a 5-month football program on perceived psychological status and body composition of overweight boys." *Scandinavian Journal of Medicine and Science in Sports, 24*(1): 10–16. doi:10.1111/sms.12268

Seabra, A. F., P. Katzmarzyk, M. J. Carvalho, A. Seabra, E. Silva, M. Coelho, S. Abreu, S. Vale, et al. 2016. "Effects of 6-month soccer and traditional physical activity programmes on body composition, cardiometabolic risk factors, inflammatory, oxidative stress markers and cardiorespiratory fitness in obese boys." *Journal of Sports Sciences, 34*(19): 1822–1829. doi:10.1080/02640414.2016.1140219

Seabra, A. F., D. M. Mendonca, M. A. Thomis, L. A. Anjos, and J. A. Maia. 2008. "Biological and socio-cultural determinants of physical activity in adolescents." *Cad Saude Publica, 24*(4): 721–736.

Shields, M., and M. S. Tremblay. 2008. "Sedentary behaviour and obesity." *Health Reports, 19*(2): 19–30.

Skoradal, M. B., E. Purkhus, H. Steinholm, M. H. Olsen, C. Orntoft, M. N. Larsen, J. Dvorak, M. Mohr, and P. Krustrup. 2018. "'FIFA 11 for Health' for Europe in the Faroe Islands: Effects on health markers and physical fitness in 10- to 12-year-old schoolchildren." *Scandinavian Journal of Medicine and Science in Sports, 28*(1): 8–17. doi:10.1111/sms.13209

Strong, W. B., R. M. Malina, C. Jr Blimkie, S. R. Daniels, R. K. Dishman, B. Gutin, A. C. Hergenroeder, et al. 2005. "Evidence based physical activity for school-age youth." *The Journal of Pediatrics, 146*(6): 732–737.

Telama, R., X. Yang, E. Leskinen, A. Kankaanpaa, M. Hirvensalo, T. Tammelin, J. S. Viikari, and O. T. Raitakari. 2014. "Tracking of physical activity from early childhood through youth into adulthood." *Medicine & Science in Sports & Exercise, 46*(5): 955–962. doi:10.1249/MSS.0000000000000181

Tremblay, M. S., A. G. Leblanc, M. E. Kho, T. J. Saunders, R. Larouche, R. C. Colley, G. Goldfield, and S. C. Gorber. 2011. "Systematic review of sedentary behaviour and health indicators in school-aged children and youth." *The International Journal of Behavioral Nutrition and Physical Activity, 8*: 98.

Uijtdewilligen, L., J. Nauta, A. S. Singh, W. Van Mechelen, J. W. Twisk, K. Van Der Horst, and M. J. Chinapaw. 2011. "Determinants of physical activity and sedentary behaviour in young people: A review and quality synthesis of prospective studies." *British Journal of Sports Medicine, 45*(11): 896–905.

Van Der Horst, K., M. J. Paw, J. W. Twisk, and W. Van Mechelen. 2007. "A brief review on correlates of physical activity and sedentariness in youth." *Medicine & Science in Sports & Exercise, 39*(8): 1241–1250.

Van Hecke, L., A. Loyen, M. Verloigne, H. P. Van Der Ploeg, J. Lakerveld, J. Brug, I. De Bourdeaudhuij, et al. 2016. "Variation in population levels of physical activity in European children and adolescents according to cross-European studies: A systematic literature review within DEDIPAC." *International Journal of Behavioral Nutrition and Physical Activity, 13*: 70. doi:10.1186/s12966-016-0396-4

Van Sluijs, E. M., A. M. Mcminn, and S. J. Griffin. 2007. "Effectiveness of interventions to promote physical activity in children and adolescents: Systematic review of controlled trials." *BMJ*, *335*(7622): 703.

Vasconcellos, F., A. Seabra, F. Cunha, R. Montenegro, J. Penha, E. Bouskela, J. F. Nogueira Neto, P. Collett-Solberg, and P. Farinatti. 2015. "Health markers in obese adolescents improved by a 12-week recreational soccer program: A randomised controlled trial." *Journal of Sports Sciences*: 1–12. doi:10.1080/02640414.2015.1064150

Vicente-Rodríguez, G. 2006. "How does exercise affect bone development during growth?" *Sports Medicine*, *36*(7): 561–569.

Weintraub, D. L., E. C. Tirumalai, K. F. Haydel, M.e Fujimoto, J. E. Fulton, and T. N. Robinson. 2008. "Team sports for overweight children: The stanford Sports to Prevent Obesity Randomized Trial (SPORT)." *Archives of Pediatrics & Adolescent Medicine*, *162*(3): 232–237.

World Health Organization. 2010. *Global Recommendations on Physical Activity for Health*. Geneva: World Health Organization.

World Health Organization. 2015. "Physical activity." *Fact Sheet*, N°385.

Chapter 6

Football for homeless and socially deprived people

Morten B. Randers, Amy Mendham, Mette K. Zebis, Jannick Marschall, Jens Jung Nielsen, Jincheng Xu and Peter Krustrup

Introduction

It is estimated that more than 1,000,000 people are homeless in the European Union and U.S., although a common definition has not been established (Fazel, Geddes, and Kushel 2014). In a given year, the European Union estimates that more than 4 million individuals experience homelessness, and sadly homelessness is on the increase in all European Union countries except Finland (FEANTSA 2017).

Homeless individuals are generally characterised by social deprivation, substance abuse, poor diet and other risk behaviours, leading to poor health profile, morbidities and premature death (Takano et al. 1999; Nordentoft and Wandall-Holm 2003; Beijer and Andréasson 2009; Feodor Nilsson et al. 2014). Compared to the general population, homeless and socially deprived people have higher morbidity and mortality rates, and for this population group, cardiovascular disease is also a leading cause of death (Barrow et al. 1999; Lee et al. 2005). Physical activity levels are reported to be markedly different in homeless and socially deprived people compared to the general population, with 65% of 38- to 44-year-old Danish homeless people reporting no participation in physical activity, versus 15% of men in the general population (Pedersen et al. 2008; Christensen et al. 2012). For homeless people in general, 69% reported no participation in physical activity (Pedersen et al. 2008), and given that physical activity is a cornerstone of the treatment and prevention of lifestyle diseases (Pedersen and Saltin 2015), greater engagement in physical activity may, for this population group in particular, be of significant importance for improving health profile and quality of life.

With the introduction of the Homeless World Cup in Austria in 2003, in which 18 countries participated, the first steps were taken to implement street football for homeless people worldwide. Under the ambitious slogan 'beating homelessness through football', the tournament has grown year on year, and July 2019, 64 teams will be heading to Cardiff, Wales. During the period in question, street football for the homeless has thus become a tool in the fight against physical inactivity and psychosocial problems in the homeless population.

Activity profile and acute physiological response during street football

Official homeless street football tournaments are played on 22×16-m pitches enclosed by 1.1-m-high boards. The goals are 4.0 m wide and 1.3 m high, and the penalty area comprises a semicircle of 4-m radius. Each team consists of up to eight players, four of whom are on the pitch at any one time: three outfield players and a goalkeeper. The goalkeeper is not allowed to leave the penalty area, while outfield players are not allowed to enter the penalty area. There are rolling substitutions, and as the focus is on inclusion—all players are expected to be given the opportunity to play for a reasonable amount of time. Each game comprises 2×7-min halves with a 1-min half-time break. The full set of rules can be found at www.homelessworldcup.org.

A number of studies have evaluated activity profile and heart rate profile during street football. The heart rate profile of 15 players from the Danish national team for homeless men was reported in a study by Randers and colleagues (2010), showing average heart rates of 83.6% of individual maximal heart rate and peak heart rates reaching 98.2% of individual maximal heart rate. These values are similar to those reported in a street football training study involving 33 homeless and socially deprived people (Randers et al. 2012). This study also reported heart rate within 80–90% of individual maximal heart rate for 44% of the playing time and higher than 90% of individual maximal heart rate for 21% of the playing time. These values are comparable to other subject groups playing 3v3 to 9v9 recreational football on grass (Krustrup et al. 2009; Randers, Nybo, et al. 2010; Randers et al. 2014; Randers, Brix, et al. 2017), but somewhat higher than reported for an English hard-to-reach population (Hulton et al. 2016). In the latter study, mean heart rate was only 75% of individual maximal heart rate and heart rate was above 90% of individual maximal heart rate for 15% of the training time. The biweekly training sessions, lasting 120 min, comprised technical training, skills/possession training and small-sided games. Mean heart rate during the small-sided games was 82% of maximal heart rate, comparable to the values reported in the previously mentioned studies (Hulton et al. 2016).

A recent study analysing heart rate during women's games at the Homeless World Cup in Amsterdam in 2015 showed even higher heart rates for women, with an average of 91.6% of individual peak heart rate and peak values reaching 98.6% (Randers et al. 2018). Heart rate was between 80 and 90% of peak heart rate for 26% of the playing time, and higher than 90% for as much as 67% of the total playing time. These values are markedly higher than observed in other types of football games for women (Krustrup et al. 2018), but it should be noted that the relative values presented in the study by Randers and colleagues (2018) were calculated using individual peak heart rates during games and not maximal individual rates obtained through incremental tests to exhaustion. Studies have shown that peak heart rates reached during football games equate to 94–99% of the maximal heart rate obtained during incremental testing, and it is therefore likely that the maximal heart rates may have been higher, resulting in less time spent in the various heart rate zones. However, a recent study involving untrained and recreationally trained healthy men showed comparable high heart rates during street football with boards keeping the ball in play (Randers, Brix, et al. 2017).

These high heart rates were obtained even though distance per minute was only 69 m min^{-1}, with only 11 and 2.4 m min^{-1} covered at 9–13 and >13 km h^{-1}, respectively, so intensity based on distance covered seems rather low (Randers et al. 2018). However, as speed rapidly changes, a number of intense accelerations, decelerations and changes of direction are performed. Moreover, only 43% of the distance covered is accounted for by forward movements, whereas 45% and 12% are accounted for by sideways or backwards movements (Randers et al. 2018). Like movements involving the ball, these specific movements, which are more frequent during street football and small-sided games due to the lower number of participants, have been shown to increase energy cost compared to normal straight-line forward running (Reilly and Ball 1984; Reilly and Bowen 1984). Thus, the activity profile, with its intermittent nature, may be one explanation for the high heart rate response observed during street football.

In homeless men, a change in activity every 2 s has been reported (Randers et al. 2012). Total distance covered during a 1-hour session was calculated as 5,534 m, equal to 92 m min^{-1}, which is higher than observed in street football for women (Randers et al. 2018) and untrained and recreationally trained men (Randers, Brix, et al. 2017) as well as in football on grass for women and men (Randers et al. 2014; Randers, Orntoft, et al. 2017; Krustrup et al. 2018). However, the higher distance covered observed in the study by Randers and colleagues (2012) with homeless men may be due to the difference in tracking method (Randers, Mujika, et al. 2010), and hence an overestimation due to the use of video time-motion. In support of this assumption, the number of steps was 5,439, resulting in a mean step length of more than 1 m, which is very unlikely (Randers et al. 2012; Helge et al. 2014).

Nevertheless, the fact that the activity pattern during street football for homeless people is comparable to the activity pattern during street football and small-sided football for untrained people implies that the exercise intensity instinctively chosen by homeless people during match-play does not differ from that of other groups of untrained individuals.

In the study involving homeless women, rating of perceived exertion (RPE) and flow were also measured. Interestingly, the women reported moderate RPE (4.8) despite the high heart rate response (Randers et al. 2018). Moreover, the RPE was lower than reported for women playing recreational 7v7 football (RPE: 5.8), although the differences in game duration and subject groups should be taken into consideration (Elbe et al. 2010). In addition, the levels of flow reported for the homeless women were higher compared to untrained women playing 7v7 (5.5 vs 5.0, respectively), and markedly higher than during football and Zumba as a workplace activity for healthcare professionals (3.5–4.3) (Elbe et al. 2016).

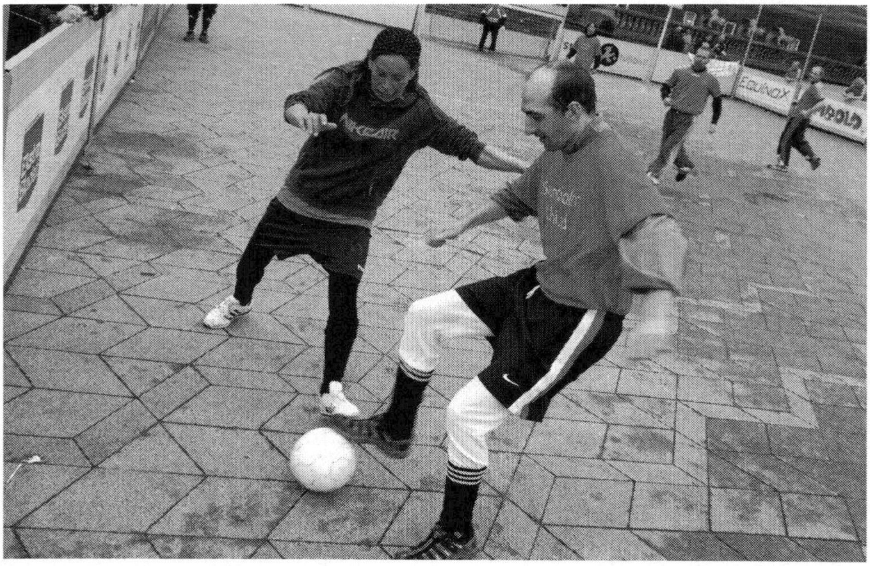

Photo 6.1 Football for Homeless, being played at the Town Square of Copenhagen.
Source: Photo Credit: The Danish homeless football organisation, Ombold.

Flow has been linked to adherence (Elbe et al. 2016), so the fact that the women experienced high flow during street football, combined with the fact that team sport has been shown to be linked to intrinsic motivation, increased network and social capital (Ottesen, Jeppesen, and Krustrup 2010; Nielsen et al. 2014; Wikman et al. 2018), makes street football interventions for homeless and socially deprived people recommendable as a physical activity with possible long-term adherence.

Health effects of football training for the homeless and socially deprived

Maximal oxygen uptake is a strong predictor of the risk of cardiovascular disease and early death (Erikssen et al. 1998; Keteyian et al. 2008; Nauman et al. 2017). The large Norwegian HUNT study showed that men with maximal oxygen uptake below the median (44.2 ml min^{-1} kg^{-1}) had an eight-times-higher risk of cardiovascular disease compared to those in the highest quartile (50.5 ml min^{-1} kg^{-1}) (Aspenes et al. 2011). For women, risk of cardiovascular disease was five times higher for those below the median (35.1 ml min^{-1} kg^{-1}) compared to those in the highest quartile (40.8 ml min^{-1} kg^{-1}), and it was shown that for every 5 ml min^{-1} kg^{-1} lowering of maximal oxygen uptake there was a 56% higher prevalence of cardiovascular risk factors (Aspenes et al. 2011).

A group of homeless and socially deprived men improved maximal oxygen uptake from 36.7 to 40.6 ml min^{-1} kg^{-1} after just one 12-week football intervention programme (Randers et al. 2012). The baseline values of this group were rather low, reinforcing the importance of physical activity programmes leading to increased cardiorespiratory fitness with a view to improving cardiovascular risk profile. The improvement in maximal oxygen uptake (3.9 ml min^{-1} kg^{-1}) reported in homeless and socially deprived men is comparable to the average change after a recreational football training programme reported in a meta-analysis by Milanović and colleagues (2015). Due to the poor postural balance reported in this group (Helge et al. 2014), the study by Randers and colleagues (2012) used an incremental cycle test to test maximal oxygen uptake. It might therefore be speculated as to whether these participants were able to exercise to exhaustion, but similar high heart rates and values for respiratory exchange ratio were reached in both pre- and post-tests. Moreover, time to exhaustion and end power output in the incremental cycle test were improved by ~8% and a 45% increase in intermittent running performance (Yo-Yo IE1) was observed, so several other test results indicate a marked increase in cardiorespiratory fitness (Randers et al. 2012).

The homeless men in the study by Randers and colleagues (2012) covered an average of 10,700 steps per day without training, with a large range (3,769–17,567 steps per day), underpinning the heterogeneity of this population. A value of 10,000 steps per day has been associated with a threshold for a healthy lifestyle, and has been suggested as a means of achieving the weekly recommended minutes of physical activity, but the value has also been questioned and seems insufficient for certain groups, e.g., children (Tudor-Locke and Bassett 2004). Lee and colleagues (2011) showed that meeting the guidelines for physical activity had no impact on mortality if cardiovascular fitness was poor, whereas high cardiovascular fitness was associated with low mortality irrespective of adherence to physical activity. Although the homeless men in question achieved more than 10,000 steps per day, their heart rate was only above 70% of HRmax for 3% of the time and only above 80% of maximal heart rate for 2–3 min per day outside training, resulting in poor cardiovascular fitness (Randers et al. 2012).

A cohort study showed similar maximal oxygen uptake between those meeting the guidelines of a minimum of 150 min of moderate-intensity activity and those with fewer accumulated minutes of physical activity provided the intensity was vigorous (75–149 min of weekly exercise) or very vigorous (<75 min per week) (Nes et al. 2012). In contrast, those who reported 75–149 min of moderate-intensity activity and those not physically active at all had markedly lower maximal oxygen uptake (Nes et al. 2012). High-intensity interval training has been shown to be more effective for improving maximal oxygen uptake than continuous moderate exercise (Nybo et al. 2010), and intensity is an important factor for reversing risk factors of metabolic syndrome (Moholdt et al. 2009; Nybo et al. 2010). As described previously, heart rate was 82% on average during street football training sessions for homeless and socially deprived men, with heart rates above 80 and 90% of maximal heart rate for 66 and 21% of total training time, respectively.

Thus, the intensity was very high during the football training, and with 2.2 hours of training per week, the street football training was the primary contributor to accumulated minutes of moderate- and vigorous-intensity activity for homeless men (Randers et al. 2012).

In contrast to other studies using recreational football as a training intervention, blood pressure was not improved after 12 weeks of street football for Danish homeless and socially deprived people (Randers et al. 2012) and in an English hard-to-reach population encompassing drug addicts and homeless people (Hulton et al. 2016). The prevalence of hypertension is higher in homeless people (Szerlip and Szerlip 2002), which fits well with the English population, whereas the baseline values in the Danish population were rather low, possibly related to the high misuse of cannabis in this subject group. In the Danish population, all eight participants with diastolic blood pressure values above 75 mmHg experienced a decline over 12 weeks of football training, though no change was found for the group as a whole. In addition, six out of nine participants with a pre-value for systolic blood pressure above 115 mmHg experienced a decrement. A meta-analysis encompassing 1 million adults showed a log-linear decrement in the risk of death from cardiovascular disease with a decrease in systolic and diastolic blood pressure down to at least 115 and 75 mmHg, respectively (Lewington 2002). A 20 mmHg decrease in systolic and a 10 mmHg decrease in diastolic blood pressure are associated with a halving of the risk of death from cardiovascular disease (Lewington 2002). Thus, the reduction in systolic and diastolic blood pressure seen for participants with elevated blood pressure prior to the street football training is of major importance, especially, given the observation that football has a good impact on blood pressure for those participants with mild to moderate hypertension (Andersen et al. 2010; Krustrup et al. 2013; Krustrup et al. 2017; Krustrup et al. 2018; Mohr et al. 2014).

Lower resting heart rate is another common finding after a football training intervention (Milanović et al. 2018), but even though resting heart rate decreased from 65 to 61 after 12 weeks of street football training, the change only tended to be different from the control group (Randers et al. 2012). In another 12-week football training study, resting heart rate decreases from 87 to 72 beats min^{-1} after 12 weeks of training (Hulton et al. 2016), but the baseline values were also markedly higher than observed in the study by Randers and colleagues (2012).

The prevalence of hyperlipidaemia is lower in the population under consideration than in the general population, but often more poorly controlled, and since cholesterol, and LDL cholesterol in particular, are strong predictors of cardiovascular disease, lowering these values is of major importance (Szerlip and Szerlip 2002; Lee et al. 2005). LDL cholesterol was lowered by 0.4 mmol L^{-1}, equal to 6%, whereas total cholesterol was unchanged. But with respect to the other parameters measured in the study by Randers and coworkers (2012), the subject group was very heterogeneous. In seven out of eight subjects with total cholesterol above 5 mmol L^{-1} prior to the football training period, total cholesterol was lower after the intervention. For LDL cholesterol, 12 of 13 with pre-values above 2.5

mmol L^{-1} had a lower LDL cholesterol concentration after the training period (Randers et al. 2012). Thus, for both total and LDL cholesterol the street football programme led to improvements for those with unfavourable pre-values. A 6% reduction in LDL cholesterol must be considered profitable given that a 1% reduction in LDL cholesterol is associated with a 2–3% lower risk of coronary heart disease (Leon and Sanchez 2001). Thus, the reduction after street football training for homeless and socially deprived men may equate to a 12–18% reduction in general, and an even higher reduction for those participants with the most unfavourable baseline values. Studies have shown that exercise training rarely results in a reduction in total cholesterol and LDL cholesterol unless body weight is reduced (Leon and Sanchez 2001; Durstine et al. 2002), but the study by Randers and colleagues (2012) observed changes even though body weight was unchanged.

Even though total body weight was unchanged, body composition was markedly improved. After 12 weeks of street football for homeless men, fat mass had been lowered by 1.6 kg (Randers et al. 2012), comparable to the 1.7 kg average fat mass change after recreational football training interventions reported in a meta-analysis (Milanović et al. 2018). However, inconsistent effects of recreational football on fat mass have been reported, and an English study involving nine hard-to-reach men did not find any changes in fat mass. In addition, the 1.6 kg change observed in Danish homeless and socially deprived men (Randers et al. 2012) is somewhat lower than the 3.0 kg observed in healthy but untrained age-matched men (Krustrup et al. 2009).

The homeless and socially deprived are a very heterogeneous group, and in the study by Randers and colleagues (2012), the difference between the highest and lowest fat percentage was 40 percentage points. Thus, both overweight and underweight are present in this subject group, even though the prevalence of obesity and the related hyperlipidaemia is lower than in the general population (Szerlip and Szerlip 2002; Lee et al. 2005).

Fat distribution, and android fat percentage in particular, has been shown to be a better indicator of cardiovascular risk profile than total body fat (Walton et al. 1995; Wu et al. 1998). For homeless men, a 2.5 percentage-point reduction in android fat percentage was found, which may be associated with an improved cardiovascular risk profile (Wiklund et al. 2008).

Another favourable change in body composition following 12 weeks of street football training was a 1.0 kg increase in lean body mass, albeit this did not differ from the control group (Randers et al. 2012). Another study by Hulton and colleagues (2016) also found a 1.0 kg higher lean body mass after 12 weeks of training, which did not reach statistical significance. Even though football training has led to increases in lean body mass in certain subject groups (Krustrup et al. 2009; Krustrup, Christensen, et al. 2010; Krustrup, Hansen, et al. 2010), a meta-analysis has shown trivial or small effects on lean body mass (Milanović et al. 2018). The lower response in homeless and socially deprived men may be related to malnutrition, which has been reported in homeless men (Darmon et al. 2001). In the study by Randers and colleagues (2012), a questionnaire revealed an estimated average protein intake of 74% of the recommended daily intake. Another factor that may have affected the response for lean body mass is the different activity profile of street football compared to larger-sided football, as described previously.

Homeless people have a 460% higher risk of being hospitalised as a result of a sudden trauma than the general population (Pedersen et al. 2008), and sudden trauma is often related to falls and bone fractures. In the elderly, muscle strength and postural balance were associated with a low frequency of falls, and bone strength was an important factor in preventing fractures when falling (Karlsson, Nordqvist, and Karlsson 2008). The ability to rapidly develop muscle force at the onset of contraction is highly important for regaining balance in situations of sudden postural perturbation, and rapid muscle force has been observed to be better in football-trained individuals compared to sedentary controls (Sundstrup et al. 2010). Superior rapid muscle force production has been observed in recreational football-trained elderly individuals compared to untrained age-matched individuals. Although rapid muscle force is a highly relevant measure in a population group that experiences higher bone fractures than the general population, rapid muscle force has not been measured in homeless people. Postural balance was, however, improved by 39–46% after 12 weeks of street football training, though the change was not significantly different from the control group (Randers et al. 2012). Bone mineral density was also unchanged after street football training in homeless subjects, but an osteogenic effect was found as a 27% increase in osteocalcin was observed (Helge et al. 2014). The activity pattern of street football, with its rapid changes of direction, accelerations, decelerations, shots and tackles, is considered a near-optimal osteogenic stimulus because ground and muscle reaction forces put strains on the bones at a high rate and in varied and unusual directions (Robling et al. 2002; Vainionpää et al. 2006; Helge et al. 2010; Jackman et al. 2013; Helge et al. 2014). However, changes in postural balance and in bone mineral density were very limited compared to the findings of previous studies (Helge et al. 2010; Krustrup et al. 2009; Randers, Nielsen, et al. 2010).

Football is an excellent activity for engaging with homeless people, the socially deprived and hard-to-reach individuals. A study of heroin users' views of sport and physical activity reported that social benefits, health and joy were key motivators for participation (Neale, Nettleton, and Pickering 2012). As previously described, football has been shown to be intrinsically motivating and leads to increased network and social capital (Ottesen, Jeppesen, and Krustrup 2010; Nielsen et al. 2014). UK studies using professional football clubs to target hard-to-reach individuals have also shown that football is an excellent arena for engaging with this challenging population group (Zwolinsky et al. 2013). A review by Hwang and colleagues (2005) concludes that coordinated treatment programmes for homeless people usually result in better health outcomes than standard care, which highlights the importance of well-planned and targeted interventions like those promoted by the Homeless World Cup Foundation and national homeless football organisations. A recently published 11-year register-based cohort study showed differences in the association between homelessness and mortality for men and women, which suggests the need for gender-tailored interventions (Feodor Nilsson et al. 2018). This is supported by a study by Bottorff and colleagues (Bottorff et al. 2015) that also highlights the importance of gender-specific health promotion strategies to effectively reach men.

Further studies are required to evaluate the effects of a training intervention on homeless women, as studies on this population group are lacking and therefore highly warranted. Moreover, it should be established whether pitch size and game format influence the osteogenic effect and hypertrophy after football training, as more activity changes are performed during 4v4 than during 7v7 training, but higher forces may be involved during larger-sided games as higher speeds are reached (Randers et al. 2010, 2014, 2017). In addition, malnutrition during the intervention period should be addressed.

In the 12-week training study by Randers and colleagues (2012), the three-times-weekly street football sessions were complemented by a one-hour session in a fitness centre. Adherence was higher for the street football training (75%) than for the fitness centre training (54%), resulting in four times as many weekly street football training sessions (2.2 vs 0.2 sessions per week). But, even though the

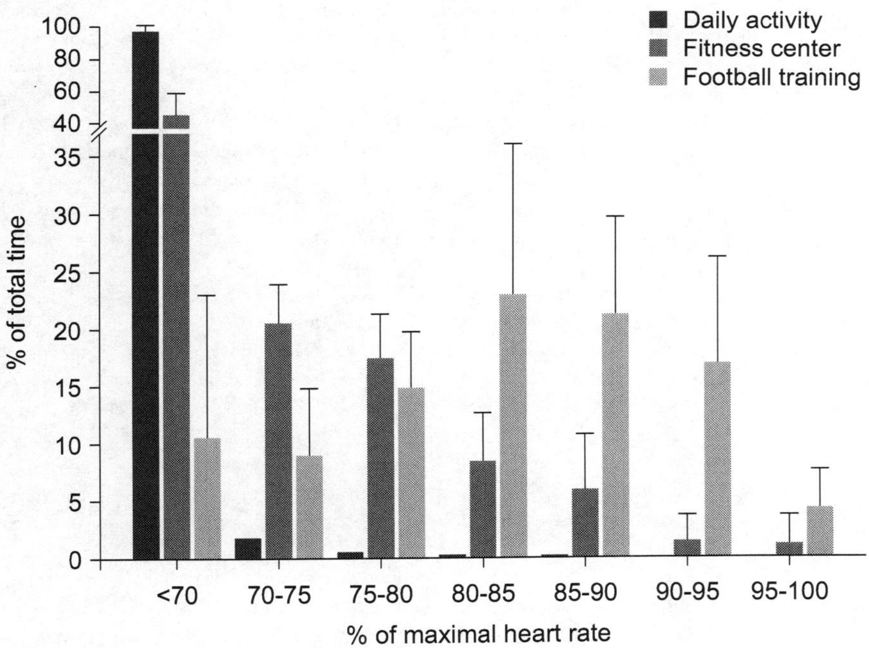

Figure 6.1 Intensity during street football, fitness centre training and everyday living for socially deprived men, expressed as the fraction of time in each of the heart rate zones from 70–100% of individual maximal heart rate.

Source: Randers et al. 2012.

frequency, volume and intensity of the street football training far exceed those of the fitness centre training, training effects cannot solely be attributed to the street football. Thus, future studies should seek to evaluate street football training alone.

References

Andersen, L. J., M. B. Randers, K. Westh, D. Martone, P. R. Hansen, A. Junge, J. Dvorak, J. Bangsbo, and P. Krustrup. 2010. "Football as a treatment for hypertension in untrained 30–55-year-old men: A prospective randomized study." *Scandinavian Journal of Medicine and Science in Sports* 20 (1):98–102. doi: 10.1111/j.1600-0838.2010.01109.x.

Aspenes, S. T., T. I. Nilsen, E. A. Skaug, G. F. Bertheussen, O. Ellingsen, L. Vatten, and U. Wisloff. 2011. "Peak oxygen uptake and cardiovascular risk factors in 4631 healthy women and men." *Medicine and Science in Sports and Exercise* 43 (8):1465–1473. doi: 10.1249/MSS.0b013e31820ca81c.

Barrow, S. M., D. B. Herman, P. Cordova, and E. L. Struening. 1999. "Mortality among homeless shelter residents in New York City." *American Journal of Public Health* 89 (4):529–534.

Beijer, U., and S. Andréasson. 2009. "Physical diseases among homeless people: Gender differences and comparisons with the general population." *Scandinavian Journal of Public Health* 37 (1):93–100.

Bottorff, J. L., C. L. Seaton, S. T. Johnson, C. M. Caperchione, J. L. Oliffe, K. More, H. Jaffer-Hirji, and S. M. Tillotson. 2015. "An updated review of interventions that include promotion of physical activity for adult men." *Sports Medicine* 45 (6):775–800. doi: 10.1007/s40279-014-0286-3.

Christensen, A. I., O. Ekholm, M. Davidsen, and K. Juel. 2012. "Sundhed og Sygelighed i Danmark 2010 & Udviklingen Siden 1987 (Health and Sickness in Denmark 2010 & Development Since 1987)." København: Statens Institut for Folkesundhed.

Darmon, N., J. Coupel, M. Deheeger, and A. Briend. 2001. "Dietary inadequacies observed in homeless men visiting an emergency night shelter in Paris." *Public Health Nutrition* 4 (2):155–161.

Durstine, J. L., P. W. Grandjean, C. A. Cox, and P. D. Thompson. 2002. "Lipids, lipoproteins, and exercise." *Journal of Cardiopulmonary Rehabilitation and Prevention* 22 (6):385–398.

Elbe, A.-M., S. Barene, K. Strahler, P. Krustrup, and A. Holtermann. 2016. "Experiencing flow in a workplace physical activity intervention for female health care workers: A longitudinal comparison between football and zumba." *Women in Sport and Physical Activity Journal* 24 (1):70–77.

Elbe, A.-M., K. Strahler, P. Krustrup, J. Wikman, and R. Stelter. 2010. "Experiencing flow in different types of physical activity intervention programs: Three randomized studies." *Scandinavian Journal of Medicine and Science in Sports* 20 (1):111–117. doi: 10.1111/j.1600-0838.2010.01112.x.

Erikssen, G., K. Liestøl, J. Bjørnholt, E. Thaulow, L. Sandvik, and J. Erikssen. 1998. "Changes in physical fitness and changes in mortality." *The Lancet* 352 (9130):759–762.

Fazel, S., J. R. Geddes, and M. Kushel. 2014. "The health of homeless people in high-income countries: Descriptive epidemiology, health consequences, and clinical and policy recommendations." *The Lancet* 384 (9953):1529–1540. doi: 10.1016/S0140-6736(14)61132-6.

FEANTSA. 2017. "Second overview of housing exclusion in Europe." 67.

Feodor Nilsson, S., C. R. Hjorthoj, A. Erlangsen, and M. Nordentoft. 2014. "Suicide and unintentional injury mortality among homeless people: A Danish nationwide register-based cohort study." *European Journal of Public Health* 24 (1):50–56. doi: 10.1093/eurpub/ckt025.

Feodor Nilsson, S., T. M. Laursen, C. Hjorthoj, and M. Nordentoft. 2018. "Homelessness as a predictor of mortality: An 11-year register-based cohort study." *Social Psychiatry and Psychiatric Epidemiology* 53 (1):63–75. doi: 10.1007/s00127-017-1456-z.

Helge, E. W., P. Aagaard, M. D. Jakobsen, E. Sundstrup, M. B. Randers, M. K. Karlsson, and P. Krustrup. 2010. "Recreational football training decreases risk factors for bone fractures in untrained premenopausal women." *Scandinavian Journal of Medicine and Science in Sports* 20 (1):31–39. doi: 10.1111/j.1600-0838.2010.01107.x.

Helge, E. W., M. B. Randers, T. Hornstrup, J. J. Nielsen, J. Blackwell, S. R. Jackman, and P. Krustrup. 2014. "Street football is a feasible health-enhancing activity for homeless men: Biochemical bone marker profile and balance improved." *Scandinavian Journal of Medicine and Science in Sports* 24 (1):122–129. doi: 10.1111/sms.12244.

Hulton, A. T., D. Flower, R. Murphy, D. Richardson, B. Drust, and K Curran. 2016. "Effectiveness of a community football programme on improving physiological markers of health in a hard-to-reach male population: The role of exercise intensity." *Soccer & Society* 17 (2):196–208.

Hwang, S. W., G. Tolomiczenko, F. G. Kouyoumdjian, and R. E. Garner. 2005. "Interventions to improve the health of the homeless: A systematic review." *American Journal of Preventive Medicine* 29 (4):311–319, e75.

Jackman, S. R., S. Scott, M. B. Randers, C. Orntoft, J. Blackwell, A. Zar, E. W. Helge, M. Mohr, and P. Krustrup. 2013. "Musculoskeletal health profile for elite female footballers versus untrained young women before and after 16 weeks of football training." *Journal of Sports Science* 31 (13):1468–1474. doi: 10.1080/02640414.2013.796066.

Karlsson, M. K., A. Nordqvist, and C. Karlsson. 2008. "Physical activity, muscle function, falls and fractures." *Food & Nutrition Research* 52 (1):1920.

Keteyian, S. J., C. A. Brawner, P. D. Savage, J. K. Ehrman, J. Schairer, G. Divine, H. Aldred, K. Ophaug, and P. A. Ades. 2008. "Peak aerobic capacity predicts prognosis in patients with coronary heart disease." *American Heart Journal* 156 (2):292–300.

Krustrup, P., J. F. Christensen, M. B. Randers, H. Pedersen, E. Sundstrup, M. D. Jakobsen, B. R. Krustrup, J. J. Nielsen, C. Suetta, L. Nybo, and J. Bangsbo. 2010. "Muscle adaptations and performance enhancements of soccer training for untrained men." *European Journal of Applied Physiology* 108 (6):1247–1258. doi: 10.1007/s00421-009-1319-8.

Krustrup, P., P. R. Hansen, M. B. Randers, L. Nybo, D. Martone, L. J. Andersen, L. T. Bune, A. Junge, and J. Bangsbo. 2010. "Beneficial effects of recreational football on the cardiovascular risk profile in untrained premenopausal women." *Scandinavian Journal of Medicine and Science in Sports* 20 (1):40–49. doi: 10.1111/j.1600-0838.2010.01110.x.

Krustrup, P., E. W. Helge, P. R. Hansen, P. Aagaard, M. Hagman, M. B. Randers, M. de Sousa, and M. Mohr. 2018. "Effects of recreational football on women's fitness and health: Adaptations and mechanisms." *European Journal of Applied Physiology* 118 (1):11–32. doi: 10.1007/s00421-017-3733-7.

Krustrup, P., J. J. Nielsen, B. R. Krustrup, J. F. Christensen, H. Pedersen, M. B. Randers, P. Aagaard, A. M. Petersen, L. Nybo, and J. Bangsbo. 2009. "Recreational soccer is an effective health-promoting activity for untrained men." *British Journal of Sports Medicine* 43 (11):825–831. doi: 10.1136/bjsm.2008.053124.

Krustrup, P., M. B. Randers, L. J. Andersen, S. R. Jackman, J. Bangsbo, and P. R. Hansen. 2013. "Soccer improves fitness and attenuates cardiovascular risk factors in hypertensive men." *Medicine and Science in Sports and Exercise* 45 (3):553–560. doi: 10.1249/MSS.0b013e3182777051.

Krustrup, P., M. B. Skoradal, M. B. Randers, P. Weihe, J. Uth, J. Mortensen, and M. Mohr. 2017. "Broad-spectrum health improvements with one year of soccer training in inactive mildly hypertensive middle-aged women." *Scandinavian Journal of Medicine and Science in Sports* 27 (12):1893–1901. doi: 10.1111/sms.12829.

Lee, D. C., X. Sui, F. B. Ortega, Y. S. Kim, T. S. Church, R. A. Winett, U. Ekelund, P. T. Katzmarzyk, and S. N. Blair. 2011. "Comparisons of leisure-time physical activity and cardiorespiratory fitness as predictors of all-cause mortality in men and women." *British Journal of Sports Medicine* 45 (6):504–510.

Lee, T. C., J. G. Hanlon, J. Ben-David, G. L. Booth, W. J. Cantor, P. W. Connelly, and S. W. Hwang. 2005. "Risk factors for cardiovascular disease in homeless adults." *Circulation* 111 (20):2629–2635. doi: 10.1161/CIRCULATIONAHA.104.510826.

Leon, A. S., and O. A. Sanchez. 2001. "Response of blood lipids to exercise training alone or combined with dietary intervention." *Medicine & Science in Sports & Exercise* 33 (6):S502–S515.

Lewington, S. 2002. "Prospective studies collaboration: Age-specific relevance of usual blood pressure to vascular mortality: A meta-analysis of individual data for one million adults in 61 prospective studies." *The Lancet* 360:1903–1913.

Milanović, Z., S. Pantelic, N. Covic, G. Sporis, and P. Krustrup. 2015. "Is recreational soccer effective for improving VO2max a Systematic review and meta-analysis." *Sports Medicine* 45 (9):1339–1353. doi: 10.1007/s40279-015-0361-4.

Milanović, Z., S. Pantelic, N. Covic, G. Sporis, M. Mohr, and P. Krustrup. 2018. "Broad-spectrum physical fitness benefits of recreational football: A systematic review and meta-analysis." *British Journal of Sports Medicine*. doi: 10.1136/bjsports-2017-097885.

Moholdt, T. T., B. H. Amundsen, L. A. Rustad, A. Wahba, K. T. Lovo, L. R. Gullikstad, A. Bye, E. Skogvoll, U. Wisloff, and S. A. Slordahl. 2009. "Aerobic interval training versus continuous moderate exercise after coronary artery bypass surgery: A randomized study of cardiovascular effects and quality of life." *American Heart Journal* 158 (6):1031–1037. doi: 10.1016/j.ahj.2009.10.003.

Mohr, M., A. Lindenskov, P. M. Holm, H. P. Nielsen, J. Mortensen, P. Weihe, and P. Krustrup. 2014. "Football training improves cardiovascular health profile in sedentary, premenopausal hypertensive women." *Scandinavian Journal of Medicine and Science in Sports* 24 (1):36–42. doi: 10.1111/sms.12278.

Nauman, J., B. M. Nes, C. J. Lavie, A. S. Jackson, X. Sui, J. S. Coombes, S. N. Blair, and U. Wisloff. 2017. "Prediction of cardiovascular mortality by estimated cardiorespiratory fitness independent of traditional risk factors: The HUNT study." *Mayo Clinic Proceedings* 92 (2):218–227. doi: 10.1016/j.mayocp.2016.10.007.

Neale, J., S. Nettleton, and L. Pickering. 2012. "Heroin users' views and experiences of physical activity, sport and exercise." *International Journal of Drug Policy* 23 (2):120–127.

Nes, B. M., I. Janszky, S. T. Aspenes, G. F. Bertheussen, L. J. Vatten, and U. Wisloff. 2012. "Exercise patterns and peak oxygen uptake in a healthy population: The HUNT study." *Medicine and Science in Sports and Exercise* 44 (10):1881–1889. doi: 10.1249/MSS.0b013e318258b443.

Nielsen, G. J. M. Wikman, C. J. Jensen, J. F. Schmidt, L. Gliemann, and T. R. Andersen. 2014. "Health promotion: The impact of beliefs of health benefits, social relations and enjoyment on exercise continuation." *Scandinavian Journal of Medicine and Science in Sports* 24 (1):66–75. doi: 10.1111/sms.12275.

Nordentoft, M., and N. Wandall-Holm. 2003. "10 year follow up study of mortality among users of hostels for homeless people in Copenhagen." *British Medical Journal* 327 (7406):81. doi: 10.1136/bmj.327.7406.81.

Nybo, L., E. Sundstrup, M. D. Jakobsen, M. Mohr, T. Hornstrup, L. Simonsen, J. Bulow, M. B. Randers, J. J. Nielsen, P. Aagaard, and P. Krustrup. 2010. "High-intensity training versus traditional exercise interventions for promoting health." *Medicine and Science in Sports and Exercise* 42 (10):1951–1958. doi: 10.1249/MSS.0b013e3181d99203.

Ottesen, L., R. S. Jeppesen, and B. R. Krustrup. 2010. "The development of social capital through football and running: Studying an intervention program for inactive women." *Scandinavian Journal of Medicine and Science in Sports* 20 (1):118–131. doi: 10.1111/j.1600-0838.2010.01123.x.

Pedersen, B. K., and B. Saltin. 2015. "Exercise as medicine: Evidence for prescribing exercise as therapy in 26 different chronic diseases." *Scandinavian Journal of Medicine and Science in Sports* 25 (3):1–72. doi: 10.1111/sms.12581.

Pedersen, P. V., A. I. Christensen, U. Hesse, and T. Curtis. 2008. "SUSY UDSAT: Sundhedsprofil for socialt udsatte i Danmark 2007," Copenhagen, Denmark.

Randers, M. B., J. Brix, M. Hagman, J. J. Nielsen, and P. Krustrup. 2017. "Effect of boards in small-sided street soccer games on movement pattern and physiological response in recreationally active young men." *Journal of Strength and Conditioning Research*. doi: 10.1519/JSC.0000000000002401.

Randers, M. B., J. Marschall, T. T. Nielsen, A. Moller, M. K. Zebis, and P. Krustrup. 2018. "Heart rate and movement pattern in street soccer for homeless women." *German Journal of Exercise and Sport Research* 48 (2):211–217. doi: 10.1007/s12662-018-0503-6.

Randers, M. B., I. Mujika, A. Hewitt, J. Santisteban, R. Bischoff, R. Solano, A. Zubillaga, E. Peltola, P. Krustrup, and M. Mohr. 2010. "Application of four different football match analysis systems: A comparative study." *Journal of Sports Sciences* 28 (2):171–182. doi: 10.1080/02640410903428525.

Randers, M. B., J. J. Nielsen, J. Bangsbo, and P. Krustrup. 2014. "Physiological response and activity profile in recreational small-sided football: No effect of the number of players." *Scandinavian Journal of Medicine and Science in Sports* 24 (1):130–137. doi: 10.1111/sms.12232.

Randers, M. B., J. J. Nielsen, B. R. Krustrup, E. Sundstrup, M. D. Jakobsen, L. Nybo, J. Dvorak, J. Bangsbo, and P. Krustrup. 2010. "Positive performance and health effects of a football training program over 12 weeks can be maintained over a 1-year period with reduced training frequency." *Scandinavian Journal of Medicine and Science in Sports* 20 (1):80–89. doi: 10.1111/j.1600-0838.2010.01091.x.

Randers, M. B., L. Nybo, J. Petersen, J. J. Nielsen, L. Christiansen, M. Bendiksen, J. Brito, J. Bangsbo, and P. Krustrup. 2010. "Activity profile and physiological response to football training for untrained males and females, elderly and youngsters: Influence of the number of players." *Scandinavian Journal of Medicine and Science in Sports* 20:14–23. doi: 10.1111/j.1600-0838.2010.01069.x.

Randers, M. B., C. Orntoft, M. Hagman, J. J. Nielsen, and P. Krustrup. 2017. "Movement pattern and physiological response in recreational small-sided football: Effect of number of players with a fixed pitch size." *Journal of Sports Sciences*:1–8. doi: 10.1080/02640414.2017.1402552.

Randers, M. B., J. Petersen, L. J. Andersen, B. R. Krustrup, T. Hornstrup, J. J. Nielsen, M. Nordentoft, and P. Krustrup. 2012. "Short-term street soccer improves fitness and cardiovascular health status of homeless men." *European Journal of Applied Physiology* 112 (6):2097–2106. doi: 10.1007/s00421-011-2171-1.

Reilly, T., and D. Ball. 1984. "The net physiological cost of dribbling a soccer ball." *Research Quarterly for Exercise and Sport* 55 (3):267–271.

Reilly, T., and T. Bowen. 1984. "Exertional costs of changes in directional modes of running." *Perceptual and Motor Skills* 58 (1):149–150.

Robling, A. G., F. M. Hinant, D. B. Burr, and C. H. Turner. 2002. "Shorter, more frequent mechanical loading sessions enhance bone mass." *Medicine and Science in Sports and Exercise* 34 (2):196–202.

Sundstrup, E., M. D. Jakobsen, J. L. Andersen, M. B. Randers, J. Petersen, C. Suetta, P. Aagaard, and P. Krustrup. 2010. "Muscle function and postural balance in lifelong trained male footballers compared with sedentary elderly men and youngsters." *Scandinavian Journal of Medicine and Science in Sports* 20 (1):90–97. doi: 10.1111/j.1600-0838.2010.01092.x.

Szerlip, M. I., and H. M. Szerlip. 2002. "Identification of cardiovascular risk factors in homeless adults." *The American Journal of the Medical Sciences* 324 (5):243–246.

Takano, T., K. Nakamura, S. Takeuchi, and M. Watanabe. 1999. "Disease patterns of the homeless in Tokyo." *Journal of Urban Health* 76 (1):73–84. doi: 10.1007/BF02344463.

Tudor-Locke, C., and D. R. Bassett. 2004. "How many steps/day are enough?" *Sports Medicine* 34 (1):1–8.

Vainionpää, A., R. Korpelainen, E. Vihriälä, A. Rinta-Paavola, J. Leppäluoto, and T. Jämsä. 2006. "Intensity of exercise is associated with bone density change in premenopausal women." *Osteoporosis International* 17 (3):455–463.

Walton, C., B. Lees, D. Crook, M. Worthington, I. F. Godsland, and J. C. Stevenson. 1995. "Body fat distribution, rather than overall adiposity, influences serum lipids and lipoproteins in healthy men independently of age." *The American Journal of Medicine* 99 (5):459–464.

Wiklund, P., F. Toss, L. Weinehall, G. Hallmans, P. W. Franks, A. Nordstrom, and P. Nordstrom. 2008. "Abdominal and gynoid fat mass are associated with cardiovascular risk factors in men and women." *The Journal of Clinical Endocrinology & Metabolism* 93 (11):4360–4366.

Wikman, J. M., P. Elsborg, G. Nielsen, K. Seidelin, M. Nyberg, J. Bangsbo, Y. Hellsten, and A.-M. Elbe. 2018. "Are team sport games more motivating than individual exercise for middle-aged women? A comparison of levels of motivation associated with participating in floorball and spinning." *Kinesiology: International Journal of Fundamental and Applied Kinesiology* 50 (1):34–42.

Wu, C.-H., W.-J. Yao, F.-H. Lu, J.-S. Wu, and C.-J. Chang. 1998. "Relationship between glycosylated hemoglobin, blood pressure, serum lipid profiles and body fat distribution in healthy Chinese." *Atherosclerosis* 137 (1):157–165.

Zwolinsky, S., J. McKenna, A. Pringle, A. Daly-Smith, S. Robertson, and A. White. 2013. "Optimizing lifestyles for men regarded as 'hard-to-reach' through top-flight football/soccer clubs." *Health Education Research* 28 (3):405–413. doi: 10.1093/her/cys108.

Chapter 7

Football and healthy ageing

Pasqualina Buono, Jesper L. Andersen, Andreina Alfieri, Annamaria Mancini, Stefania Orrù, Marie Hagman and Peter Krustrup

Ageing is characterised by a progressive decline in the function of all organs and organ systems, albeit at different rates, between individuals. Actually, it is a common opinion that organs/systems developed certain capacities to react to perturbations and return to homeostasis, a concept that has been defined as an 'organ reserve' (Neustadt and Pieczenik, 2008). This reserve decreases with age and could explain the functional deterioration of the various organs/systems that occurs during ageing. In fact, it has been calculated that the reserve capacity in a healthy young adult is 7–11 times higher than the demand, whereas at 85 years, the organ reserve is reduced by 50% compared to its original capacity (Neustadt and Pieczenik, 2008). The physiological modifications associated with ageing that occur in the cardiovascular system (CV) are some of the most clinically relevant. The morphological and functional CV alterations dramatically reduce functional capacity during ageing: at the age of 75, more than half of CV functional capacity, defined by maximum oxygen consumption (VO_2 max), has been lost (Hawkins and Wiswell, 2003). VO_2max is considered the international reference standard for physical fitness: a reduction in VO_2max is strictly associated with CV disease and increased all-cause mortality, including metabolic non-communicable diseases (Bangsbo et al., 2015; Krustrup et al., 2010a). Furthermore, low cardiorespiratory capacity is considered a strong and independent predictor of mortality risk (this is discussed in detail in Chapter 1). Moreover, poor cardiorespiratory fitness is strongly associated with a reduction in many physical abilities, leading to reduced performance in activities of daily living (ADL) (Sundstrup et al., 2016).

The musculoskeletal system also shows strong functional impairment during ageing; this decline leads to *sarcopenia*, a complex syndrome characterised by loss of skeletal muscle mass, leading to muscle weakness and impaired performance (Nascimento et al., 2018). The prevalence of sarcopenia can vary from 4% up to 27% depending on gender and race (Tyrovolas et al., 2016). The main changes occurring in skeletal muscle during ageing are related to the loss of muscle mass, something that is more pronounced in the lower limbs. In the ageing process, a progressive decrease (up to 30–40%) in the number of muscle fibres is observed (Kalyani et al., 2014). Moreover, the muscle fibre composition is affected by ageing: in fact, a muscle fibre type transformation towards a higher relative number of slow fibres is observed during the earlier stages of ageing (Andersen, 2003). Alongside these specific changes in fibre type, an age-related remodelling of the motor units is also observed during ageing, resulting in reduced force-generating capacity and slowing of skeletal muscle (Nascimento et al., 2018; Miljkovic et al., 2015; Frontera, Zayas, and Rodriguez, 2012). Furthermore, sarcopenia is also associated with a decline in mitochondrial biogenesis and function. In particular, the accumulation of mitochondrial DNA mutations and the increased oxidative damage induced by reactive oxygen species (ROS) strongly compromise the integrity and function of mitochondria in the elderly, leading to reduced oxidative capacity (Chistiakov et al., 2018). Together, the alterations contributing to muscle ageing are responsible for general physical disability, increased risk of falls and reduced quality of life (QoL) typically observed in elderly people (Cruz-Jentoft et al., 2010; Fajemiroye et al., 2018).

In order to achieve an increased lifespan, and especially an extension of healthy ageing, we need to expand our knowledge of the cellular and molecular events controlling cell growth and senescence pathways, and try to understand how age-related dysregulation induces cellular senescence. Physical ageing decline is associated with important modifications in transcriptional regulation and protein synthesis, mitochondrial function and oxidative metabolism, and DNA repair mechanisms (DiLoreto and Murphy, 2015). These aspects have recently been investigated in skeletal muscle from lifelong football-trained elderly subjects, as discussed below.

In the past decade, growing scientific evidence strongly suggested that a sedentary lifestyle is an independent risk factor for chronic cardiovascular and metabolic diseases (Pedersen and Saltin, 2006), whereas active lifestyle promotes healthy ageing, in terms of both prevention and management of chronic non-communicable diseases (Kim et al., 2007; Ostergard et al., 2006). It is well described that recreational football training promotes positive effects on several health-related parameters, i.e. improvement in VO_2max, muscle strength and muscle mass, and bone mineral density in both unhealthy and elderly male and female subjects (Hagman et al., 2018; Helge et al., 2014; de Sousa et al., 2014; Krustrup et al., 2010a, 2010b, 2013, 2018; Krustrup and Krustrup, 2018; L.J. Andersen et al., 2014; T.R. Andersen et al., 2014; Randers et al., 2012; Schmidt et al., 2013; Milanović et al., 2018; Møller et al., 2018; Skoradal et al., 2018a, 2018b; Uth et al., 2018). In addition, it has been described how just one hour of recreational football training 2–3 times a week for 12 weeks induced cardiovascular and musculoskeletal improvements that were maintained even after a long-term training period with reduced training frequency (Randers et al., 2012).

The effects induced by long-term football training on the expression of various muscle biomarkers related to health were discussed in a recent study. The authors observed an increase in the mRNA expression levels of key biomarkers directly or indirectly involved in energy balance, mitochondrial biogenesis and oxidative metabolism, including PPARγ, AMPKα1/α2, TFAM, NAMPT, PGC1α and SIRT1, in skeletal muscle tissue from young long-term trained subjects (Alfieri et al., 2015). This increase positively correlates with the improvement in cardiovascular fitness, body composition, blood glucose and lipid profile in the trained subjects, thereby reducing the risk of developing metabolic diseases (Alfieri et al., 2015; Randers et al., 2010).

Similarly, lifelong football training positively affects clinical and physiological biomarkers related to healthy ageing. A clinical study conducted in elderly subjects demonstrated an improvement in cardiovascular function (i.e. VO_2max and microvascular endothelial function) and body composition (healthier body composition) in a group of lifelong football-trained veterans compared to age-matched untrained elderly subjects (Schmidt et al., 2015). However, despite a wealth of physiological and clinical evidence on the positive effects of football training in elderly subjects, there are so far no studies focusing on the mRNA/protein expression of key molecular markers involved in healthy longevity pathways in the muscle of elderly subjects. Very recently, mRNA and/or protein expression of AMPKα1/α2, NAMPT, TFAM and PGC1α, key markers in mitochondrial biogenesis and oxidative metabolism, was found to be enhanced in muscle from lifelong football-trained elderly subjects compared to age-matched active healthy untrained subjects (Mancini et al., 2017). The authors show that lifelong football training counteracts the decline in oxidative capacity in muscle mitochondria in football veterans, a peculiar feature of the ageing process, as we previously discussed. In particular, the authors reported an increase in mRNA and protein expression of AMPK (AMPKα1/α2), key markers involved in mitochondrial biogenesis and oxidative metabolism, together with increased mRNA expression of downstream markers of the oxidative pathway PGC1α, TFAM and NAMPT in muscle from veterans compared to untrained subjects (Fig. 7.1). All the above evidence, supported by increased activity of mitochondrial citrate synthase, another hallmark of muscle oxidative capacity, fits nicely with the increased VO_2max observed in football veterans compared to age-matched untrained active elderly subjects (Gerhart-Hines et al., 2007; Short et al., 2003).

Lifelong football training also positively affects the expression of biomarkers involved in DNA repair mechanisms and in senescence suppression pathways, as demonstrated by the increased expression levels of key proteins belonging to these pathways, i.e. p42–44 mitogen-activated protein kinase-MAPK (Erk1/2), AKT serine/threonine kinase 1 (AKT), mammalian target of rapamycin (mTOR) and Forkhead box M1 (FoxM1), in football veterans compared to active untrained age-matched elderly subjects. In particular, the increase of Erk1/2 proteins, which regulate proliferation and differentiation of muscle cells playing an important role in the myogenic response to exercise, is interesting in this context (Parkington et al., 2004). AKT, which is involved in the growth and hypertrophy of skeletal muscle, could be involved in the senescence suppression pathway, but the mechanisms are not well understood (Bodine et al., 2001; Pallafacchina et al., 2002). Nevertheless, it is interesting that AKT at the protein level was increased in skeletal muscle from football veterans (Mancini et al., 2017), which is in line with another finding obtained in trained versus untrained young subjects (Frosig et al., 2007). mTOR is another crucial regulator of cell growth and longevity pathways (Harrison et al., 2009; Katewa and Kapahi, 2011); its expression was found to be upregulated in skeletal muscle of elderly mice compared with young mice (Lamming et al., 2012). The role of mTOR in human muscle ageing has not been completely elucidated. It regulates protein synthesis in response to environmental stimuli such as nutrients (i.e., amino acid) and growth factors (i.e. insulin and insulin-like growth factor 1) (Li et al., 2012). Similarly to AMPK, mTOR also responds to mechanical stimuli (i.e. muscle contraction) in humans. In fact, some studies have reported that resistance exercise acutely activates AMPK and mTOR signalling (Dreyer et al., 2010; Koopman et al., 2006; Watson and Baar, 2014), but it is not clear whether chronic/long-term resistance training could lead to an activation of these signal cascades. The expression levels of mTOR protein did not show significant changes in muscle from veterans compared to active untrained elderly subjects, as reported in Mancini et al. (2017), which is in line with a previous study indicating no variation in mTOR protein expression in muscle from active and sedentary young and elderly subjects, probably due to high interindividual variability (Sandri et al., 2013). FoxM1 transcription factor regulates several biological functions, including cell proliferation, cell cycle progression and differentiation, playing a pivotal role in the senescence suppression pathway and in DNA repair mechanisms (Behrens et al., 2014). Increased FoxM1 transcription factor expression has been associated with senescence suppression (Bella et al., 2014); both FoxM1 mRNA and protein expression levels were increased in muscle from veterans compared to untrained elderly subjects (Mancini et al., 2017).

Very recently, it has been demonstrated that lifelong football training positively affects the expression of genes and proteins involved in auto-lysosomal and proteasome (RAD23A, HSPB6, RAB1B, TRAP1, SIRT2 and HSBPB1, in cell growth and differentiation (RPL1, RPL4, RPL36, MRLP37) and in autophagy pathways (Bcl-2, HSP70, HSP90, PSMD13 and ATG5-ATG12 protein complex) in skeletal muscle of football-trained veterans compared to age-matched untrained elderly subjects. These results suggest that lifelong football training promotes skeletal muscle longevity (Mancini et al. 2019).

Many studies over the past decade have found that football as an exercise modality is close to optimal in combining different types of exercise into one when it comes to increasing general health status in the elderly. Nevertheless, it is also clear that at this point in time, very few studies of good quality have been conducted to try to reveal the molecular mechanisms behind the beneficial physiological adaptations observed. There is thus a significant need for more studies to address this issue.

In conclusion, lifelong football training induces upregulation in muscle of key molecular markers involved in mitochondrial biogenesis, oxidative metabolism, DNA repair promotion and senescence suppression. Furthermore, lifelong football training affects the protein quality control and exercise-induced autophagy in skeletal muscle, thus promoting healthy ageing. These *omics* adaptations support improvement in body composition, cardiovascular function and metabolic profile, thus promoting healthy ageing in lifelong football-trained elderly subjects. In this context, implementation of sports facilities at the local level should be encouraged in order to improve the practice of football even in the elderly. Furthermore, future research should be carried out to obtain a consensus on the minimum volume of training required to achieve metabolic improvement in the elderly, including in terms of metabolic non-communicable disease prevention.

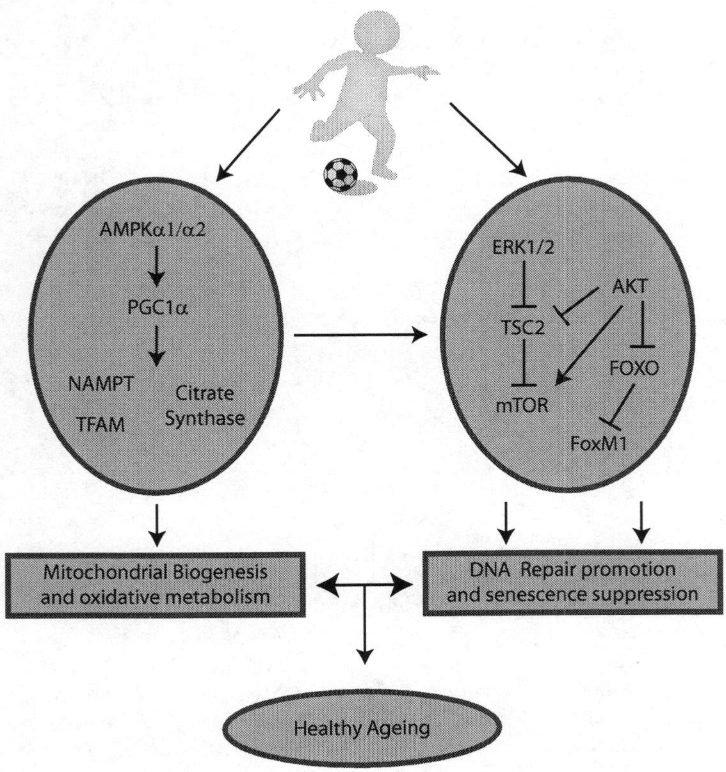

Figure 7.1 Lifelong football training effects on the expression of molecular markers associated with healthy ageing in skeletal muscle. Lifelong football training induces upregulation of key markers involved in the mitochondrial biogenesis and oxidative metabolism pathways (AMPKα1/α2, PGC1α, NAMPT, TFAM and citrate synthase activity) and in DNA repair promotion and senescence suppression (ERK1/2, AKT, mTOR and FoxM1).

Source: Adapted from Mancini et al. (2017).

References

Alfieri, A., Martone, D., Randers, M.B., Labruna, G., Mancini, A., Nielsen, J.J., Bangsbo, J., Krustrup, P., Buono, P. 2015. Effects of long-term football training on the expression profile of genes involved in muscle oxidative metabolism. *Molecular and Cellular Probes* 29:43–47. doi: 10.1016/j.mcp.2014.11.003.

Andersen, J.L. 2003. Muscle fibre type adaptation in the elderly human muscle. *Scandinavian Journal of Medicine & Science in Sports* 13(1):40–47.

Andersen, L.J., Randers, M.B., Hansen, P.R., Hornstrup, T., Schmidt, J.F., Dvorak, J., Søgaard, P., et al. 2014. Structural and functional cardiac adaptations to 6 months of football training in untrained hypertensive men. *Scandinavian Journal of Medicine & Science in Sports* 24(Suppl. 1):27–35. doi: 10.1111/sms.12237.

Andersen, T.R., Schmidt, J.F., Thomassen, M., Hornstrup, T., Frandsen, U., Bredsgaard, Randers M, et al. 2014. A preliminary study e effects of football training on glucose control, body composition and performance in men with type 2 diabetes. *Scandinavian Journal of Medicine & Science in Sports* 24(Suppl. 1):43–56. doi: 10.1111/sms.12259.

Bangsbo, J., Hansen, P.R., Dvorak, J., Krustrup, P. 2015. Recreational football for disease prevention and treatment in untrained men: A narrative review examining cardiovascular health, lipid profile, body composition, muscle strength and functional capacity. *British Journal of Sports Medicine* 49(9):568–76. doi: 10.1136/bjsports-2015-094781.

Behrens, A., van Deursen, J.M., Rudolph, K.L., Schumacher, B. 2014. Impact of genomic damage and ageing on stem cell function. *Nature Cell Biology* 16:201–207. doi: 10.1038/ncb2928.

Bella, L., Zona, S., de Moraes, G.N., Lam, E.W. 2014. FOXM1: A key oncofoetal transcription factor in health and disease. *Seminars in Cancer Biology* 29:32–39. doi: 10.1016/j.semcancer.2014.07.008.

Bodine, S.C., Stitt, T.N., Gonzalez, M., Kline, W.O., Stover, G.L., Bauerlein, R., Zlotchenko, E., Scrimgeour, A., Lawrence, J.C., Glass, D.J. et al. 2001. Akt/mTOR pathway is a crucial regulator of skeletal muscle hypertrophy and can prevent muscle atrophy in vivo. *Nature Cell Biology* 3:1014–1019.

Chistiakov, D.A., Sobenin, I.A., Revin, V.V., Orekhov, A.N., Bobryshevc, Y.V. 2018. Mitochondrial aging and age-related dysfunction of mitochondria. *BioMed Research International* 2014:238463. doi: 10.1155/2014/238463.

Cruz-Jentoft, A.J., Baeyens, J.P., Bauer, J.M., Boirie, Y., Cederholm, T., Landi, F., Martin, F.C., et al. 2010. Sarcopenia: European consensus on definition and diagnosis: Report of the European working group on sarcopenia in older people. *Age Ageing* 39(4):412–423. doi: 10.1093/ageing/afq034.

de Sousa, M.V., Fukui, R., Krustrup, P., Pereira, R.M., Silva, P.R., Rodrigues, A.C., de Andrade, J.L., et al. 2014. Positive effects of football on fitness, lipid profile, and insulin resistance in Brazilian patients with type 2 diabetes. *Scandinavian Journal of Medicine & Science in Sports* 2(S1):57–65. doi: 10.1111/sms.12258.

DiLoreto, R., Murphy, C.T. 2015. The cell biology of aging. *Molecular Biology of the Cell* 26(25):4524–4531. doi: 10.1091/mbcE14-06-1084.

Dreyer, H.C., Fujita, S., Glynn, E.L., Drummond, M.J., Volpi, E., Rasmussen, B.B. 2010. Resistance exercise increases leg muscle protein synthesis and mTOR signalling independent of sex. *Acta Physiologica (Oxford)* 199(1):71–81. doi: 10.1111/j.1748-1716.2010.02074.x.

Fajemiroye, J.O., da Cunha, L.C., Saavedra-Rodríguez, R., Rodrigues, K.L., Naves, L.M., Mourão, A.A., da Silva, E.F., et al. 2018. Aging-induced biological changes and cardiovascular diseases. *BioMed Research International* 2018:7156435. doi: 10.1155/2018/7156435.

Frontera, W.R., MD, Zayas, A.R., Rodriguez, N. 2012. Aging of human muscle: Understanding at the single muscle cell level. *Physical Medicine & Rehabilitation Clinics of North America* 23(1):201–207. doi: 10.1016/j.pmr.2011.11.012.
Frosig, C., Sajan, M.P., Maarbjerg, S.J., Brandt, N., Roepstorff, C., Wojtaszewski, J.F., Kiens, B., Farese, R.V., Richter, E.A. 2007. Exercise improves phosphatidylinositol-3,4,5-trisphosphate responsiveness of atypical protein kinase C and interacts with insulin signalling to peptide elongation in human skeletal muscle. *The Journal of Physiology* 582:1289–1301.
Gerhart-Hines, Z., Rodgers, J.T., Bare, O., Lerin, C., Kim, S.H., Mostoslavsky, R., Alt, F.W., Wu, Z., Puigserver, P. 2007. Metabolic control of muscle mitochondrial function and fatty acid oxidation through SIRT1/PGC-1α. *The EMBO Journal* 26:1913–1923.
Hagman, M., Helge, E.W., Hornstrup, T., Fristrup, B., Nielsen, J.J., Jørgensen, N.R., Andersen, J.L., Helge, J.W., Krustrup, P. 2018. Bone mineral density in lifelong trained male football players compared with young and elderly untrained men. *Journal of Sport and Health Science* 7(2):159–168. doi: 10.1016/j.jshs.2017.09.009.
Harrison, D.E., Strong, R., Sharp, Z.D., Nelson, J.F., Astle, C.M., Flurkey, K., Nadon, N.L. et al. 2009. Rapamycin fed late in life extends lifespan in genetically heterogeneous mice. *Nature* 460:392–395. doi: 10.1038/nature08221.
Hawkins, S.A., Wiswell, R.A. 2003. Rate and mechanism of maximal oxygen consumption decline with aging implications for exercise training. *Sports Medicine* 33(12): 877–888.
Helge, E.W., Andersen, T.R., Schmidt, J.F., Jorgensen, N.R., Hornstrup, T., Krustrup, P., Bangsbo, J. 2014. Recreational football improves bone mineral density and bone turnover marker profile in elderly men. *Scandinavian Journal of Medicine & Science in Sports* 24(Suppl1):98–104. doi: 10.1111/sms.12239.
Kalyani, R.R., Corriere, M., Ferrucci, L. 2014. Age-related and disease-related muscle loss: The effect of diabetes, obesity, and other diseases. *The Lancet Diabetes & Endocrinology* 2(10):819–829. doi: 10.1016/S2213-8587(14)70034-8.
Katewa, S.D., Kapahi, P. 2011. Role of TOR signaling in aging and related biological processes in Drosophila melanogaster. *Experimental Gerontology* 46:382–390. doi: 10.1016/j.exger.2010.11.036.
Kim, E.S., Im, J.A., Kim, K.C., Park, J.H., Suh, S.H., Kang, E.S., Kim, S.H., et al. 2007. Improved insulin sensitivity and adiponectin level after exercise training in obese Korean youth. *Obesity (Silver Spring)* 15:3023–3030. doi: 10.1038/oby.2007.360.
Koopman, R., Zorenc, A.H., Gransier, R.J., Cameron-Smith, D., van Loon, L.J. 2006. Increase in S6K1 phosphorylation in human skeletal muscle following resistance exercise occurs mainly in type II muscle fibers. *American Journal of Physiology: Endocrinology and Metabolism* 290:E1245–E1252.
Krustrup, P., Aagaard, P., Nybo, L., Petersen, J., Mohr, M., Bangsbo, J. 2010a. Recreational football as a health promoting activity: A topical review. *Scandinavian Journal of Medicine & Science in Sports* 20(Suppl1):1–13. doi: 10.1111/j.1600-0838.2010.01108.x.
Krustrup, P., Christensen, J.F., Randers, M.B., Pedersen, H., Sundstrup, E., Jakobsen, M.D., Krustrup, B.R., et al. 2010b. Muscle adaptations and performance enhancements of soccer training for untrained men. *European Journal of Applied Physiology* 108:1247–1258. doi: 10.1007/s00421-009-1319-8.
Krustrup, P., Krustrup, B.R. 2018. Football is medicine: It is time for patients to play! *British Journal of Sports Medicine* (June 9). pii: bjsports-2018–099377. doi: 10.1136/bjsports-2018-099377.
Krustrup, P., Randers, M.B., Andersen, L.J., Jackman, S.R., Bangsbo, J., Hansen, P.R. 2013. Soccer improves fitness and attenuates cardiovascular risk factors in

hypertensive men. *Medicine & Science in Sports & Exercise* 45(3):553–560. doi: 10.1249/MSS.0b013e3182777051.

Krustrup, P., Williams, C.A., Mohr, M., Hansen, P.R., Helge, E.W., Elbe, A.M., de Sousa, M., et al. 2018. The "football is medicine" platform-scientific evidence, large-scale implementation of evidence-based concepts and future perspectives. *Scandinavian Journal of Medicine & Science in Sports* 28(Suppl 1):3–7. doi: 10.1111/sms.13220.

Lamming, D.W., Ye, L., Katajisto, P., Goncalves, M.D., Saitoh, M., Stevens, D.M., Davis, J.G., et al. 2012. Rapamycin-induced insulin resistance is mediated by mTORC2 loss and uncoupled from longevity. *Science* 335:1638–1643. doi: 10.1126/science.1215135.

Li, M., Verdijk, L.B., Sakamoto, K., Ely, B., van Loon, L.J., Musi, N. 2012. Reduced AMPK-ACC and mTOR signaling in muscle from older men, and effect of resistance exercise. *Mechanisms of Ageing and Development* 133(11–12):655–664. doi: 10.1016/j.mad.2012.09.001.

Mancini, A., Vitucci, D., Labruna, G., Imperlini, E., Randers, M.B., Schmidt, J.F., Hagman, M., et al. 2017. Effect of lifelong football training on the expression of muscle molecular markers involved in healthy longevity. *European Journal of Applied Physiology* 117(4):721–730. doi: 10.1007/s00421-017-3562-8.

Mancini, A., Vitucci, D., Randers, M.B., Schmidt, J.F., Hagman. M., Andersen, T.R., Imperlini, E., et al. 2019. Lifelong football training: Effects on autophagy and healthy longevity promotion. *Frontiers in Physiology*. Feb 19;10:132.

Milanović, Z., Pantelić, S., Čović, N., Sporiš, G., Mohr, M., Krustrup, P. 2018. Broad-spectrum physical fitness benefits of recreational football: A systematic review and meta-analysis. *British Journal of Sports Medicine* pii: bjsports-2017-097885. doi: 10.1136/bjsports-2017-097885.

Miljkovic, N., Lim, J.Y., Miljkovic, I., Frontera, W.R. 2015. Aging of skeletal muscle fibers. *Annals of Rehabilitation Medicine* 39(2):155–162. doi: 10.5535/arm.2015.39.2.155.

Møller, T.K., Nielsen, T.T., Andersen, R., Lundager, I., Hansen, H.F., Ottesen, L., Krustrup, P., Randers, M.B. 2018. Health effects of 12 weeks of team-sport training and fitness training in a community health centre for sedentary men with lifestyle diseases. *BioMed Research International* 2018:1571807. doi: 10.1155/2018/1571807.

Nascimento, C.M., Ingles, M., Salvador-Pascual, A., Cominetti, M.R., Gomez-Cabrera, M.C., Viña, J. 2018. Sarcopenia, frailty and their prevention by exercise. *Free Radical Biology and Medicine* pii: S0891-5849(18)31499-0. doi: 10.1016/j.freeradbiomed.2018.08.035.

Neustadt, J., Pieczenik, S. 2008. Organ reserve and healthy aging. *Integrative Medicine* 7(3):50–52.

Ostergard, T., Nyholm, B., Hansen, T.K., Rasmussen, L.M., Ingerslev, J., Sorensen, K.E., Botker, H.E., Saltin, B., Schmitz, O. 2006. Endothelial function and biochemical vascular markers in first-degree relatives of type 2 diabetic patients: The effect of exercise training. *Metabolism* 55:1508–1515.

Pallafacchina, G., Calabria, E., Serrano, A.L., Kalhovde, J.M., Schiaffino, S. 2002. A protein kinase B-dependent and rapamycin-sensitive pathway controls skeletal muscle growth but not fiber type specification. *Proceedings of the National Academy of Sciences* 99:9213–9218.

Parkington, J.D., LeBrasseur, N.K., Siebert, A.P., Fielding, R.A. 2004. Contraction-mediated mTOR, p70S6k, and ERK1/2 phosphorylation in aged skeletal muscle. *Journal of Applied Physiology* 97:243–248.

Pedersen, B.K., Saltin, B. 2006. Evidence for prescribing exercise as therapy in chronic disease. *Scandinavian Journal of Medicine & Science in Sports* 16 (Suppl 1):3–63.

Randers, M.B., Nielsen, J.J., Krustrup, B.R., Sundstrup, E., Jakobsen, M.D., Nybo, L., Dvorak, J., Bangsbo, J., Krustrup, P. 2010. Positive performance and health effects of a football training program over 12 weeks can be maintained over a 1-year period with reduced training frequency. *Scandinavian Journal of Medicine & Science in Sports* 20(Suppl 1):80–9. doi: 10.1111/j.1600-0838.2010.01091.x.

Randers, M.B., Petersen, J., Andersen, L.J., Krustrup, B.R., Hornstrup, T., Nielsen, J.J., Nordentoft, M., Krustrup, P. 2012. Short-term street soccer improves fitness and cardiovascular health status of homeless men. *European Journal of Applied Physiology* 112:2097–2106. doi: 10.1007/s00421-011-2171-1.

Sandri, M., Barberi, L., Bijlsma, A.Y., Blaauw, B., Dyar, K.A., Milan, G., Mammucari, C., et al. 2013. Signalling pathways regulating muscle mass in ageing skeletal muscle: The role of the IGF1-Akt-mTOR-FoxO pathway. *Biogerontology* 14:303–323. doi: 10.1007/s10522-013-9432-9.

Schmidt. J.F., Andersen, T.R., Andersen, L.J., Randers, M.B., Hornstrup, T., Hansen, P.R., Bangsbo, J., Krustrup, P. 2015. Cardiovascular function is better in veteran football players than age-matched untrained elderly healthy men. *Scandinavian Journal of Medicine & Science in Sports* 25:61–69. doi: 10.1111/sms.12153.

Schmidt, J.F., Andersen, T.R., Horton, J., Brix, J., Tarnow, L., Krustrup, P., Andersen, L.J., Bangsbo, J., Hansen, P.R. 2013. Soccer training improves cardiac function in men with type 2 diabetes. *Medicine & Science in Sports & Exercise* 45:2223–2233. doi: 10.1249/MSS.0b013e31829ab43c.

Short, K.R., Vittone, J.L., Bigelow, M.L., Proctor, D.N., Rizza, R.A., Coenen-Schimke, J.M., Nair, K.S. 2003. Impact of aerobic exercise training on age-related changes in insulin sensitivity and muscle oxidative capacity. *Diabetes* 52:1888–1896.

Skoradal, M.B., Helge, E.W., Jørgensen, N.R., Mortensen, J., Weihe, P., Krustrup, P., Mohr, M. 2018a. Osteogenic impact of football training in 55- to 70-year-old women and men with prediabetes. *Scandinavian Journal of Medicine & Science in Sports* 28(Suppl 1):52–60. doi: 10.1111/sms.13252.

Skoradal, M.B., Weihe, P., Patursson, P., Mortensen, J., Connolly, L., Krustrup, P., Mohr, M. 2018b. Football training improves metabolic and cardiovascular health status in 55- to 70-year-old women and men with prediabetes. *Scandinavian Journal of Medicine & Science in Sports* 28(Suppl 1):42–51. doi: 10.1111/sms.13081.

Sundstrup, E., Jakobsen, M.D., Andersen, L.L., Andersen, T.R., Randers, M.B., Helge, J.W., Suetta, C., et al. 2016. Positive effects of 1-year football and strength training on mechanical muscle function and functional capacity in elderly men. *European Journal of Applied Physiology* 116(6):1127–1138. doi: 10.1007/s00421-016-3368-0.

Tyrovolas, S., Koyanagi, A., Olaya, B., Ayuso-Mateos, J.L., Miret, M., Chatterji, S., Tobiasz-Adamczyk, B., et al. 2016. Factors associated with skeletal muscle mass, sarcopenia, and sarcopenic obesity in older adults: A multi-continent study. *Journal of Cachexia, Sarcopenia and Muscle* 7(3):312–21. doi: 10.1002/jcsm.12076.

Uth, J., Fristrup, B., Haahr, R.D., Brasso, K., Helge, J.W., Rørth, M., Midtgaard, J., Helge, E.W., Krustrup, P. 2018. Football training over 5 years is associated with preserved femoral bone mineral density in men with prostate cancer. *Scandinavian Journal of Medicine & Science in Sports* 28(Suppl 1):61–73. doi: 10.1111/sms.13242.

Watson, K., Baar, K. 2014. mTOR and the health benefits of exercise. *Seminars in Cell & Developmental Biology* 36:130–139.

Chapter 8

Motivational aspects of Football as Medicine

Johan M. Wikman, Knud Ryom, Paulina S. Melby, Peter Elsborg, Anne-Marie Elbe

Introduction

The other chapters of this book have outlined that football is effective as medicine for a plethora of lifestyle diseases in a wide variety of participant groups. Furthermore, football also seems to be an effective way of increasing emotional and physical well-being (e.g. Friedrich & Mason, 2017). However, in order for football as medicine to work, people need to engage in it on a regular basis. A prerequisite for regular physical activity is motivation. Motivation can be defined as a person's desire to achieve a certain goal or perform a certain action (e.g. wanting to participate in regular football practice to improve one's fitness). Following Heckhausen (2010), a person's motivation to achieve a certain goal is determined by personal as well as situational factors. Personal factors pertain to motives, needs or goals whereas situational factors refer to the (sporting) environment. In this chapter, we will apply the most frequently used theories in the physical activity context to explore the motivational aspects of football. The Self-Determination Theory (Deci & Ryan, 1985) and the concept of flow (Csikszentmihalyi & Csikszentmihalyi, 1988) will be applied to investigate the sources of motivation that are personal rather than situational, while the Achievement Goal Theory (Nicholls, 1984) will be used to investigate the sources of motivation that are situational rather than personal.

Personal motivational factors

The Self-Determination Theory

The Self-Determination Theory (SDT) distinguishes between intrinsically and extrinsically motivated behaviour. 'Intrinsically motivated behaviours are those that are freely engaged out of interest without the necessity of separable consequences' (Deci & Ryan, 2000, p. 233). Hence, an intrinsically motivated individual will participate in an activity for the sake of the activity itself, because he/she finds it enjoyable, fun or otherwise giving in some way. An extrinsically motivated individual, on the other hand, participates in an activity for the expected positive consequences (Deci & Ryan, 1985; Ryan & Deci, 2000; Vallerand, 2000). Using these descriptions of intrinsic and extrinsic motivation in football, an intrinsically motivated individual will play football because it is perceived as enjoyable, while an extrinsically motivated individual will play football because of the expected health benefits, for example, that are expected to follow.

According to SDT, intrinsic motivation is rooted in three basic psychological needs, and when they are satisfied, the individual will thrive psychologically and experience wellbeing (Deci & Ryan, 2000). The need for autonomy is the need to feel like a causal agent in one's own life, and to act based on one's integrated sense of self. The need for competence is the need to feel capable and effective in dealing with the challenges, small or large, that one encounters in life. The need for relatedness is the need to have positive social connections with others (Deci & Vansteenkiste, 2004). Since these needs are inherent for all healthy human beings, a person will naturally attempt to engage in activities that lead to experiences and feelings of autonomy, competence and relatedness to others (Deci & Ryan, 2000; Deci & Vansteenkiste, 2004). The motivation to pursue such activities is intrinsic (Deci & Ryan, 1985; Ryan & Deci, 2000; Vallerand, 2000).

Research suggests that while both intrinsic and extrinsic motivation can lead to regular participation in sport, it seems that intrinsic motivation is favourable over extrinsic, when it comes to regular participation (e.g. Ntoumanis, 2005; Ryan & Deci, 2007). Therefore, as intrinsic motivation is connected to well-being and thriving through the three basic psychological needs, and is better for regular participation, it seems that activities which induce high levels of intrinsic motivation hold an advantage over activities that do not.

Flow

A state of absolute intrinsic motivation is flow. Flow is defined as a psychological state 'in which the person feels simultaneously cognitively efficient, motivated and happy' (Moneta & Csikszentmihalyi, 1996, p. 277). It is characterised by being completely immersed in the activity (Csikszentmihalyi & Rathunde, 1992). According to Csikszentmihalyi and Csikszentmihalyi (1988), people need to experience an optimal match between personal skills and external challenges, and if this is achieved, flow can be experienced in any activity. Flow has been widely researched in many areas of life, including football and other sports (e.g. Elbe et al., 2010; Jackson & Csikszentmihalyi, 1999).

The benefits of flow are manifold. Schüler and Brunner (2009) put forward that experiencing flow might contribute to the long-term adherence to physical activity because individuals that experience flow are rewarded for their activity and are likely to seek out this activity again. Furthermore, experiencing flow has been linked to increased well-being (Haworth, 1993) and an improved self-concept (Jackson et al., 2001) and therefore, could contribute to long-term beneficial health effects, which are especially relevant for the physical activity context. Experiences of flow have also been suggested to reduce psychological distress, such as post traumatic stress disorder, especially in team sport interventions (Ley et al., 2017). Experiencing flow could, therefore, contribute to the individual's immediate well-being and also contribute to long-term beneficial health effects. In order for an individual to be intrinsically motivated, the three basic psychological needs should be fulfilled, and in order for an individual to experience flow, there should be a match between challenge and skill. In the following sections, we argue that football and team sports in general hold certain advantages compared to individual physical activity when it comes to eliciting intrinsic motivation and flow.

Are team sports such as football more intrinsically motivating than individual sports?

A number of studies suggest that team sports, including football, are more advantageous with regard to eliciting motivation than individual sports. Team sports can be characterised as 'a physical activity, in which the individuals of at least one group consisting of two or more, work together to achieve a common goal, in spite of resistance embedded in the rules of that activity' (Wikman, Elsborg, & Ryom, 2018, p. 134), whereas individual sports are physical activities in which an individual does not work together with anyone to achieve the goal of the activity.

Nielsen et al. (2014) used interviews to investigate why elderly men participating in football had much better adherence rates compared to elderly men who participated in spinning and crossfit. They found that football elicited more intrinsic motivation than spinning/crossfit and argued that this was the reason for the higher adherence to football. In an intervention study comparing the effects of elderly men's participation in floorball and petanque, respectively, Wikman et al. (2017) conducted interviews and reported that the men in the floorball group voiced experiences of intrinsic motivation and enjoyment to a higher degree than the men in the petanque group. In another intervention study, Wikman et al. (2018) used questionnaires to compare motivation for floorball and spinning in middle-aged women, and found that floorball elicited higher intrinsic motivation, and that this predicted continuation after the intervention. Similarly, Pedersen et al. (2017) found in their comparison of the effects of team training (team sports adjusted to the sample) and resistance training in elderly men and women that the participants in the team training group expressed a higher degree of intrinsic motivation and enjoyment than the resistance training group. Lastly, Hornstrup et al. (2018) found an increase in intrinsic motivation in the intervention group over a three-month handball intervention period compared to a control group. So, it seems that team games, and presumably football, have a higher potential for creating intrinsic motivation than individual sports.

This is corroborated when looking at studies investigating flow. Elbe et al. (2010) found that men experienced lower levels of worrying thoughts, which counteract the development of flow, in football than in running. The women in the study, however, experienced higher rates of flow in running than in football, which could be related to them having more difficulties with having their skills meet the challenge of the game than the males. Elbe et al. (2016) found that in a physical activity intervention for female health care workers, football elicited higher flow values at the beginning of the intervention than the individual sport activity Zumba. The results are in line with research on the high flow levels experienced in teams (Bakker et al., 2011), as well as with recent studies suggesting that team sport athletes experience total flow at a higher level than individual athletes (Boyd et al., 2018).

All in all, when it comes to intrinsic motivation and flow, team sports seem to have an advantage over individual physical activities. In the next section, we will discuss the reasons for why football and other team sports seem to be more motivating than individual physical activity.

Why is football more motivating?

Basic need satisfaction

One reason why football is more motivating is that it to a higher degree satisfies the basic psychological needs. For example, Nielsen et al. (2014) found that older inactive men, participating in an intervention with recreational football, experienced that the social interactions that occurred during the game itself were most important to adherence and enjoyment. Corroborating these findings, both Wikman et al. (2017) and Pedersen et al. (2017) found that the social interaction was the main reason for why the participants found the floorball and team sports, respectively, so enjoyable. Similarly, Ottesen, Jeppesen, and Krustrup (2010) argue that football holds an advantage over individual sports when it comes to bonding during the activity itself. The competitive element is also mentioned in several studies as a source of relatedness (Lozano-Sufrategui et al., 2017). A study of homeless men with addiction and mental health problems stressed the importance of the competitive element and physical contact in floorball, which provided opportunities to develop empathetic relationships and collective solidarity (Holt, Scherer, & Koch, 2015).

The basic need for competence also seems to be satisfied in football. Nielsen et al. (2014) found that football participants to a higher degree than spinning/crossfit participants found enjoyment in improving their skills and performing on the pitch. If teams were unfair, they changed them to create better competition. Improvement and performance in challenging situations satisfied their basic psychological need for competence. Similarly, Wikman et al. (2017) found that the competitive game of floorball satisfied the need for competence in their sample of elderly men, and that this contributed to enjoyment of the activity. Lastly, it is possible that a team game provides the participant with more influence on how he/she engages in the activity. Elbe et al. (2016) argue that their football participants had more influence on the challenge they chose, while in Zumba, this is more strongly determined by the pace the instructor sets. Hence, it could also be that football satisfies the basic psychological need for autonomy more than a group fitness activity as well.

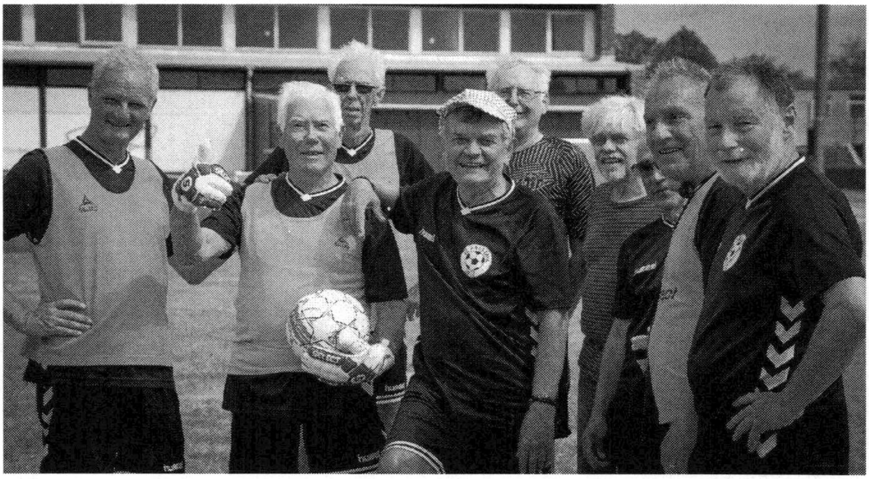

Photo 8.1 Motivational aspects of football. Team Spirit of the FC Prostate 2012 team.
Source: Photo Credit: Bo Kousgaard, University of Southern Denmark.

In summary, the interactive nature of football, as is the case with other team-based activities, possesses a social element that is lacking in individual sports. The social interactions that occur during football seem to contribute to the enjoyment among participants in a positive and rewarding manner that are conducive for eliciting intrinsic motivation. Moreover, it seems the varied technical and tactical demands in football provide the participating individual the opportunity of satisfying the basic need for competence, and that the degree of influence over one's engagement can satisfy the basic need for autonomy, although these suggestions need to be investigated further. All in all, the results of the studies presented in this chapter, viewed through the lens of the SDT, suggest that participating in football holds a significant potential for developing intrinsic motivation.

Social relations

In addition to the basic need for relatedness that is satisfied during the activity, there is an additional social perspective in football, namely the positive social aspects that participants outlined as positive consequences of the activity, and this affects participants' extrinsic motivation. It has been argued that the playing aspect of football is closely related to the social nature of team sport, such as cooperation and face-to-face interaction (Lozano-Sufrategui et al., 2017; Ottesen, Jeppesen, & Krustrup, 2010). Additionally, the physical contact during team sport seems to foster a feeling of connectedness, confidence, and thus a feeling of collectivity and a positive mutual interdependency emerging from playing together (Bruun et al.,

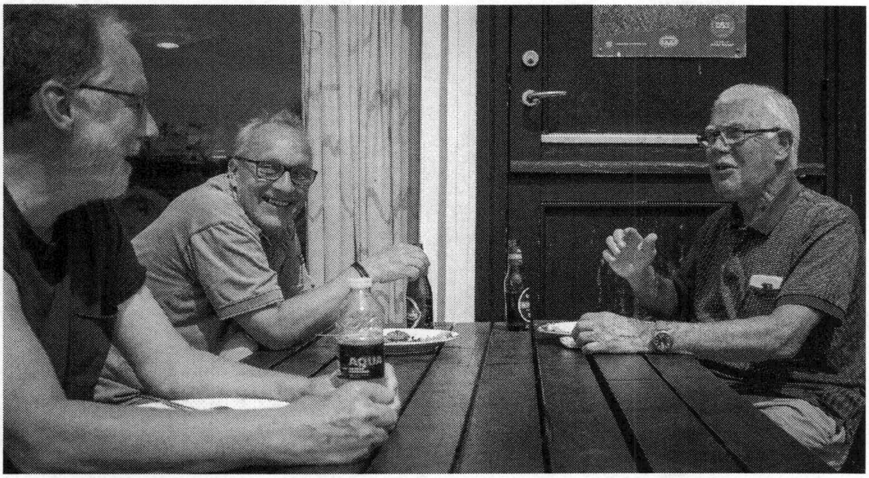

Photo 8.2 Motivational aspects of football. Building social capital in the third half.
Source: Photo Credit: Bo Kousgaard, University of Southern Denmark.

2014; Pedersen et al., 2017). This collective and social context of a team sport seems to be crucial for motivation and adherence in a plethora of different participants (Holt, Scherer, & Koch, 2015; Kirby & Kluge, 2013; Lozano-Sufrategui et al., 2017; Mynard, Howie, & Collister, 2009).

Strengthening this point, when compared to individual resistance training, untrained older adults participating in a team sport expressed to a higher degree how the social environment was a prominent reason to adhere to the activity (Pedersen et al., 2017). In the individual resistance training groups, elements related to health and fitness benefits were more prominent (Pedersen et al., 2017). Similarly, when Nielsen et al. (2014) compared the experiences of a football group with experiences of a spinning/crossfit group, new friendships created between the participants in the football group were mentioned as an important social aspect. For participants in both types of exercise, the social interactions that took place just before or after the activity were experienced as a positive aspect of the activity. But only the football group mentioned friendships and comradery connected to the activity, indicating a stronger social aspect of football. Hence, the positive social relations formed as a consequence of the activity contribute to individuals experiencing extrinsic motivation to participate.

Better situations that create flow?

There are several possible explanations as to why team sports and football have advantages with regard to eliciting flow. Kowal and Fortier (1999) identified higher flow levels in team members that also felt socially connected, and Jackson (1996) found that a good interaction between teammates helps individuals to attain flow. Therefore, it seems that positive team interactions are a prerequisite for experiencing flow and these are easily achieved in football. Furthermore, Elbe et al.'s (2010) study indicated that males had fewer worrying thoughts when they played football than when they ran, which is also an important prerequisite for experiencing flow. Last, the goals in football are very clear and football offers easy opportunities to receiving immediate feedback (e.g. was the pass successful, did the opponent score or did we score a goal?). Thus, the 'nature' of football provides immediate feedback, which is conjured with specific characteristic of the flow state (Swann et al., 2012).

Revisiting the explanations of Csikszentmihalyi and Csikszentmihalyi (1988), it is important that the participants perceive the challenge and his/her available skills as aligned, so that the highly intrinsically motivated state of flow is experienced. From the positive results from football, the opportunities for finding this balance between the challenge of the task and personal skills and abilities might be greater in football than other sports (Elbe et al., 2016). However, Elbe et al.'s (2010) study indicated that it was easier for previously inactive females to achieve flow in running than in football, which could be an indication that their skill level did not match the challenge of the game.

Situational motivational factors

Achievement Goal Theory

The Achievement Goal Theory (Nicholls, 1984) describes individuals' motives related to achievement situations and categorises them as either task or ego oriented. Task-oriented individuals wish to develop mastery, improvement or learning and the demonstration of their ability is self-referenced and not other-referenced. Task orientation can lead to individuals orienting themselves on their personal standards, being less afraid of failure and also being able to experience high levels of competence. A high task orientation is associated with greater joy, intrinsic interest and satisfaction, less fear of failure, greater commitment to practice and learning, and greater effort (Nicholls, 1984). Furthermore, for individuals with a high task orientation, cooperation with others is an important aspect of sporting success (Duda & Nicholls, 1992) and they perceive their social connections as positive.

Ego-oriented individuals are motivated by outperforming others and by demonstrating their ability relative to others. Whether something was a success or a failure is determined by a comparison with the performance of others (Ntoumanis & Biddle, 1999). However, if the opponent's performance is better, which is very likely in sport and cannot be controlled, this can lead to disappointment, frustration and loss of motivation.

How can football activities be conducted in a motivating way?

It has been described above that football has certain advantages over individual sport activities for creating intrinsic and extrinsic motivation, and also for eliciting flow experiences. However, barriers for participation in football exist, such as the competitive nature of the game, fixed practice times and that a certain number of other players are required, as well as low football skills of inexperienced participants. The goal of this section is to outline how football can be conducted in a motivating way for participants of all skill levels, ages and for both genders.

Motivational climate

A very important aspect when conducting a football physical activity intervention is the motivational climate in which it takes place. The concept of motivational climate used in this chapter is based on the above-described theory of achievement goals (Nicholls, 1984), and distinguishes between a mastery or performance climate (Ames, 1992a). In short, the mastery climate encourages task-oriented behaviour in participants, while the performance climate encourages ego-oriented behaviour. Research suggests that a mastery climate is associated with a range of adaptive motivational outcomes such as perceived competence, self-esteem, objective performance, intrinsic forms of motivational regulation, affective states, practice and competitive strategies and moral attitudes, and the experience of flow (Harwood et al., 2015; Ntoumanis & Biddle, 1999). In contrast, a performance climate is associated with extrinsic regulation and amotivation, negative affect, maladaptive strategy use, antisocial attitudes and perfectionism (Harwood et al., 2015; Ntoumanis & Biddle, 1999).

Numerous studies conducted in football corroborate these findings, like that a mastery climate is associated with adaptive personal characteristics and perceptions (Smith, Balaguer, & Duda, 2006), such as positive peer relations (Ommundsen et al., 2005), self-efficacy (Zourbanos et al., 2016) as well as vitality and passion (Ommundsen et al., 2013), while a performance climate is either unrelated or negatively associated. All in all, mastery climate, or rather participants' perception of a mastery climate, seems to be facilitating for psychological consequences of and participation in football.

It is comforting to see, that, overall, coaches seem to be more mastery-oriented than performance-oriented. However, due to the fact that competition is an important element of the game of football, a performance climate cannot be completely avoided. This is underlined by the findings of Ryska and Yin (1999), where recreational teams reported a greater degree of mastery climate compared to competitive teams. Similarly, it seems that a performance climate is more prevalent in a competition than in a training setting (van de Pol & Kavussanu, 2012), and is determined by the coach's behaviour (Smith et al., 2017). Therefore, it seems prudent that coaches, instructors and other facilitators of football activities consider the motivational climate in the activity and pay attention to reducing the performance climate for physical activity intervention.

One concept that promotes football in a mastery rather than a performance-oriented way is Football Fitness. Football Fitness (Bennike, Wikman, & Ottesen, 2014) aims at attracting new user groups not familiar with the football context with training sessions in which the competition element is absent and which emphasises training and fun. In addition, the Football Fitness concept is a concept that accommodates the interplay between physical activity participation and leisure time, family life and work life (Thing, Hybholt, Jensen, & Ottesen, 2017).

Approaches to intervene on motivational climate

Other theoretically based interventions for improving motivational climate are the TARGET framework (Ames, 1992a, 1992b; Epstein, 1988) and the concept of Empowering Coaching (Duda & Appleton, 2016). The TARGET framework gives specific recommendations for how a mastery climate can be created, namely by impacting the structure of the activity and the instructors' behaviour. TARGET is an acronym referring to Task (design of activities), Authority (location of decision-making), Recognition (manner of distributing rewards such as praise), Grouping (criteria for selecting working groups), Evaluation (standards of performance considered important) and Time (pace of learning). A mastery climate can be created by 1) giving challenging tasks, as opposed to repetitive tasks, 2) giving participants influence over the activity, as opposed to controlling all aspects of decision-making, 3) providing recognition privately, as opposed to publicly, 4) working with mixed ability groups, as opposed to grouping by ability, 5) giving positive evaluation for personal improvement, as opposed to ability, and by 6) accommodating variability in pace of learning, as opposed to not allowing slow learners enough time (Braithwaite, Spray, & Warburton, 2011). The TARGET framework seems to provide a framework for effective interventions in physical education (Braithwaite et al., 2011) and for student athletes (Cecchini et al., 2014), and could be a promising model to adhere to when designing football for medicine interventions.

Empowering Coaching is a concept that has been applied in a wide variety of settings and participants groups, including youth football. It is based on SDT and the Achievement Goal Theory, and assumes that sport participation can be enhanced when youths have positive experiences in sport and can develop intrinsic motivation to exercise. In this program, coaches learn how to create a mastery climate and how to satisfy the young participants' basic psychological needs. The Promoting Adolescent Physical Activity (PAPA) (Duda et al., 2013) project involved thousands of coaches and athletes all over Europe, and collected motivational as well as physical activity data of participants, confirming that the program achieves the expected goals of creating intrinsically motivated exercise behaviour.

Such programs, with a solid theoretical background and evidenced positive effects, should be used to inform coach education in football. This will positively impact the motivational climate which is decisive for how participants engage in football and will contribute to improving their motivation for continued participation.

Conclusion

Playing football is beneficial for physical and psychological health as well as well-being for participants of all ages, skill levels and both genders. Furthermore, football seems to have specific characteristics and advantages over individual sport activities that can positively impact participants' motivation to play. It is therefore important that football for medicine activities are conducted in a way that creates a positive motivational climate so that it can impact participants' willingness to return to practice on a regular basis. Only if we can ensure that participants enjoy playing, are intrinsically motivated and come to practice on a regular basis, can the positive health effects be achieved. The programs outlined in this chapter on how a positive motivational climate can be created can lay the foundation for football as medicine interventions.

References

Ames, C. (1992a). Classrooms: Goals, structures, and motivation. *Journal of Educational Psychology*, *84*, 261–271.

Ames, C. (1992b). Achievement goals and the classroom motivational climate. In D. Schunk & J. Meece (Eds.), *Student perceptions in the classroom* (pp. 327–348). Hillsdale, NJ, England: Lawrence Erlbaum Associates.

Bakker, A. B., Oerlemans, W., Demerouti, E., Slot, B. B., & Ali, D. K. (2011). Flow and performance: A study among talented Dutch soccer players. *Psychology of Sport and Exercise*, *12*, 442–450. doi:10.1016/j.psychsport.2011.02.003

Bennike, S., Wikman, J. M., & Ottesen, L. S. (2014). Football Fitness: A new version of football? A concept for adult players in Danish football clubs. *Scandinavian Journal of Medicine & Science in Sports*, *24*, 138–146. https://doi.org/10.1111/sms.12276

Boyd, J. M., Schary, D. P., Worthington, A. R., & Jenny, S. E. (2018). An examination of the differences in flow between individual and team athletes. *Physical Culture and Sport: Studies and Research*, *78*(1), 33–40.

Braithwaite, R., Spray, C. M., & Warburton, V. E. (2011). Motivational climate interventions in physical education: A meta-analysis. *Psychology of Sport and Exercise*, *12*(6), 628–638. https://doi.org/10.1016/j.psychsport.2011.06.005

Bruun, D. M., Krustrup, P., Hornstrup, T., Uth, J., Brasso, K., Rørth, M., . . . Midtgaard, J. (2014). 'All boys and men can play football': A qualitative investigation of recreational football in prostate cancer patients. *Scandinavian Journal of Medicine & Science in Sports*, *24*(Suppl 1), 113–121. doi: 10.1111/sms.12193

Cecchini, J. A., Fernandez-Rio, J., Mendez-Gimenez, A., Cecchini, C., & Martins, L. (2014). Epstein's TARGET framework and motivational climate in sport: Effects of a field-based, longterm intervention program. *International Journal of Sport Science & Coaching*, *9*, 1325–1340. doi:10.1260/1747-9541.9.6.1325

Csikszentmihalyi, M., & Csikszentmihalyi, I. S. (1988). *Optimal experience: Psychological studies of flow in consciousness*. Cambridge: Cambridge University Press. doi:10.1017/CBO9780511621956

Csikszentmihalyi, M., & Rathunde, K. (1992). The measurement of flow in everyday life: Toward a theory of emergent motivation. In R. Dienstbier & J. E. Jacobs (Eds.), *Nebraska symposium on motivation: Developmental perspectives on motivation* (Vol. 40, pp. 57–97). Lincoln and London: University of Nebraska Press.

Deci, E. L., & Ryan, R. M. (1985). *Intrinsic motivation and self-determination in human behavior*. New York, NY: Plenum Publishing.

Deci, E. L., & Ryan, R. M. (2000). The 'what' and 'why' of goal pursuits: Human needs and the self-determination of behavior. *Psychological Inquiry*, *11*(4), 227.

Deci, E. L., & Vansteenkiste, M. (2004). Self-determination theory and basic need satisfaction: Understanding human development in positive psychology. *Ricerche Di Psicologia*, *1*, 23–41.

Duda, J. L., & Appleton, P. (2016). Empowering and disempowering coaching behaviors: Conceptualization, measurement considerations, and intervention implications. In M. Raab, P. Wylleman, R. Seiler, A.-M. Elbe, & A. Hatzigeorgiadis (Eds.), *Sport and exercise psychology research: From theory to practice* (pp. 373–388). London: Elsevier.

Duda, J. L., & Nicholls, J. G. (1992). Dimensions of achievement motivation in schoolwork and sport. *Journal of Educational Psychology*, *84*(3), 290–299.

Duda, J. L., Quested, E., Haug, E., Samdal, O., Wold, B., Balaguer, I., . . . Cruz, J. (2013). Promoting Adolescent health through an intervention aimed at improving the quality of their participation in Physical Activity (PAPA): Background to the project and main trial protocol. *International Journal of Sport and Exercise Psychology*, *11*(4), 319–327. https://doi.org/10.1080/1612197X.2013.839413

Elbe, A.-M., Barene, S., Strahler, K., Krustrup, P., & Holtermann, A. (2016). Experiencing flow in a workplace physical activity intervention for female health care workers: A longitudinal comparison between football and zumba. *Women in Sport and Physical Activity Journal*, *24*(1), 70–77. https://doi.org/10.1123/wspaj.2015-0011

Elbe, A.-M., Strahler, K., Krustrup, P., Wikman, J., & Stelter, R. (2010). Experiencing flow in different types of physical activity intervention programs: Three randomized studies. *Scandinavian Journal of Medicine & Science in Sports*, *20*(Supp 1), 111–117. https://doi.org/10.1111/j.1600-0838.2010.01112.x

Epstein, J. (1988). Effective schools or effective students? Dealing with diversity. In R. Haskins & B. MacRae (Eds.), *Policies for America's public schools Norwood* (pp. 89–126). Norwood, NJ: Ablex.

Friedrich, B., & Mason, O. J. (2017). "What is the score?" A review of football-based public mental health interventions. *Journal of Public Mental Health*, *16*(4), 144–158. https://doi.org/10.1108/JPMH-03-2017-0011

Harwood, C. G., Keegan, R. J., Smith, J. M. J., & Raine, A. S. (2015). A systematic review of the intrapersonal correlates of motivational climate perceptions in sport and physical activity. *Psychology of Sport and Exercise*, *18*, 9–25. https://doi.org/10.1016/j.psychsport.2014.11.005

Haworth, J. (1993). Skills-challenge relationships and psychological wellbeing in everyday life. *Society & Leisure*, *16*, 115–128.

Heckhausen, J., & Heckhausen, H. (2010). Motivation and action: Introduction and overview. In *Motivation and action* (2nd ed., pp. 1–9). Berlin, Heidelberg: Springer-Verlag.

Holt, N. L., Scherer, J., & Koch, J. (2015). Using masculine capital to understand the role of a sport program in the lives of men from a Western Canadian inner city. *Journal of Sport and Exercise Psychology, 37*(5), 523–533. https://doi.org/10.1123/jsep.2015-0109

Hornstrup, T., Wikman, J. M., Fristrup, B., Póvoas, S., Helge, E. W., Nielsen, S. H., . . . Krustrup, P. (2018). Fitness and health benefits of team handball training for young untrained women: A cross-disciplinary RCT on physiological adaptations and motivational aspects. *Journal of Sport and Health Science, 7*(2), 139–148. https://doi.org/10.1016/j.jshs.2017.09.007

Jackson, S. A. (1996). Toward a conceptual understanding of the flow experience in elite athletes. *Research Quarterly for Exercise & Sport, 1*, 76–90. doi:10.1080/02701367.1996.10607928

Jackson, S. A., & Csikszentmihalyi, M. (1999). *Flow in sports: The keys to optimal experiences and performances*. Champaign, IL: Human Kinetics Publishers.

Jackson, S. A., Thomas, H., Marsh, H., & Smethurst, C. (2001). Relationships between flow, self-concept, psychological skills, and performance. *Journal of Applied Sport Psychology, 13*, 129–153. doi:10.1080/104132001753149865

Kirby, J. B., & Kluge, M. A. (2013). Going for the gusto: Competing for the first time at age 65. *Journal of Aging and Physical Activity, 21*(3), 290–308.

Kowal, J., & Fortier, M. S. (1999). Motivational determinants of flow: Contributions from self-determination theory. *Journal of Social Psychology, 3*, 355–368. doi:10.1080/00224549909598391

Ley, C., Krammer, J., Lippert, D., & Barrio, M. R. (2017). Exploring flow in sport and exercise therapy with war and torture survivors. *Mental Health and Physical Activity, 12*, 83–93.

Lozano-Sufrategui, L., Pringle, A., Carless, D., & McKenna, J. (2017). 'It brings the lads together': A critical exploration of older men's experiences of a weight management programme delivered through a Healthy Stadia project. *Sport in Society, 20*(2), 303–315. https://doi.org/10.1080/17430437.2016.1173912

Moneta, G. B., & Csikszentmihalyi, M. (1996). The effect of perceived challenges and skills on the quality of subjective experience. *Journal of Personality, 2*, 275–310. doi:10.1111/j.1467-6494.1996.tb00512.x

Mynard, L., Howie, L., & Collister, L. (2009). Belonging to a community-based football team: An ethnographic study. *Australian Occupational Therapy Journal, 56*(4), 266–274. https://doi.org/10.1111/j.1440-1630.2008.00741.x

Nicholls, J. G. (1984). Achievement motivation: Conceptions of ability, subjective experience, task choice, and performance. *Psychological Review, 91*(3), 328.

Nielsen, G., Wikman, J. M., Jensen, C. J., Schmidt, J. F., Gliemann, L., & Andersen, T. R. (2014). Health promotion: The impact of beliefs of health benefits, social relations and enjoyment on exercise continuation. *Scandinavian Journal of Medicine & Science in Sports, 24*, 66–75. https://doi.org/10.1111/sms.12275

Ntoumanis, N. (2005). A prospective study of participation in optional school physical education using a self-determination theory framework. *Journal of Educational Psychology, 97*(3), 444–453. https://doi.org/10.1037/0022-0663.97.3.444

Ntoumanis, N., & Biddle, S. J. H. (1999). A review of motivational climate in physical activity. *Journal of Sports Sciences, 17*(8), 643–665. https://doi.org/10.1080/026404199365678

Ommundsen, Y., Lemyre, P.-N., Abrahamsen, F., & Roberts, G. C. (2013). The role of motivational climate for sense of vitality in organized youth grassroots football players: Do harmonious and obsessive types of passion play a mediating role? *International Journal of Applied Sports Sciences, 25*(2), 102–117.

Ommundsen, Y., Roberts, G. C., Lemyre, P.-N., & Miller, B. W. (2005). Peer relationships in adolescent competitive soccer: Associations to perceived motivational climate, achievement goals and perfectionism. *Journal of Sports Sciences*, *23*(9), 977–989. https://doi.org/10.1080/02640410500127975

Ottesen, L., Jeppesen, R. S., & Krustrup, B. R. (2010). The development of social capital through football and running: Studying an intervention program for inactive women. *Scandinavian Journal of Medicine & Science in Sports*, *20*, 118–131. https://doi.org/10.1111/j.1600-0838.2010.01123.x

Pedersen, M. T., Vorup, J., Nistrup, A., Wikman, J. M., Alstrøm, J. M., Melcher, P. S., . . . Bangsbo, J. (2017). Effect of team sports and resistance training on physical function, quality of life, and motivation in older adults. *Scandinavian Journal of Medicine & Science in Sports*, *27*(8), 852–864. https://doi.org/10.1111/sms.12823

Ryan, R. M., & Deci, E. L. (2000). Self-determination theory and the facilitation of intrinsic motivation, social development, and well-being. *American Psychologist*, *1*(55), 68–78.

Ryan, R. M., & Deci, E. L. (2007). Self-determination theory and the promotion and maintenance of sport, exercise, and health. In M. S. Hagger & N. L. D. Chatzisarantis (Eds.), *Intrinsic motivation and self-determination in exercise and sport* (pp. 1–20). Champaign, IL: Human Kinetics.

Ryska, T. A., & Zenong Yin. (1999). Dispositional and situational goal orientations as discriminators among recreational and competitive league athletes. *Journal of Social Psychology*, *139*(3), 335–342.

Schüler, J., & Brunner, S. (2009). The rewarding effect of flow experience on performance in a marathon race. *Psychology of Sport and Exercise*, *1*, 168–174. doi:10.1016/j.psychsport.2008.07.001

Smith, A. L., Balaguer, I., & Duda, J. L. (2006). Goal orientation profile differences on perceived motivational climate, perceived peer relationships, and motivation-related responses of youth athletes. *Journal of Sports Sciences*, *24*(12), 1315–1327. https://doi.org/10.1080/02640410500520427

Smith, N., Quested, E., Appleton, P. R., & Duda, J. L. (2017). Observing the coach-created motivational environment across training and competition in youth sport. *Journal of Sports Sciences*, *35*(2), 149–158. https://doi.org/10.1080/02640414.2016.1159714

Swann, C., Keegan, R. J., Piggott, D., & Crust, L. (2012). A systematic review of the experience, occurrence, and controllability of flow states in elite sport. *Psychology of Sport and Exercise*, *13*, 807–819.

Thing, L. F., Hybholt, M. G., Jensen, A. L., & Ottesen, L. (2017). 'Football fitness': Constraining and enabling possibilities for the management of leisure time for women. *Annals of Leisure Research*, *20*, 427–445.

Vallerand, R. J. (2000). Deci and Ryan's self-determination theory: A View from the hierarchical model of intrinsic and extrinsic motivation. *Psychological Inquiry*, *11*(4), 312–318.

van de Pol, P. K. C., Kavussanu, M., & Ring, C. (2012). Goal orientations, perceived motivational climate, and motivational outcomes in football: A comparison between training and competition contexts. *Psychology of Sport and Exercise*, *13*(4), 491–499. https://doi.org/10.1016/j.psychsport.2011.12.002

Wikman, J. M., Elsborg, P., Nielsen, G., Seidelin, K., Nyberg, M., Bangsbo, J., . . . Elbe, A.-M. (2018). Are team sport games more motivating than individual exercise for middle-aged women? A comparison of levels of motivation associated with participating in floorball and spinning. *Kinesiology*, *50*(1).

Wikman, J. M., Elsborg, P., & Ryom, K. (2018). Psychological benefits of team sport. In D. Parnell & P. Krustrup (Eds.), *Sport and health* (pp. 132–146). New York, NY: Routledge.
Wikman, J. M., Nistrup, A., Vorup, J., Pedersen, M. T., Melchor, P. S., Bangsbo, J., & Pfister, G. (2017). The effect of floorball training on health status, psychological health and social capital in older men. *Aimsph 2017*, 4, 364–382. https://doi.org/10.3934/publichealth.2017.4.364
Zourbanos, N., Haznadar, A., Papaioannou, A., Tzioumakis, Y., Krommidas, C., & Hatzigeorgiadis, A. (2016). The relationships between athletes' perceptions of coach-created motivational climate, self-talk, and self-efficacy in youth soccer. *Journal of Applied Sport Psychology*, *28*(1), 97–112. https://doi.org/10.1080/10413200.2015.1074630

Chapter 9

Fitness and health effects of other team sports

'Recreational team sports – the motivational medicine'

Carlo Castagna, Susana Póvoas, Ioannis Fatouros, Fabio Serpiello, Therese Hornstrup and Don Kirkendall

Introduction

Exercise, nutrition and psychological mindset are the main variables that can be manipulated with the aim to positively affect the health, wellness and social interaction of the world population. Despite the collected evidence and global consensus about the importance and positive effect of the implementation of these actions, governments are still reluctant to support vast campaigns for exercise promotion. Inconsistent health policies, coupled with social constraints and lack of motivation to regularly exercise, urge the necessity of novel strategies to decrease peoples' resistance to exercise. In this regard, exercise-centered rather than work-centered societies should be conceived, given the reported evidence of a positive return, in terms of health benefits, public health care cost and productivity, that investment in physical activities may have.

Motivation is an independent variable that may affect resistance to engage in exercise programs. Activities that may result in enjoyment while providing the physiological and psychological benefits associated with current guidelines for health and wellness improvements are warranted.

Team sports played at competitive level have been reported to induce physiological demands that are in the range of those suggested to maintain and improve cardiovascular fitness in the general population. Additionally, the high-intensity intermittent nature of team sports practice involving sudden changes of direction coupled with decision-making has been reported to affect players' neuromuscular and cognitive functions. The physical and physiological improvements reported in team sports players are the result of plurennial training (either physically or technical-tactically) and participation in competitions. Injury rates in team sports are among the highest in competitive sports, with matches being the condition registering the highest rate of contact and non-contact incidents. It is estimated that team sports, as a whole, attract the interest of most of the active and inactive people in the world.

Given the amount of people active in and potentially attracted by team sports, the interest in regular or adapted forms of ball activities deserve keen attention on part of sport scientists, exercise physiologists, medical doctors and policy makers. It is assumed that the formulation of team sports paradigms (coded or adapted) collating the benefit usually obtained from performing diverse exercise activities (i.e. aerobic and resistance training) with the social interaction naturally associated with ball games may result in a viable strategy to reduce individuals' resistance to exercise. In accordance with this, research should provide clear indications about the best practice to help health professionals to prescribe aggregating enjoyable, feasible, effective and safe ball sports or drills to various populations.

Descriptive and training studies have provided compelling evidence about the effectiveness of low doses (i.e. weekly and short-term) of recreational football for contrasting the side effects of the sedentary lifestyle of western countries such as cardiovascular disease risk factors, diabetes-related effectors, high-blood pressure, obesity and metabolic syndrome. Although waiting for large-scale confirmation studies, the body of knowledge collected for recreational football encouraged the aphorism 'Football is Medicine', suggesting the extension of the interest on other coded team sports. The scenario provided by non-football team sports participation is stunning, with an estimated 100 million basketball players, 70 million team handball players and an additional audience brought from other coded team sports like volleyball, rugby union, field hockey, futsal and floorball that complement the 500 million of footballers. In what follows, we will review the published evidence that promotes the use of recreational non-football team sports as a potential new "drug" for lifestyle diseases. The reported wide-range effects on physical, physiological and psychosocial domains of non-football team sports practice will be outlined and critically discussed in this chapter.

Cardiorespiratory fitness and aerobic performance

Competitive team handball is an intermittent high-intensity exercise mode that, in contrast to football, heavily involves upper limbs in explosive actions (one-on-one situations, passes and throws) reiterated across the match. Furthermore, lower limbs are involved in sudden stops, changes of direction, jumps and one-on-one situations, heavily stressing the skeletal and neuromuscular domain. Like in other competitive team sports, team handball players exercise at 80–90% of their individual maximal heart rate, significantly taxing the aerobic and anaerobic pathways. With the aim to explore the possibility to include team handball among the interventions helpful in attracting previously sedentary people to enroll in systematic exercise programs, Povoas et al. (2017) examined the physical and physiological demands of recreational team handball played as official format matches (60 min duration; 7v7). The results evidenced the high-intensity nature of team handball played at a recreational level with cardiovascular (82 ± 6% of maximal heart rate), skeletal and neuromuscular demands that resulted in relatively similar or slightly lower than those reported in the competitive matches and within the range shown to potentially improve the participants' health and physical fitness. A later training study confirmed the interest of recreational team handball practice (7v7 or 6v6 for 60 min) in male sedentary participants formerly experienced in the sport (33–55 years), reporting practically interesting improvements in physiological and health-related variables (Povoas et al., 2018). Indeed, in just 12 weeks and with a reported small training attendance (i.e. 2.2 ± 0.7 days per week) the studied participants improved their maximal oxygen uptake by ~14%. Recreational team handball players' intermittent high-intensity performance improved by an outstanding 80% (i.e. Yo-Yo Intermittent Endurance Level 2). A training intervention with younger men (20–30 years) who attended a recreational team handball program in the form of training sessions based on small-sided games (SSG; 4v4 or 3v3), resulted in similar aerobic fitness improvements even though the participants had no experience with the sport (Hornstrup et al., 2019). Indeed, attending training sessions just 1.7±0.3 times per week over a 12-week period improved participants' maximal oxygen uptake by 11 ± 6% and allowed them to cover 32% longer distance in the Yo-Yo Intermittent Endurance Level 1 test post-intervention. Furthermore, time to exhaustion during a treadmill test used to assess maximal oxygen uptake increased significantly (+16%). Similarly to the Portuguese study, the participants spontaneously attained the 84% of their individual maximal heart rate during training and for 21% of the match time the heart rates were >90% HRmax. Muscle biopsy analysis revealed a marked increase in key mitochondrial enzymes such as citrate synthase (+22%), suggesting that peripheral adaptations contributed to improvements in aerobic fitness (Hornstrup et al., 2019). The same training protocol delivered (12 weeks) in previously untrained young women (20–30 years) consisting of SSG-based training (19x14 m court, 4x10 min SSG) sessions 1.9±0.3 times per week was ineffective in improving treadmill maximal oxygen uptake (Hornstrup et al., 2018). However, the competitive nature of play and the reported attendance were sufficient to improve participants' time to exhaustion in the Yo-Yo Intermittent Endurance Level 1 test (+35%, $p<0.001$) and in an incremental treadmill test (+11.5%, $p=0.003$). The intensity of the training protocol and participants' pre-intervention physical status, in association with their chronological age (<30 years), might be the reason for the unexpected resistance to changes in maximal oxygen uptake in this cohort. Indeed, the considered SSG produced an average match intensity corresponding to 85 ± 6% of individual maximal heart rate, with as much as 35% of the playing time spent above 90% of their individual maximal heart rate. Since the authors reported that the training sessions's HR was recorded only occasionally during the intervention, an overestimation of the average match intensity could have actually occurred as a result of the Hawthorne effect (being under control bias). The fact that male former team handball players' improved their aerobic fitness in the face of a lower average match heart rate (80 ± 7%), time spent above 90% of maximal heart rate (~24%) and longer session duration (60 vs 40 min) compared to the female intervention supports this speculation. Moreover, this observation indicates that training session volume and not only training intensity may play a role in recreational team handball induced VO_2max adaptations. Maximal oxygen uptake is as a key variable in aerobic fitness and relates to longevity and morbidity (Nes, Vatten,

Nauman, Janszky, & Wisloff, 2014). As such, more studies are needed to examine the optimal dose of team handball-based SSGs to trigger practical changes of VO_2max in the range of those reported with male former players.

Three months of recreational basketball in the form of SSG (i.e. 3v3) was effective in improving maximal oxygen uptake (1.6–2.4%) and treadmill time to exhaustion (4.6–8.0%) in untrained men (aged 20–42 years). Interestingly, the magnitude of the reported training effects was greater in those participants who played full-court recreational basketball (3v3 with two baskets, 20×12 m) compared to their half-court counterparts (3v3 with one basket, 10×12 m). These results are lower than the values reported by recreational football and team handball interventions, apparently suggesting a more anaerobic profile for recreational basketball. However, the reported difference might be to some extent be explained by the moderately lower baseline maximal oxygen uptake level of team handball players (40.1 ± 8.4 mL/min/kg) and age-matched football players compared to the recreational basketball players in the Randers et al. (2018) study (43.7–44.7 mL/min/kg). However, the 4×12-min basketball sessions were reported to elicit mean exercise heart rates in the range of those observed in football and team handball exercise interventions (83.8–84.5% of maximal heart rate), irrespective of the court mode (i.e. full or half court with 2 or 1 baskets, respectively) used. Recreational basketball participants maintained their exercise heart rate above 90% of their maximal heart rate for approximately 25% of their match time, suggesting that exercise intensity was not probably the cause of the reduced effect of this exercise mode on maximal oxygen uptake (Randers et al., 2018).

Basketball practice produced significant changes in cardiovascular fitness-related variables such as blood lactate concentration and exercise heart rate at arbitrarily selected treadmill speeds (28–32% and 7–11%, respectively). Together with a significant 5–8% (half vs. full court, respectively) increment in time to exhaustion during the maximal oxygen uptake treadmill test, these changes demonstrate the positive effect on cardiovascular fitness of recreational basketball SSG in young adult. Additionally, the Randers et al. (2018) study points to an accurate prescription of the drills to achieve the targeted physiological results, starting from the choice of court dimensions.

Floorball is the indoor version of field hockey, or the court version of ice hockey, that was set to competitive rules in early 1980s in Sweden. Surprisingly, the published literature revealed that more recreational than competitive versions of floorball have been investigated. The documented interest is a clear demonstration of the perceived sustainability of this novel team sport as a health-enhancing exercise mode. Attending recreational floorball training sessions twice a week (40 min per session) for 26 months was not sufficient to provide improvement or maintenance of maximal oxygen uptake in elderly participants (age 65–76 years) (Pedersen, Vorup, & Bangsbo, 2018). However, the observed decrements in maximal aerobic power were lower (~7 vs ~18%) than that observed in the control group included in the training study. In accordance of this study outcome, Vorup et al. (2017) reported no training-related changes in maximal aerobic power in men aged 65–76 years that trained for 12 weeks. This study participants were playing adapted floorball in sessions of 3–5 6-min bouts, resulting a total exposure of 18–30 min and a 1:1 work-to-rest ratio. The evidence from these floorball studies suggest an inadequacy for either short- or long-term interventions of the proposed training volume in the elderly when the aim is the development of cardiorespiratory fitness. However, floorball for aerobic fitness should not be discouraged, as 1 MET reduction in maximal oxygen uptake may result in a 20% reduction in cardiovascular mortality risk (Nes et al., 2014). Indeed, activities enabling conservation or reduction in age-related decrement in maximal aerobic power should be regarded with great practical interest. A different outcome was revealed when a 12-week floorball training program was implemented in pre-menopause and post-menopause women (48–52 years) using a larger training volume (60 min twice a week, 30 min floorball warm-up plus 30 min floorball SSG) (Nyberg et al., 2014; Seidelin et al., 2017). The greater training exposure produced significant improvements in maximal aerobic power (4.4–5.5%) and in the Yo-Yo Intermittent Endurance Level 1 test (40.6–42.5%). Although significant, these changes are lower than those reported in recreational football and male team handball. Interestingly, the extension of the training period to 40 weeks with just 1 training session per week maintained the improvements in maximal aerobic power and the Yo-Yo Intermittent Endurance Level 1 test achieved after 12 weeks of more intensive floorball practice (Seidelin et al., 2017). Given the interest and the perceived exercise enjoyment reported by participants during floorball participation, future research should focus on the dose-response variables in order to maximise training achievements in aerobic fitness in different populations (Wikman et al., 2017). Particular interest should be devoted to the study of court dimensions, as the use of bats may potentially limit players' displacements to tackle the ball.

Rugby union is a collision sport with a reported high injury rate when played at amateur and professional level (Yeomans et al., 2018). Recreational versions of rugby union which discard tackling (touch rugby) in the form of SSGs (6v6) have been proposed as a safe exercise paradigm to promote more enjoyable high-intensity exercise in the general population (Mendham, Coutts, & Duffield, 2012; Mendham et al., 2016). Participants involved in non-contact rugby SSGs exercised at 80–85% (average of 83%) of their theoretical maximal heart rate reporting a work rate of 67–79 m·min^{-1} to cover approximately a total of 2,700–3,200 m during a 40-min match (4×10 min with 2 min of passive recovery). Interestingly, ~5% of the total distance was covered at speeds above 14 km·h^{-1}, considered as high-intensity activity in middle-aged (38–49 years) obese (28–31% body fat) participants (n=19) (Mendham et al., 2016).

Descriptive studies using touch rugby SSGs as an exercise paradigm provide evidence of acute upregulation of mitochondrial biogenesis and oxidative metabolism enzymes (i.e. PGC-1α and AMPK) that were higher than in response to continuous cycling (Mendham et al., 2016). The positive effects of touch rugby on aerobic fitness were confirmed by a randomised controlled training study in which participants trained 3 days per week for 8 weeks (total distance ~3,100 m per session, 200 m^2 per player) (Mendham et al., 2015; Mendham, Duffield, Marino, & Coutts, 2014). Oxygen uptake and peak power output at the end of submaximal exercise (80% of maximal heart rate) increased by 17% and 18% respectively. Surprisingly, there were no significant changes in SIRT1, p53 or PGC-1α protein suggesting longer training intervention (>8 weeks) may be needed to realize a rise in mitochondrial biogenesis biomarkers using touch rugby. Interestingly, the effects reported for touch rugby were not superior to those in the exercise control group performing cycling for the same volume and intensity (Mendham et al., 2015, 2014).

Futsal is the indoor version of football (soccer) played as 5v5 including a goalkeeper. The competitive version of futsal is quite popular all over the world and organised in national, confederation and world championships across ages and sexes (Castagna, D'Ottavio, Granda Vera, & Barbero Alvarez, 2009). The potential of indoor 5-a-side football played at a recreational level was originally proposed as an optional exercise mode to improve cardiovascular fitness in students (Castagna et al., 2007). Recreational futsal proved to induce exercise intensities in the range of those proposed to improve aerobic fitness in moderately trained or sedentary individuals. A 2×20-min session of recreational futsal activated post-exercise protein signalling in skeletal muscle similar to those induced by the same average intensity (i.e. first ventilatory threshold) and duration of continuous running (Serpiello et al., 2014). Given the reported acute effect of recreational futsal on molecules linked to muscle adaptations that are supposed to provide a reduction of risk in developing chronic lifestyle diseases, training studies carried out in different populations are warranted (Serpiello et al., 2014).

Training methods using a variety of progressive and alternated drills with the same physiological aim is considered an effective strategy to improve performance. Alternating different team sports (football, team handball, basketball, volleyball and floorball) during a training intervention did not result in changes in aerobic fitness in 61-year-old participants presenting lifestyle diseases over 12–16 weeks (Moller et al., 2018). This was probably the result of a lower average training intensity (75% estimated maximal heart rate) and that only 10% of the total time was spent at heart rates above 90% of estimated maximal heart rate. Interestingly, the control group performing a typical physical fitness protocol (aerobic cycling plus strength training) reported changes in VO_2max (+8%, $p = 0.05$). Training intensity was not constantly checked during the training intervention suggesting that training load control should be performed when using a combination of team sports as an effective training intensity prescription.

Body composition

Compartmental body fat and lean body mass levels are associated with health status. Prolonged aerobic exercise and resistance training are usually prescribed to patients with the aim of modifying body composition to improve health status. Recreational team handball practice implemented as 2 training sessions per week produced significant changes in body composition in young female participants with a 2.1% increase in total muscle mass (+0.9 kg) and a 2.2% non-significant decrease in body fat after 12 weeks (Hornstrup et al., 2018). Using the same protocol, male players (20–30 years) experienced a 7% decrease in total fat mass, but no changes in muscle mass compared to baseline values (Hornstrup et al., 2019).

Similarly, 3v3 basketball practice extended for 12 weeks was effective in significantly reducing body fat by 0.9–1.6% and increasing lean body mass by 0.8–1.3 kg. Eight weeks of non-contact rugby training provided a ~4% decrease in fat mass and ~2% increase in fat free mass in obese men (Mendham et al., 2015, 2014).

Long-term floorball training provided sufficient anabolic stimuli to maintain muscle mass in elderly subjects (66–78 years). Pedersen et al. (2018) reported no significant variation in lean body mass in 73-year-old floorball recreational players during a 26-month intervention. This finding should be regarded with great interest, as a loss of 0.7% of muscle mass is usually observed in this age span. Interestingly, that study's age-matched active lifestyle control group reported a 1.5% reduction in lean body mass, which is in line with the average population predictive data. Floorball training sessions twice per week (36–60-min weekly exposure) were successful in significantly decreasing total body and visceral body fat by 5% and 14%, respectively, in elderly male participants (65–76 years) (Vorup, Pedersen, Melcher, et al., 2017). Nevertheless, the higher training volume was not effective in modifying lean body mass, probably because of the short training exposure of this study (12 weeks).

A recent study suggested post-exercise protein supplementation (0–3h post) may increase muscle mass in previously untrained male subjects (72 years) who were included in a randomised control trial using team sport SSGs in the form of floorball and cone ball as training interventions (Vorup, Pedersen, Brahe, et al., 2017). Given the interest and the effect on health of nutrition strategies and often contrasting information emerging from nutrition interventions on exercise outcome and the nature of the cited study, further confirmation studies are strongly warranted before nutrition prescription in recreational team sports is considered.

In post-menopause women (52 years), recreational floorball interventions revealed a ~3.6% increment in lean body mass. However, a change in lean body mass (+1.6–1.9%) was evident in the active control group of pre-menopause women (48 years) revealing a population-specific effect of recreational floorball on lean body mass (Nyberg et al., 2014; Seidelin et al., 2017). Leg muscle mass increased post-floorball intervention by 2.5–4.6% with apparently no clear trend due to the pre-post menopause status using the same floorball training protocol. Interestingly, the lean body mass increased in post-menopause women despite a lower expression in mTOR, a protein considered a key central regulator of skeletal muscle hypertrophy (Seidelin et al., 2017).

Bone density has a key role in the prognosis of osteoporotic status in the elderly and post-menopausal women. Recreational floorball was shown to produce a selective increase (~2%) of leg bone mineral density in middle-aged women

(48–52 years) independent of their menopause status (Nyberg et al., 2014; Seidelin et al., 2017). Playing recreational team handball produced a significant effect on the bone osteogenic variables with significant positive changes in proximal femur bone mass density in both male and female participants (20–30 years) (Hornstrup et al., 2018, 2019). Interestingly, in the bone of male participants, the adaptations were equally distributed between upper and lower limbs suggesting a homogeneous bone stress in response to recreational team handball protocols (Hornstrup et al., 2019). This data supports the interest of recreational floorball training in contrasting the negative effect of osteoporosis in populations prone to this disease.

Metabolic health

High blood pressure, elevated cardiovascular risk factors, obesity and propensity to type II diabetes are the health challenges of a growing proportion of the population. The search for sustainable strategies to prevent, control or cure these health threats is of great social and economic concern for most governments' welfare. Surprisingly, the solution reveals itself to be simpler and more at reach than previously thought and is, luckily, potentially non-pharmacological. And the icing on the cake – more enjoyable and socially rewarding. Indeed, those are the evidence-based benefits that can be brought to the citizens with just dribbling, hitting, bouncing, passing and throwing a ball with easy-to-follow and enjoyable rules on a regular basis a few times a week in the form of friendly games.

Recreational team handball, floorball and touch rugby training interventions proved effective in lowering some cardiometabolic risk factors that are associated with cardiac dysfunctions, arterosclerosis, type II diabetes and sudden mortality.

BLOOD PROFILE

Recreational team handball played in the form of 7v7 and 6v6 games and not as 4v4 or 3v3, were effective in lowering total cholesterol (–10%), LDL cholesterol (–14%) and triglycerides (–15%) with a beneficial increase (+11%) of HDL cholesterol fraction (Hornstrup et al., 2018, 2019; Povoas et al., 2018). The floorball SSG increased the HDL cholesterol (+6%) in post-menopausal women, but had no effect in other cholesterol-related variables. In the elderly (65–76 years), floorball practice lowered LDL cholesterol by 11% and triglycerides by 8% (Vorup, Pedersen, Melcher, et al., 2017). No effect on blood lipids was reported by touch rugby studies carried out with male middle-aged participants reported to be prone to obesity (Mendham et al., 2014, 2015).

Blood pressure

Systolic blood pressure was decreased by 2.8 mmHg in non-hypertensive participants who participated in team sports at a recreational level (Moller et al., 2018). The changes, although not impressive and lower than those reported for recreational football, should be viewed with interest, as they were observed in citizens at risk of developing lifestyle diseases. Participants' baseline values were probably the reason why no significant changes were observed in blood pressure values after a team handball intervention in 20–30 years men (111 and 67 mmHg for systolic and diastolic blood pressure, respectively) and women (103 and 69 mmHg for systolic and diastolic blood pressure, respectively) (Hornstrup et al., 2019; Hornstrup et al., 2018). In recreational basketball players of a similar age (20–42 years) with baseline blood pressure levels (121–122 and 72–73 mmHg for systolic and diastolic blood pressure, respectively), changes in systolic and diastolic blood pressure were court-dimension dependent (Randers et al., 2018). Indeed, participants that trained on a full court experienced a 3.9 and 6.4 mmHg decrease in systolic and diastolic blood pressure, respectively, compared to the corresponding 1.3 and 4.8 mmHg recorded in the group training on a half court. The court-dimension effect was confirmed by the decline reported in mean arterial pressure in the post-training assessment in the full-court group but not in the half-court groups. Interestingly, comparable reductions of blood pressure (–4 mmHg) were reported for male recreational team handball players who trained for 12 weeks on a full court with those reported by training studies that used SSGs (Povoas et al., 2018). These results again suggest an effect of court dimension on the potential physiological and metabolic training outcomes.

Studies on non-hypertensive elderly (70 years, 139 and 83 mmHg) using floorball as an exercise mode, reported no changes in blood pressure variables (Vorup, Pedersen, Melcher, et al., 2017). Significant changes in diastolic but not systolic blood pressure were reported in pre- and post-menopausal women (–2.8 and –3.9 mmHg) playing floorball for 12 weeks. Interestingly, a trend toward a higher diastolic blood pressure was found in post-menopausal women compared to their pre-menopausal counterparts (Nyberg et al., 2014).

DIABETES

Recreational basketball training over 12 weeks did not change the fasting blood glucose and plasma insulin levels in male players (Randers et al., 2018). Póvoas et al. (Povoas et al., 2018) reported lower fasting blood glucose (–6.6%) and plasma insulin (–33.6%) after a team handball training intervention. Similar (moderate to large) changes during oral glucose tolerance tests (2 h) were also evident for blood glucose and plasma insulin concentrations (–17 and –50%). Vorup et al. (Vorup, Pedersen, Melcher, et al., 2017) found a ~9% decrease in insulin resistance in recreational floorball players. Over a similar training duration, a recreational floorball intervention carried out on pre- and early post-menopausal women did not bring favorable changes in blood glucose levels (Seidelin et al., 2017). However, the prolongation of the training intervention from 12 to 40 weeks resulted in a general improvement in regulatory function of glucose. This suggests a time effect on variables related to insulin resistance in response to recreational team sports interventions in disease-prone populations. Favorable changes in insulin resistance related variables were seen in obese males who trained with intermittent high-intensity activity in the form of non-contact rugby SSGs, as evidenced by changes in glucose disposal (Mendham et al., 2015). The reported increase in lean body mass evidenced in non-football team sports add to the direct effect of these casually intermittent high-intensity forms of exercise on insulin/glucose sensitivity and uptake mechanisms that are beneficial in preventing development of type II diabetes (Srikanthan & Karlamangla, 2011). Although no changes were noted in glycosylated haemoglobin, team sport protocols appeared to increase lean body mass in another study (Hornstrup et al., 2018).

Physical function

Despite the pandemic diffusion of sedentary lifestyles, daily life activities still introduce physical challenges which require physical independence. An active way to look at daily life activities is to train citizens to cope with the physical challenges that work, domestic chores and leisure tasks may require across the stages of life. Given that, the construct of physical functionality may be the development and or maintenance of the physical prerequisites that are supposed to be helpful in tackling daily-life motor tasks. Training involving the selection of critical recurrent task-oriented movements (global approach) are supposed to be a viable strategy to improve physical functions and to warrant social independency and movement efficiency.

Time-motion analyses has provided evidence of the random high-intensity intermittent nature of team handball, street basketball, floorball, futsal and touch rugby played at a recreational level in different populations. Team sports are deemed to improve physical functions as a result of their unpredictable nature during recreational matches. Improvements in postural balance in the range of ~30% have been reported as result of a 12-week recreational team handball intervention (Povoas et al., 2018). In older (65–76 years) participants, recreational floorball improved physical performance in motor tests mimicking ADL such as timed motor tasks and muscle strength (+8%) (Vorup, Pedersen, Melcher, et al., 2017).

Conclusions and future directions

The published evidence supports the interest of exercise science on team sports practice in the form of spontaneous matches or training beyond the bulk of literature on fitness and wellness of recreational football. The current knowledge has enabled us to affirm that ball activities in the form of friendly confrontation as a training paradigm should be considered as a valid strategy in counteracting the effects associated with lifestyle diseases that threaten and negatively affect the modern population. The beneficial effects on health from regular participation in recreational team sports are similar to, and in some cases superior to, that reported for programs that follow a defined prescription for improving fitness and for the development and maintenance of health. Recreational team sports have the added benefit of being enjoyable, socially rewarding and with fewer psychological demands. Team sports may be considered a resource for humanity to gain quality of life and independency. The interest of the benefits provided and potentially brought by recreational team sports warrant future studies examining the dose-response effect of sustainable training paradigms in order to disclose the hormetic nature of this novel, non-pharmacological approach. The health benefits of recreational team sports, which are known to occur in smaller scale studies, need to be investigated in larger-scale population projects in order to justify to decision-makers the need for committing to the necessary economic, human resource, and infrastructure improvements. Particular attention should be devoted to the injury prevention issue that logically comes in to play when dealing with unpredictable intermittent high-intensity activities like recreational team sports. Nevertheless, the current reported evidence suggests that recreational team sports have a low injury rate even when spontaneously practiced. With the aim to optimise intervention responses, training intensities should be monitored in order to avoid ineffective results. The large proportion of citizens potentially using this form of exercise mode should attract more investments to fund high-quality research (i.e. large-scale RCT) from local, national, international and world organisations, municipalities and governments.

References

Castagna, C., Belardinelli, R., Impellizzeri, F. M., Abt, G. A., Coutts, A. J., & D'Ottavio, S. (2007). Cardiovascular responses during recreational 5-a-side indoor-soccer. *Journal of Science and Medicine in Sport*, *10*(2), 89–95.

Castagna, C., D'Ottavio, S., Granda Vera, J., & Barbero Alvarez, J. C. (2009). Match demands of professional Futsal: A case study. *Journal of Science and Medicine in Sport*, *12*(4), 490–494. doi:S1440-2440(08)00068-6 [pii] 10.1016/j.jsams.2008.02.001

Hornstrup, T., Løwenstein, F. T., Larsen, M. A., Helge, E. W., Póvoas, S. C., Helge, J. W., . . . Krustrup, P. (2019). Cardiovascular, muscular, and skeletal adaptations to recreational team handball training: A randomized controlled trial with young adult untrained men. *European Journal of Applied Physiology*, *119*(2):561–573.

Hornstrup, T., Wikman, J. M., Fristrup, B., Povoas, S., Helge, E. W., Nielsen, S. H., . . . Krustrup, P. (2018). Fitness and health benefits of team handball training for young untrained women-A cross-disciplinary RCT on physiological adaptations and motivational aspects. *Journal of Sport & Health Science*, *7*(2), 139–148. doi:10.1016/j.jshs.2017.09.007

Mendham, A. E., Coutts, A. J., & Duffield, R. (2012). The acute effects of aerobic exercise and modified rugby on inflammation and glucose homeostasis within Indigenous Australians. *European Journal of Applied Physiology*, *112*(11), 3787–3795. doi:10.1007/s00421-012-2361-5

Mendham, A. E., Duffield, R., Coutts, A. J., Marino, F., Boyko, A., & Bishop, D. J. (2015). Rugby-specific small-sided games training is an effective alternative to stationary cycling at reducing clinical risk factors associated with the development of type 2 diabetes: A randomized, controlled trial. *PLoS One*, *10*(6), e0127548. doi:10.1371/journal.pone.0127548

Mendham, A. E., Duffield, R., Coutts, A. J., Marino, F. E., Boyko, A., McAinch, A. J., & Bishop, D. J. (2016). Similar mitochondrial signaling responses to a single bout of continuous or small-sided-games-based exercise in sedentary men. *Journal of Applied Physiology (1985)*, *121*(6), 1326–1334. doi:10.1152/japplphysiol.00289.2016

Mendham, A. E., Duffield, R., Marino, F., & Coutts, A. J. (2014). Small-sided games training reduces CRP, IL-6 and leptin in sedentary, middle-aged men. *European Journal of Applied Physiology*, *114*(11), 2289–2297. doi:10.1007/s00421-014-2953-3

Moller, T. K., Nielsen, T. T., Andersen, R., Lundager, I., Hansen, H. F., Ottesen, L., . . . Randers, M. B. (2018). Health effects of 12 weeks of team-sport training and fitness training in a community health centre for sedentary men with lifestyle diseases. *Biomedical Research International*, *2018*, 1571807. doi:10.1155/2018/1571807

Nes, B. M., Vatten, L. J., Nauman, J., Janszky, I., & Wisloff, U. (2014). A simple nonexercise model of cardiorespiratory fitness predicts long-term mortality. *Medicine & Science in Sports and Exercise*, *46*(6), 1159–1165. doi:10.1249/MSS.0000000000000219

Nyberg, M., Seidelin, K., Andersen, T. R., Overby, N. N., Hellsten, Y., & Bangsbo, J. (2014). Biomarkers of vascular function in premenopausal and recent postmenopausal women of similar age: Effect of exercise training. *American Journal of Physiology: Regulatory, Integrative & Comparative Physiology*, *306*(7), R510–517. doi:10.1152/ajpregu.00539.2013

Pedersen, M. T., Vorup, J., & Bangsbo, J. (2018). Effect of a 26-month floorball training on male elderly's cardiovascular fitness, glucose control, body composition, and functional capacity. *Journal of Sport & Health Science*, *7*(2), 149–158. doi:10.1016/j.jshs.2017.12.002

Povoas, S. C. A., Castagna, C., Resende, C., Coelho, E. F., Silva, P., Santos, R., . . . Krustrup, P. (2017). Physical and physiological demands of recreational team handball for adult untrained men. *BioMed Research International*, *2017*, 6204603. doi:10.1155/2017/6204603

Povoas, S. C. A., Castagna, C., Resende, C., Coelho, E. F., Silva, P., Santos, R., . . . Krustrup, P. (2018). Effects of a short-term recreational team handball-based programme on physical fitness and cardiovascular and metabolic health of 33–55-year-old men: A pilot study. *BioMed Research International*, *2018*, 4109796. doi:10.1155/2018/4109796

Randers, M. B., Hagman, M., Brix, J., Christensen, J. F., Pedersen, M. T., Nielsen, J. J., & Krustrup, P. (2018). Effects of 3 months of full-court and half-court street basketball training on health profile in untrained men. *Journal of Sport & Health Science*, *7*(2), 132–138. doi:10.1016/j.jshs.2017.09.004

Seidelin, K., Nyberg, M., Piil, P., Jorgensen, N. R., Hellsten, Y., & Bangsbo, J. (2017). Adaptations with intermittent exercise training in post- and premenopausal women. *Medicine & Science in Sports and Exercise*, *49*(1), 96–105. doi:10.1249/MSS.0000000000001071

Serpiello, F. R., McKenna, M. J., Coratella, G., Markworth, J. F., Tarperi, C., Bishop, D., . . . Schena, F. (2014). Futsal and continuous exercise induce similar changes in specific skeletal muscle signalling proteins. *International Journal of Sports Medicine*. doi:10.1055/s-0034-1367045

Srikanthan, P., & Karlamangla, A. S. (2011). Relative muscle mass is inversely associated with insulin resistance and prediabetes: Findings from the third National Health and Nutrition Examination Survey. *Journal of Clinical Endocrinology and Metabolism*, *96*(9), 2898–2903. doi:10.1210/jc.2011-0435

Vorup, J., Pedersen, M. T., Brahe, L. K., Melcher, P. S., Alstrom, J. M., & Bangsbo, J. (2017). Effect of small-sided team sport training and protein intake on muscle mass, physical function and markers of health in older untrained adults: A randomized trial. *PLoS One*, *12*(10), e0186202. doi:10.1371/journal.pone.0186202

Vorup, J., Pedersen, M. T., Melcher, P. S., Dreier, R., & Bangsbo, J. (2017). Effect of floorball training on blood lipids, body composition, muscle strength, and functional capacity of elderly men. *Scandinavian Journal of Medicine & Science in Sports*, *27*(11), 1489–1499. doi:10.1111/sms.12739

Wikman, J. M., Nistrup, A., Vorup, J., Pedersen, M. T., Melchor, P. S., Bangsbo, J., & Pfister, G. (2017). The effect of floorball training on health status, psychological health and social capital in older men. *AIMS Public Health*, *4*(4), 364–382. doi:10.3934/publichealth.2017.4.364

Yeomans, C., Kenny, I. C., Cahalan, R., Warrington, G. D., Harrison, A. J., Hayes, K., . . . Comyns, T. M. (2018). The incidence of injury in amateur male rugby union: A systematic review and meta-analysis. *Sports Medicine*, *48*(4), 837–848. doi:10.1007/s40279-017-0838-4

Chapter 10

Football at the workplace

Svein Barene, Gertrud Pfister, Peter Krustrup

Introduction

The beneficial health effects from sufficient levels of physical activity are highly recognised (Lee et al., 2012; Tolonen, Rahkonen, & Lahti, 2017). However, over the past decades there has been a decline in the levels of physical activity during leisure time in the population worldwide (Love, Adams, van Sluijs, Foster, & Humphreys, 2018) leading to a decrease of cardiovascular fitness (VO_2max), elevated blood pressure and an unhealthy blood serum lipid profile (cholesterol, LDL and HDL) as well as obesity, which are well-documented risk factors for several non-communicable diseases (Love et al., 2018). Based on a previous study by Lee et al. (2012), physical inactivity was suggested to be responsible for more than 5 million deaths each year (Lee et al., 2012), and is hence recognised as a global pandemic that requires global action (Ding et al., 2016). The direct costs of physical inactivity in Western countries are estimated to be approximately 1.5–3.8% of the total health care expenditure (Tolonen et al., 2017).

Work is suggested to have a beneficial influence on both physical and mental health, as well as on wellbeing (Waddell & Burton, 2006). However, according to a longitudinal study by Church et al. (2011), there has been a decrease in jobs requiring moderate-intensity physical activity during the past 5 decades in the U.S. from at least 50% in the early 1960s to less than 20% today (Church et al., 2011). Despite the fact that occupations with primarily physically demanding, albeit often monotonous work tasks still exist (e.g. in health care and construction work), there has been enormous development in work-efficient machinery during the industrial revolution until today in most professions. This development has led to predominantly sedentary work tasks, usually characterised by sustained strain, high mental stress and low intensity, which in turn has led to a reduction in the individuals' total energy metabolism during working time (Toomingas, Mathiassen, & Tornqvist, 2016).

In combination with an unhealthy lifestyle, this most likely will lead to negative effects on the health and wellbeing of the individual, such as musculoskeletal disorders, decreased work ability, productivity loss, as well as more sick days (Rongen, Robroek, van Lenthe, & Burdorf, 2013; Strijk, Proper, van

Mechelen, & van der Beek, 2013). Previous research has suggested that both physical activity level (Henriksen, Rayce, Melkevik, Due, & Holstein, 2016; Johnsen, Toftager, Melkevik, Holstein, & Rasmussen, 2017) and occupational class (Kivimäki et al., 2015) are strongly interrelated with socioeconomic status. In this regard, occupation and the living conditions connected with it are suggested as an indicator of socioeconomic position (Lahelma, Martikainen, Laaksonen, & Aittomäki, 2004).

A high socioeconomic position is associated with material resources, positive health and lifestyle, as well as social and economic influence within the hierarchical society (Sumanen, Lahelma, Pietiläinen, & Rahkonen, 2017). In contrast, the members of lower occupational classes have limited opportunities for in-work development, flexibility to balance work and family life, protection from adverse working conditions, etc., which are strongly associated with increased sickness absence (Marmot & Bell, 2012; Sumanen et al., 2017) and causes substantial costs for employers (Ding et al., 2016). In Western countries, the indirect costs from sickness absence and productivity loss have been estimated to be 3.6–3.9% of total health care expenditures (Tolonen et al., 2017).

Based on the aforementioned challenges associated with insufficient physical activity level of people both in leisure and working time, as well as adverse working conditions, implementation of regular physical activity at the workplace may be beneficial both with regard to employees' physical and psychological health and work ability, and with regard to the employers who gain from an increase of productivity and a decrease of sickness absence.

Given that approximately 65% of the world's population above 15 years of age is part of the work force (OECD, 2019), the workplace provides access to a large and diverse intersection of society (WHO, 2008; Malik, Blake, & Suggs, 2014). Furthermore, given that most full-time workers spend more than 35 hours per week at work (Proper et al., 2003), and that education, income, health and working conditions work as stratification into certain labour market sectors (Goetzel & Ozminkowski, 2008; Sorensen et al., 2011), the workplace is suggested as an appropriate arena for reaching high-risk groups to promote public health (Christensen et al., 2011).

Health care workers are engaged in promotion, protection or improvement of health in the population, and are predominantly female. The work tasks are characterised by relatively high physical demands, such as patient handling and other manual tasks, in addition to considerable walking and standing in awkward postures. Moreover, these workers are reported to have a high prevalence of low cardiovascular fitness and obesity, making this occupational group particularly vulnerable to various work-related physical and psychosocial health challenges. Hence, health care workers represent an occupational group that will benefit from health improvement and should be motivated to increase their physical activity level. However, the combination of a physically exhausting job and an extensive 'second shift' at home may influence their energy and motivation for performing recreational physical activity (Lenneis, 2016).

Football in a workplace setting – opportunities and challenges of a physical activity intervention with middle-aged female hospital employees

Football is a popular sport with approximately 500 million active players worldwide of which 60% are registered in football clubs (Krustrup et al., 2009), which is the highest participation rate of all sports (Dunning, 1999). The game attracts not only millions as players but also many more people as fans, who enjoy the games in the stadium and/or follow their teams via various media. But football is more than a sport. The teams seem to represent their club, their city or their country, and they produce 'sites of memory', i.e. remembrances which mirror the aims and values of their communities and also their nations.

It goes without saying that it is not the game, per se, which gains so much attention, but it is men's football that triggers identification and stirs up emotions. Although some women played similar games in some countries and cultures, the 'inventors' of 'real' football were boys and men who participated in aggressive folk games in the Middle Ages and later played the game in English boarding schools. In the course of the 20th century, men's football became the most popular sport worldwide, with an estimated 500 million playing football and with billions of fans watching the matches. The Football World Cup even exceeds the Olympic Games in popularity; in 2006, the World Cup had a total cumulative television audience of more than 26 billion viewers. The final match attracted an audience of 715 million.

In a historical perspective, women's football is relatively young. In spite of its positive development regarding both quality and status in recent years, women's football has struggled to achieve legitimacy compared to the game of the men (Hermann & Vollmeyer, 2016), which may partly be explained by differences with regard to speed and strength which influence football performances. However, it can be assumed that environmental factors, such as the socialisation of players and interest of mass media, may have an important influence on the discrepancies between men's and women's football (Chalabaev, Sarrazin, Fontayne, Boiché, & Clément-Guillotin, 2013). It can be assumed that boys experience more positive support from parents for participation in football than girls (Fredricks & Eccles, 2005), and that girls have a number of negative experiences with playing the game, e.g. they may not be taken seriously and/or be laughed at when playing matches (Slater & Tiggemann, 2011).

Gender differences in sport participation can be a result of socialisation and the internalisation of gender stereotypes (Hermann & Vollmeyer, 2016), which have a negative influence on the motivation to play football. Doubts about their skills and prejudices with regard to female players may also play a role (Hively & El-Alayli, 2014). Moreover, previous studies have suggested that the gender stereotypes are maintained, maybe even augmented, by media coverage of female players and teams (Schmidt, 2016), and by gender stereotyping of judges (Coulomb-Cabagno, Rascle, & Souchon, 2005) and sponsors, which makes it difficult to find financial support for women's football players and for events (Hardin, Simpson, Whiteside, & Garris, 2007).

In addition to improving health, football is reported to be highly motivating, at least for boys and men, and creates team spirit among the participants who may emulate the star players (Nielsen et al., 2014). Therefore, it can be assumed that the game is an excellent choice for a workplace physical activity intervention. However, it is men's football which is in the center of public attention and we do not know if or how much the female participants identify with male football stars. Although there is a growing women's football movement – currently 1.270 million women are registered footballers in Europe (UEFA, 2017) – the women are not playing in the limelight. Although women's football has experienced a continuous upsurge, there are still large differences in popularity between the men's and the women's game, and it is an open question if and how fandom influences participation in the sport or in the intervention.

Also, we do not know if and how the form of activity in a workplace intervention influences the engagement of the participants and prevents drop-out. In one of our previous projects with female cleaners from Turkey, in interviews we found that they liked playing because it was not boring and they could enjoy the sport together with their colleagues and friends. Other projects of the 'Copenhagen Center for Team Sport and Health' also used the fun of playing to keep participants, e.g. seniors (men), engaged and active. Psychological tests supported these insights derived from observation and qualitative interviews: There was evidence that playing team sports had positive influences and instigated a decrease of anxiety and depression among the participants (Wikman et al., 2017). However, we have to be aware that using football as an activity for a workplace intervention may also cause problems – not the least because football is still a men's game and women may not feel comfortable participating in an activity which makes them look masculine and clumsy.

Having the designs and results of previous interventions in mind, we aimed to examine the potential health effects of playing football on female hospital employees by implementing training at a Norwegian Hospital in 2011. Our primary outcome variables were cardiovascular fitness (VO_2max), body weight, bone mineral content (BMC), bone mineral density (BMD), osteocalcin (bone marker), isometric strength, musculoskeletal pain intensity and duration, as well as work ability and the rating of perceived exertion (RPE) during work.

Scientific approach to football at the workplace

Participants

An inquiry was directed to the director of personnel at a large hospital in the northern part of Norway comprising 752 female employees, whereof 548 worked as nurses or nursing assistants and 204 in other occupations, such as bioengineers, environmental workers, occupational therapists, etc. A total of 161 female employees enrolled in the study and completed a screening questionnaire prior to the baseline measurements. This large interest indicates that the employees were aware of the health benefits of physical activity and that they appreciated the opportunity to train after their working hours. Of these, 127 were nurses or nursing assistants, whereas the remaining 35 were bioengineers who we chose to include for implementation purposes in a working setting. Due to an unforeseen administrative challenge with the project application to the Regional Committees for Medical and Health Research Ethics, there was a 10-week delay for the scheduled start-up during the autumn of 2010, and we chose to postpone the intervention to January 2011. This delay may be the main reason for 53 drop-outs prior to the baseline measurements.

Randomised grouping

Based on the participant's affiliation with different departments and units at the hospital, 28 employees were defined as cluster 1 with regard to their close proximity at work, followed by construction of two almost equal sized clusters, i.e. cluster 2 (n = 27) and 3 (n = 28), matched on age, body mass index and work seniority. The remaining consenters were assigned into three smaller clusters; cluster A (n = 7), B (n = 8) and C (n = 9) matched on the same variables as mentioned above. In the next step, clusters 1–3 and A–C, respectively, were randomly selected into either the football, Zumba or control group as follows: the football group: cluster 3+C (n = 37), the Zumba group: cluster 2+B (n = 35) and the control group: cluster 1+A (n = 35).

The intervention was conducted between January and October of 2011, and comprised several physiological measurements at baseline (January), after 12 weeks (follow-up test 1, April) and 40 weeks (follow-up test 2, October). Based on the subject of this book, we will only refer to the football intervention in the following sections.

Measurement procedures pre- and post-intervention

The measurements were conducted over three weeks and comprised four elements: 1) an electronic questionnaire containing self-reported information on muscle pain intensity and duration, work ability and Borg's Rating of Perceived Exertion (RPE) during work; 2) fasting blood samples; 3) DXA scan; 4) blood pressure and maximal oxygen consumption; and 4) isometric muscle strength and postural sway.

For examining the intensity and duration of muscle pain in different regions of the body, the Nordic Musculoskeletal Questionnaire (Kuorinka et al., 1987) was used comprising the two following questions: 'Please indicate the pain intensity in the [body] region the past 7 days' with response categories from 0 to 10 (0 = no pain, 10 = maximal pain) on a Likert scale, and 'Please indicate the number of days with pain in the [body] region the past 3 months'. The body regions were the neck-shoulder and the lower back, respectively. To measure work ability, a single item from the Work Ability Index (WAI) was used: 'Please indicate your current work ability compared with lifetime best on a scale from 0 to 10' (0 = completely unable to work, 10 = work ability at its best) (Ahlstrom, Grimby-Ekman, Hagberg, & Dellve, 2010; Ilmarinen, 2007). RPE during work was measured with the following question: 'Please indicate the level of perceived physical exertion during work on a 15 category scale from 6 to 20' (6 = no exertion at all, 20 = maximal exertion) (Borg, 1970).

The football intervention

Throughout the first 12 weeks (January–March), the football intervention was conducted outside working hours three days a week between 4.00–6.00 a.m. in the hospital's gymnastic hall (10 × 20 m) and comprised of three-a-side or four-a-side football matches. To be able to facilitate the training for all, the football participants were divided into two groups who played 60 min from 4.00 to 5.00 and 5.00 to 6.00 p.m, respectively. To accommodate those employees with shift work, two additional 60-min training sessions were offered between 10.00–11.00 a.m. In these sessions, the participants played five-a-side, six-a-side or seven-a-side football matches in a municipal sports hall (20 × 40 m). Each training was supervised by an instructor. The sessions started with 5-min low-intensity warm-up exercises and included a 5-min half-time break. Due to the participants limited experience and skills in football, the first two weeks included an additional 30-min individual basic technical training prior to the games.

During the last 28 weeks (March–October), the training was organised outside on a grass football pitch (15 × 20 m) as five-a-side, six-a-side or seven-a-side matches. In contrast to the first 12 weeks, in this part of the project the participants were given the responsibility to organise the football sessions and there was no encouragement to attend the training. In this way we gained information about the participants' compliance – without the pressure of a supervisor.

Measurement procedures during the intervention

The attendance rate was recorded by the project leader throughout the first 12 weeks, and by the participants themselves via their Facebook group during the last 28 weeks. The intensity was determined during weeks 1–2, 6–7, 11–12, 22–23 and 39–40 by heart rate (HR) measurements (Polar Team System, Polar Electro Oy, Kempele, Finland). In addition, the participants completed a short questionnaire measuring the rating of perceived exertion (RPE) on a 100 mm visual analogue scale (VAS) immediately prior to and after the respective sessions. Lastly, in-depth interviews were conducted at baseline and after 12 weeks with five participants with the aim to examine their experiences with the project and the perceived influences of the intervention on the working environment and, in general, on their lives.

Main results

Adherence to the intervention and intensity during training

Out of the 37 female hospital employees who were randomised to the football group, 4 (11%) chose to withdraw prior to the intervention. Out of the remaining 33 who started playing football, 7 participants (19%) dropped out within 6 weeks. Based on this, 26 participants (70%) completed intervention period 1 (1–12 weeks). However, 12 of these (32%) chose to withdraw from the study prior to intervention period 2, implying that 14 participants (38%) continued training. Of these, 2 participants dropped out before 25 weeks, whereas 1 dropped out between 25 and 35 weeks. From this, a total of 11 participants (30%) completed the 40-week intervention period.

During intervention period 1 (January–March), a total of 36 training sessions, i.e. an average of 3 weekly training sessions, were defined as 100% adherence. The corresponding number completed training sessions were 28.6 ± 6.3 (2.4 ± 0.5 per week). During intervention period 2 (April–October), a total of 37 training sessions, i.e. an average of 1.5 weekly training sessions, were defined as 100% adherence. The total number completed training sessions were 11.9 ± 12.7 (0.5 ± 0.5 per week). Due to summer vacation, there was a 4-week period without training.

During intervention period 1, the average HR was 148 ± 11 bpm (78.3 ± 4.4% of maximal heart rate [HRmax]) with a corresponding average HR during intervention period 2, i.e. 148 ± 11 bpm (78.6 ± 3.2% HRmax).

Intervention effects

Cardiovascular fitness

Maximal oxygen uptake (VO_2max)

From baseline to 12 weeks follow-up, the ITT analyses revealed a significant increase in VO_2max in the football group (32.8 ± 5.5 to 33.8 ± 5.8 ml/kg/min, P = 0.02) compared to the control group (33.1 ± 6.7 to 32.6 ± 6.8 ml/kg/min) (Table 10.1). From baseline to the 40-week follow-up, only a tendency for increase (P = 0.08) was revealed in the football group (Table 10.1).

Average HR at a submaximal workload of 100 W

From baseline to the 12-week follow-up, the football group significantly reduced HR at 100W (149.4 ± 14.3 to 139.7 ± 14.6 bpm, P = 0.01) compared to the control group (147.3 ± 14.3 to 144.0 ± 15.7 bpm), but no significant intervention effects were observed with regard to HR at 100W submaximal workload after 40 weeks (Table 10.1).

Table 10.1 Changes in VO_2 max and HR at submaximal workload (100W) based on the intention-to-treat principle from baseline to the 12- and 40-week follow-up, respectively

Characteristics	*Football group (n = 37)*			
	Follow-up Week	*Diff.**	*95% CI*	*Sig.*
VO_2 max (ml/kg/min)	12	1.5	0.3 to 2.8	0.02
	40	1.1	−0.2 to 2.4	0.08
VO_2 max (l/min)	12	0.08	−0.03 to 0.21	0.11
	40	0.05	−0.05 to 0.14	0.32
Time to exhaustion (s) during the VO_2 max-test	12	11.0	0.0 to 21.9	0.05
	40	4.0	−7.9 to 15.9	0.51
Power output (W) at exhaustion during the VO_2 max-test	12	7.6	0.3 to 14.9	0.04
	40	6.6	−0.5 to 13.8	0.07
Submax HR (bpm; 100W)	12	−6.7	−11.6 to −1.9	0.01
	40	−1.4	−6.0 to 3.3	0.56

* Diff. refers to the contrast estimate for the outcome (based on the Ancova analyses adjusted for baseline body mass index [BMI]).

Body composition

Fat percentage

From baseline to the 12-week follow-up, the football group significantly reduced (34.7 ± 6.1 to 33.2 ± 6.4%, P = 0.002) their total body fat percentage compared to the control group (36.3 ± 6.4 to 35.9 ± 6.4%) (Table 10.2). From baseline to the 40-week follow-up, the football group (34.7 ± 6.1 to 34.0 ± 6.4%, P = 0.01) significantly reduced their total body fat percentage compared to the control group (36.3 ± 6.4 to 36.9 ± 6.6%) (Table 10.2).

Fat mass

From baseline to the 12-week follow-up, the football group significantly reduced their total body fat mass (22.4 ± 6.4 to 21.3 ± 6.6 kg, P=0.001) compared to the control group (24.4 ± 7.5 to 24.2 ± 7.6 kg) (Table 10.2). From baseline to the 40-week follow-up, the football group (22.4 ± 6.4 to 21.9 ± 6.5 kg, P = 0.004) revealed a corresponding reduction in total body fat mass compared to the control group (24.4 ± 7.5 to 25.1 ± 7.9 kg) (Table 10.2).

Body weight

From baseline to the 12-week follow-up, the football group significantly reduced body weight (69.2 ± 9.2 to 68.8 ± 9.0 kg, P=0.02) compared to the control group (71.4 ± 11.5 to 71.7 ± 11.8 kg), but from baseline to 40 weeks, the football group (69.2 ± 9.2 to

Table 10.2 Changes in body composition (body weight, BMI, body fat percentage, fat mass, bone mineral content [BMC], bone mineral density [BMD], osteocalcin and leptin) based on the intention-to-treat principle from baseline to the 12- and 40-week follow-up, respectively

Characteristics	*Football group (n=37)*			
	Follow-up Week	*Diff.**	*95% CI*	*Sig.*
Weight (kg)	12	−0.8	−1.4 to −0.1	0.02
	40	−1.1	−2.4 to −0.1	0.08
BMI (kg/m²)	12	−0.3	−0.5 to −0.0	0.03
	40	−0.3	−0.7 to 0.1	0.17
% fat (total)	12	−1.1	−1.8 to −0.4	0.00
	40	−1.2	−2.1 to −0.3	0.01
Total fat mass (kg)	12	−1.0	−1.6 to −0.4	0.00
	40	−1.2	−2.1 to −0.4	0.00
Total BMD (g/cm²)	12	−0.01	−0.02 to 0.01	0.38
	40	0.01	−0.01 to 0.02	0.39
Lower limb BMD (g/cm²)	12	0.03	−0.01 to 0.06	0.09
	40	0.05	0.02 to 0.09	0.00
Total body BMC (g)	12	35.2	4.0 to 66.5	0.03
	40	39.2	3.2 to 75.4	0.03
Lower limb BMC (g)	12	11.6	−1.7 to 24.9	0.09
	40	22.1	8.1 to 36.0	0.00
Osteocalcin (μg/L)	12	5.3	2.7 to 7.9	0.00
	40	6.6	2.2 to 11.0	0.00
Leptin (μg/L)	12	−2.7	−7.3 to 1.9	0.25
	40	−6.6	−12.5 to −0.7	0.03

** Diff. refers to the contrast estimate for the outcome (based on the Ancova analyses adjusted for baseline BMI).*

69.0 ± 8.9 kg, P=0.08) revealed only a tendency for reduction compared to the control group (71.4 ± 11.5 to 72.1 ± 11.7 kg) (Table 10.2).

Body mass index (BMI)

From baseline to the 12-week follow-up, the football group (24.7 ± 3.1 to 24.6 ± 3.1 kg/m^2, P = 0.03) significantly reduced their BMI compared to the control group (25.9 ± 3.6 to 26.0 ± 3.6 kg/m^2), with no significant difference (P=0.165) observed from baseline to the 40-week follow-up (Table 10.2).

Bone mineral content and bone mineral density

From baseline to the 12-week follow-up, a significant difference in total body BMC was observed between the football group (2270 ± 257 to 2270 ± 259 g, P=0.03) and the control group (2246 ± 320 to 2211 ± 313 g), which was also the case from

0 to 40 weeks when comparing football (2270 ± 257 to 2272 ± 269 g, $P < 0.05$) with the control group (2246 ± 320 to 2211 ± 324 g) (Table 10.2). Moreover, a significant difference was observed in lower limb BMC for the football group from 0 to 40 weeks (813 ± 93 to 813 ± 100 g, P=0.002) in comparison to the control group (827 ± 121 to 804 ± 117 g) (Table 10.2).

After 12 weeks, no intervention effects were observed either in total body BMD or lower limb BMD (Table 10.2). However, the football group significantly increased the lower limb BMD (2.24 ± 0.18 to 2.29 ± 0.19 g/cm^2, P=0.004) from 0 to 40 weeks compared to the control group (2.29 ± 0.21 to 2.28 ± 0.23 g/cm^2) (Table 10.2).

Plasma bone markers

From baseline to the 12-week follow-up, the football group significantly increased the plasma osteocalcin (19.3 ± 7.0 to 23.3 ± 9.7 μg/L, P<0.001) compared to the control group (20.8 ± 9.4 to 19.4 ± 8.6 μg/L) (Table 10.2). From 0 to 40 weeks, a corresponding significant increase was observed in plasma osteocalcin for the football group (19.3 ± 7.0 to 24.9 ± 11.3 μg/L, P=0.004) in comparison to the control group (20.8 ± 9.4 to 19.4 ± 67.9 μg/L) (Table 10.2).

No intervention effects were found for plasma leptin after 12 weeks, however, from baseline to the 40-week follow-up, the football group significantly decreased (18.7 ± 12.9 to 14.0 ± 10.6 μg/L, P=0.03) the plasma leptin compared to the control group (28.3 ± 20.9 to 29.5 ± 21.1 μg/L) (Table 10.2).

Other variables

No intervention effects were observed in blood pressure, blood glucose, plasma lipids or triglycerides, neither after 12 or 40 weeks.

Muscle pain and work-related outcome measures

Muscle pain intensity

From baseline to the 12-week follow-up, the football group significantly reduced their muscle pain intensity (2.6 ± 2.2 to 1.8 ± 2.2, P=0.001), on a Likert scale from 0 to 10 in the neck-shoulder region compared to the control group (1.8 ± 2.0 to 2.4 ± 2.0) (Table 10.3). From 0 to 40 weeks, the football group revealed a corresponding significant reduction (2.6 ± 2.2 to 1.8 ± 2.0, P=0.002) in muscle pain intensity in the neck-shoulder compared to the control group (1.8 ± 2.0 to 2.3 ± 2.2) (Table 10.3).

Muscle pain duration

From baseline to the 12-week follow-up, the football group (22.0 ± 29.7 to 16.2 ± 27.4 days, P=0.10) revealed a numerical, but insignificant reduction in numbers of days with pain in the neck-shoulder region the past 3 months compared to

Table 10.3 Changes in muscle pain intensity (on a Likert scale from 0–10) and duration of pain (in the neck/shoulder and the lower back region), work ability and rating of perceived physical exertion (RPE) based on the intention-to-treat principle from baseline to the 12- and 40-week follow-up, respectively

Characteristics	*Football group (n = 37)*		
	*Diff.**	*95% CI*	*Sig.*
Pain intensity (0–10)			
Neck-shoulder region			
0–12 weeks	−1.9	−3.0 to −0.8	0.00
0–40 weeks	−1.9	−3.2 to −0.7	0.00
Lower back region (0–10)			
0–12 weeks	−0.1	−1.1 to −0.8	0.82
0–40 weeks	−0.5	−1.5 to 0.4	0.42
Duration of pain (number of days with pain the past 3 months)			
Neck-shoulder region			
0–12 weeks	−9.2	−20.0 to 1.6	0.10
0–40 weeks	−16.4	−29.6 to −3.2	0.00
Lower back region			
0–12 weeks	5.8	−4.3 to 15.9	0.26
0–40 weeks	−7.0	−18.8 to 4.8	0.24
Work ability (0–10)			
0–12 weeks	0.1	−0.6 to 0.8	0.84
0–40 weeks	−0.0	−0.7 to 0.7	0.91
RPE during working hours (0–10)			
0–12 weeks	0.3	−1.2 to 1.9	0.69
0–40 weeks	−0.2	−1.9 to 1.6	0.86

* Diff. refers to the contrast estimate for the outcome (based on the Ancova analyses adjusted for baseline BMI and cluster affiliation).

the control group (17.6 ± 23.1 to 19.7 ± 26.8 days) (Table 10.3). From baseline to the 40-week follow-up, the football group significantly reduced their muscle pain duration the past 3 months in the neck-shoulder region (22.0 ± 29.7 to 16.4 ± 29.5 days, P=0.02) compared to the control group (17.6 ± 23.1 to 24.7 ± 32.9 days) (Table 10.3).

No intervention effects were observed in pain intensity in the lower back region, work ability or rating of perceived exertion (RPE) during work, neither after 12 or 40 weeks (Table 10.3).

Discussion

The main results of this randomised controlled workplace physical activity intervention were significant short-term increases in the maximal oxygen uptake (VO_2max) in the football group compared to the control group after 12 weeks.

Both after 12 and 40 weeks, the football group revealed a significant reduction in body weight, total body fat mass and fat percentage compared to the control group. In addition, the football group revealed a reduction in muscle pain intensity in the neck-shoulder region after both 12 and 40 weeks, with a corresponding reduction in the duration of muscle pain in the neck-shoulder region after 40 weeks. No intervention effects were observed in self-reported work ability nor the rate of perceived physical exertion (RPE) at work.

This chapter is divided into four parts. The first part comprises a discussion of the main findings of the study on the primary (i.e. VO_2max) and secondary outcomes (i.e. body composition, biomarkers in blood, blood pressure, muscle pain, BMC/BMD, work ability and rate of perceived physical exertion at work). Due to the generally reported challenges associated with implementation of workplace health-promoting initiatives, the second part will focus on the recruitment process, adherence and dropout throughout the present study. The third part will discuss limitations of the study, whereas the last part will elucidate practical implications from the study.

Primary and secondary outcomes

Maximal oxygen uptake (VO_2max)

After 12 weeks, the football group revealed a 5% improvement in the relative VO_2max compared to the control group. However, due to a corresponding 1.5% decrease in VO_2max for the control group, the increase in the football group corresponds to 3.2%. The increase is rather modest compared to a previous intervention study by Krustrup et al. (2010) demonstrating a 15% increase in VO_2max among untrained females after 1-hour twice-weekly football training for 16 weeks (Krustrup, Hansen, Randers, et al., 2010). To examine whether the modest improvements in VO_2max observed for the football group in the present study were due to the conservative ITT analyses, additional per-protocol analyses were conducted. However, the per-protocol analyses revealed only a 4.2% increase in VO_2max for the football group compared to the control group. The modest effect on cardiovascular fitness from the present study may be explained by either lower training intensity or lower training frequency compared to intervention studies demonstrating higher increases in VO_2max after short-term football training. In the present study, the average HR for the football group was 78% HRmax, whereas the reported average intensity level in studies showing larger effects in VO_2max were between 80–85% HRmax (Krustrup, Aagaard, et al., 2010; Krustrup, Hansen, Randers, et al., 2010; Krustrup et al., 2009; Randers, Nybo, et al., 2010). These findings are in accordance to Gormley et al. (2008) who suggests that high-intensity physical activities are more effective for increasing the VO_2max compared to activities comprising lower intensities, even when the lower intensity exercise is performed with a sufficient duration to accomplish the same total amount of work (Gormley et al., 2008). As the average number of training sessions for the football group in the present study was higher than in the abovementioned study by Krustrup et al. (2010), i.e. 2.4 (Barene, Krustrup, Jackman, Brekke, & Holtermann, 2014a) vs. 1.8 (Krustrup, Hansen, Randers, et al., 2010) sessions per week, this indicates that training intensity may be more crucial for improving the VO_2max compared to the training frequency. After 40 weeks, the football group revealed no significant increase in the relative VO_2max compared to the control group. In fact, from the baseline to the 40-week follow-up test there was a 1.7% decrease in the football group with a corresponding 4.9% decrease in the control group. The decrease in VO_2max after 40 weeks contradicts the findings from two previous long-term intervention studies on football among untrained males (Randers, Nielsen, et al., 2010) and premenopausal females (Krustrup, Hansen, Andersen, et al., 2010). Randers et al. (2010) demonstrated that improvements in VO_2max obtained after 12 weeks of football training might be maintained after 52 weeks, despite of a reduced training frequency during the last 40 weeks, i.e. from 2.4 (between 0 and 12 weeks) to 1.3 (between 12 and 64 weeks) sessions per week (Randers, Nielsen, et al., 2010). Furthermore, a 16-month intervention study by Krustrup et al. (2010) demonstrated that a 14% improvement in VO_2max obtained after 4 months was improved by another 2% after 16 months despite of reduced training frequency, i.e. from 1.9 (between 0 and 4 months) to 1.7 (between 4 and 16 months) weekly sessions (Krustrup, Hansen, Andersen, et al., 2010). In the present study, the lack of improvement in VO_2max in the football group may be explained both by insufficient training frequency and insufficient intensity levels. The average training frequency for the football group in the present study was lower compared to the abovementioned long-term studies, i.e. 0.5 (Barene, Krustrup, Brekke, & Holtermann, 2014b) vs. 1.3 (Randers, Nielsen et al., 2010) and 1.7 (Krustrup, Hansen, Andersen et al., 2010) sessions per week. According to Mujika (1998), a minimum of training frequency seems to be necessary to improve the VO_2max (Mujika, 1998). Hence, the lack of effect in VO_2max after 40 weeks for the football group in the present study may be explained by the relatively low training frequency during the last 28 weeks (Barene, Krustrup Brekke et al., 2014b). Furthermore, as the average intensity level among the participants for the football group in the present study was lower compared to the abovementioned long-term studies, i.e. 79% HRmax (Barene, Krustrup, Brekke, et al., 2014b) vs. 82% HRmax (Krustrup, Hansen, Andersen et al., 2010; Randers, Nielsen et al., 2010), this may represent an additional explanation to the lack of improvement in VO_2max in the football group. To evaluate if the modest effects on the VO_2max after 40 weeks could be explained by the conservative ITT analyses, additional per-protocol analyses were conducted. Based on per-protocol analyses, including only the participants who completed training throughout the 40 weeks, there was a 0.1 ($P=0.061$) increase in VO_2max in the football group ($n=9$), with a 7.1% decrease in the control group ($n=23$). Hence, we may suggest that the additional per-protocol analyses support the tendencies revealed from the ITT analyses. In summary, the present study indicates that workplace-initiated, twice-weekly football training improves the cardiovascular fitness among female hospital employees after 12 weeks.

Body composition

After 12 weeks, the football group significantly reduced their body weight (–0.8 kg), BMI (–1.0%), total body fat mass and fat percentage compared to the control group. These findings indicate that football training may be beneficial with regard to short-term effects on fat mass reduction among female hospital employees. These results are in accordance with findings from previous studies on 16 weeks of football training for women (Krustrup, Hansen, Randers, et al., 2010) and 12 weeks of football training for men (Krustrup et al., 2009), which showed a reduction of 1.4 and 2.7 kg in total body fat mass, respectively.

After 40 weeks, the football group revealed significant reductions in total fat mass and fat percentage compared to the control group, with a sustained fat loss from 12 to 40 weeks. This is consistent with Randers et al. (2010), who found a significant decrease in both total fat mass and fat percentage after 64 weeks of football among untrained males (Randers, Nielsen et al., 2010), as well as with a study by Krustrup et al (2010), demonstrating a significant decrease in gynoid fat mass after 64 weeks of football among untrained premenopausal females (Krustrup, Hansen, Andersen et al., 2010). Moreover, after 40 weeks the football group significantly reduced plasma leptin (–6.6 μg/L) compared to the control group. Leptin is considered to be important in the control of body mass by its adjustment of food intake when energy balance is altered (Dirlewanger et al., 1999). Because plasma leptin increases in obese persons, subcutaneous fat is suggested to be a major determinant of plasma leptin levels (Yadav, Kataria, Saini, & Yadav, 2013).

Bone mineral content (BMC) and bone mineral density (BMD)

After 12 weeks, the football group showed a significant difference in total body BMC compared to the control group, with a corresponding insignificant tendency for difference in lower-limb BMC. Because there was no change in total body or lower-limb BMC in the football group from baseline to 12 weeks follow-up, the significant differences are explained by reductions in the control group, i.e. –1.6% in both total body and lower-limb BMC. Based on a previous 1-year prospective study among 20 men, Premkumar et al. (2013) suggests that decreased solar radiation exposure may cause reductions in BMC (Premkumar, Sable, Dhanwal, & Dewan, 2013). This aspect, in combination with lower levels of physical activity during winter time for the participants in the present study, may have caused the tendency for reductions in BMC in the control group. The maintained levels of BMC in the football group may be due the high-impact movements in football involving forceful muscle actions that may have offset a reduction of BMC in the football group (Krustrup, Aagaard et al., 2010).

After 40 weeks, the football group increased both the total body BMC (by 39.3 g), the lower-limb BMC (by 22.1 g), and the lower limb BMD (by 0.05 g/cm^2) compared to the control group. However, as the football group revealed no significant changes in neither BMC nor BMD between baseline and 40 weeks follow-up, the significant differences compared to the control group are mainly explained by reductions in the control group. The clinical relevance of those findings is therefore likely to be modest. A possible explanation to the reductions in BMC and BMD in the control group may be reduced levels of physical activity during the last 28 weeks of the intervention period. After 40 weeks, the football group surprisingly revealed reductions in lumbar-spine BMC compared to the control group, which may be explained by low strain in specific skeletal regions during football training (Calbet, Dorado, Diaz-Herrera, & Rodriguez-Rodriguez, 2001). However, this potential explanation needs to be examined more thoroughly in future studies.

After 12 weeks, the football group (21%) significantly increased the plasma level of osteocalcin compared to the control group. This is in accordance to Woitge et al. (1998), who reported a 15% increase in osteocalcin level in healthy young men after eight weeks of endurance training with three sessions per week, and intensity level between 60–85% HRmax (Woitge et al., 1998). Moreover, a recent study by Jackman et al. (2013) revealed a 37% increase in plasma osteocalcin in untrained women after 16 weeks of football training (Jackman et al., 2013). Due to earlier studies claiming that osteogenic stimulus depends on the presence of mechanical impact posing strain on bone (Turner & Robling, 2003; Vainionpaa et al., 2006), the present results indicate that football training involves sufficiently intensive movements and high-impact actions for improving bone mineral content.

After 40 weeks, the football group significantly increased plasma osteocalcin (6.6 μg/L) compared to the control group. This improvement corresponds to an absolute increase of 29% and might therefore be considered of clinical relevance with regard to an increased bone turnover, and may hence have a preventive effect for future osteoporosis (Calbet et al., 2001; Creighton, Morgan, Boardley, & Brolinson, 2001). This finding indicates that the short-term increase in osteocalcin observed after 12 weeks of football training may be maintained for months in spite of reduced training frequency. The improvements in BMD, BMC and plasma osteocalcin indicate that football training might be a health-beneficial activity for female hospital employees.

No intervention effects were found in S-Glucose, plasma lipids, triglycerides or blood pressure. Based on previous intervention studies demonstrating positive physiological health effects on plasma lipids and blood pressure both after 12 and 16 weeks of football training among untrained males (Krustrup et al., 2009) and females (Krustrup, Hansen, Randers et al., 2010), respectively, effects on these indicators of health was expected. The lack of effects on plasma lipids and blood pressure in the present study may be explained by a better health status with lower average blood pressure in the present population compared to the other two studies. To the best of our knowledge, no previous intervention studies have observed effects on S-Glucose after football training.

Muscle pain intensity and duration

In the present study, the football group reduced pain intensity in the neck-shoulder region both after 12 (−68%) and 40 (−62%) weeks compared to the control group.

These improvements were observed when including all participants in the football group (i.e. both those with and without pain at baseline) in an intention-to-treat analysis. This finding provides a relatively strong documentation that football leads to reduced pain intensity of the neck-shoulder region among female hospital employees. These findings are in accordance with previous workplace health promotion studies observing positive effects on neck-shoulder pain intensity from strengthening and/or stretching exercises among different occupational groups (Andersen et al., 2010; Pedersen, Andersen, Zebis, Sjogaard, & Andersen, 2013; Ylinen et al., 2003, 2006).

With regard to muscle pain duration, the football group significantly (P=0.02) decreased the number of days (−13 days) with pain during the past 30 days in the neck-shoulder region after 40 weeks compared to the control group. It is suggested that physical activity may induce transient elevations in pain threshold in non-exercised parts of the body in healthy subjects, and that muscle activity in one part of the body potentially may influence on distant muscles as well (Andersen et al., 2008). Other potential explanations to the positive effects observed in the present study on neck-shoulder pain intensity and duration may be an increase of anti-inflammatory serum biomarkers (Ortega et al., 2009; Strohacker, Wing, & McCaffery, 2013), beneficial stimulation of sensory and effective pain networks in the central nervous system (Ellingson, Colbert, & Cook, 2012), improved vascular adaption and blood flow to neck-shoulder muscles (Sogaard et al., 2012; Strom, Knardahl, Stanghelle, & Roe, 2009), or general improvements in physical capacity reducing the relative physical workload during working tasks (Holtermann et al., 2010). No intervention effects were observed in muscle pain intensity or duration of the lower back after 12 or 40 weeks, which is in accordance to previous workplace physical intervention studies (Christensen et al., 2011; Daltroy et al., 1997; Horneij, Hemborg, Jensen, & Ekdahl, 2001; Yu et al., 2013). The findings from the present study indicate that football training may reduce muscle pain intensity and duration in the neck-shoulder region among female hospital employees, with no effects observed in the lower-back region.

Work ability

The football group revealed no significant change in work ability compared to the control group. Apart from a previous intervention study demonstrating that strength training may prevent deterioration of work ability (Sundstrup et al., 2014), no previous randomised controlled workplace physical training intervention study has observed improvements in work ability after 12 weeks. The combination of low cardiovascular fitness and high physical work demands is considered to influence on the work ability (Arvidson, Borjesson, Ahlborg, Lindegard, & Jonsdottir, 2013), and hence it is suggested that an improvement of the cardiovascular fitness may increase the work ability (Capodaglio et al., 2010). However, despite of an improvement VO_2max in the football group after 12 weeks (Barene, Krustrup,

Jackman, Brekke, & Holtermann, 2014a), no corresponding improvement was observed in work ability.

Rating of perceived physical exertion (RPE)

The football group revealed no significant improvement in perceived physical exertion during work compared to the control group, neither after 12 or 40 weeks. An explanation to this may be the relatively moderate perceived physical exertion at work that was reported by the participants prior to the intervention in both groups (average score of 10 on a scale from 6 to 20). Based on an increased VO_2max in the football group after 12 weeks, a corresponding reduction in the relative workload was expected. However, the lack of effect on RPE in the present study is in accordance to a previous workplace training intervention study, which also demonstrated improvement in cardiovascular fitness among construction workers (Gram, Holtermann, Sogaard, & Sjogaard, 2012). Hence, apart from one previous workplace physical training intervention study showing improvement in RPE among female nurses after 12-month follow-up (Horneij et al., 2001), it may seem that workplace training intervention studies do not improve perceived physical exertion at work, even in workgroups characterised by high physical work demands. Possible explanations to the lack of effect on RPE despite of improvements in VO_2max may be the many other factors at work also influencing RPE, as well as the possibility that the workers increase the tempo during work when improving their cardiovascular fitness.

Strengths and weaknesses of the study

The strength of the present study was the cluster-randomised controlled design with intention-to-treat evaluation, which is considered to be the gold standard in evaluating interventions (Schulz, Altman, & Moher, 2011). The study was conducted in a relatively large, healthy working population in natural environmental circumstances. Other strengths were the high rates of participation to the physiological tests pre- and post-intervention, as well as the high response rates to the questionnaire at baseline (95%) and after 12 (84%) and 40 (64%) weeks. Additional strengths were the high adherence to the training intervention during the first 12 weeks. The regular day-to-day recording of training participation, as well as the close follow-up and comprehensive registrations of adherence to intensity level and self-perceived exertion of the participants during different phases throughout the intervention period also strengthens the study.

Limitations of the study are the lack of information about employees not willing to participate in the study and those who chose to drop-out from the study in the time between the recruitment of participants to the initiation of the intervention. These limitations may decrease the generalizability of the findings of the study. Further possible weaknesses may be seasonal variations related to temperature and rain/snow that may have influenced motivation for participating, as well as decreased solar radiation throughout the follow-up period that may have led to changes in D-vitamin uptake and bone mineral content that may have biased the results from the DXA-scans. Another limitation of the study is the relatively moderate adherence to training between 12 and 40 weeks. Furthermore, the lack of information about both the leisure-time physical activity and eating habits in general and throughout the intervention period may constitute potential biases to the results on VO_2max, biomarkers in blood and body composition. Moreover, information about muscle pain intensity and duration, work ability and perceived physical exertion may have been influenced by a bias caused by self-reporting.

Conclusions

The present study indicated that workplace initiated twice-weekly football training sessions conducted outside working hours improved maximal oxygen uptake and lowered the fat mass in female hospital employees after 12 weeks. The football training also lowered the work load during submaximal exercise. Furthermore, the training significantly increased the plasma level of osteocalcin, indicating that football activity involve a sufficient degree of intensive, high-impact movements providing osteogenic stimuli. The 40-week effects of football training with an approximately 50% reduction in training frequency after 12 weeks suggests that the exercise may promote long-term physiological health among female hospital employees. Furthermore, the training resulted in significant long-term decreases in fat mass, significant improvements in lower limb BMD/BMC, as well as plasma levels of osteocalcin and leptin. The present study also shows that one-hour, twice-weekly football training at the workplace may alleviate pain in the neck-shoulder region after just 12 weeks of training. Overall, this study indicates that football in a workplace context may be health beneficial for female hospital employees.

Practical implications

Because of the growing incidence of obesity in the Western population and the increasing rates of lifestyle diseases such as cardiovascular disease and diabetes (Blair & Church, 2004; Han, Richmond, Avenell, & Lean, 1997) as well as osteoporosis (Deng, Xu, Davies, Heaney, & Recker, 2002; Helge et al., 2010), the workplace may represent an appropriate arena to promote physical activity in the prevention of these and other diseases. This study about a workplace physical activity intervention demonstrates that 40 weeks of football training taking place outside the working hours may have beneficial effects on aerobic fitness and on cardiovascular health, as well as promising effects on musculoskeletal health, both in a short- and a long-term perspective. Considering that the combination of high prevalence of high work demands, low cardiovascular fitness (VO_2max) and overweight/obesity among health care workers may increase the risk of musculoskeletal pain, impaired work ability and high RPE during work, this study indicates that football may be an appropriate activity for improving the cardiovascular fitness and reducing the muscle pain among female hospital employees. Based on the overall assessment of the study, we suggest that health promotion via physical activity in form of football can be implemented successfully in a workplace, even outside the working hours. Despite a 3 km geographical distance from the workplace to the training facilities, the adherence to training was relatively high during the first 12 weeks, with a reduction of adherence during the last 28 weeks. To obtain acceptable/sufficient adherence to physical activity outside working hours, we suggest that the training sessions should be organised immediately after work.

Interview with five of the participants

During the first training week, interviews were conducted with five of the participants (age range of 34–63 years). The same women took part in follow-up interviews after 12 weeks.

The experience of being drawn to the football team

With the exception of one of the participants who had limited experience with playing football with colleagues at her previous job, none of the five women had previous experience with football. Moreover, all of them expressed that they would have preferred to be allocated to the second intervention group who participated in Zumba. At the same time, all interviewees were happy that they were not drawn to the control group.

Previous experience with exercise and physical activity

Female 1 (34) was an active handball player until she was 24 years old, but has performed sporadic strength and aerobics training at the local fitness centre after that. Even though she perceived her own football skills as very limited, she was willing to participate in the football group. Female 2 (45) claimed to have no football skills at all, but did not worry about that as long as she participated only to have fun, to sweat and gain energy. She had no goal of becoming a good football player. Female 3 (47) had never played football as a child, but participated for a period in a mixed company football team at her previous workplace, which was not in a hospital nor as a health worker. Even though she neither particularly wanted to participate in the football group nor perceived her own football skills as good, she enjoyed watching football on television and highlighted in that regard the Norwegian national team's legendary 2–1 victory against Brazil in 1998. Female 4 (53) had no previous experience with football. In addition to being afraid of the ball she had a painful knee, probably osteoarthritis, which she was anxious about exposing to external trauma. Female 5 (63) said she enjoyed being physically active by walking in the forest, as well as by cycling to and from work in the summer time, and emphasised that training gives energy to her everyday life. However, she had never played football before, but she enjoyed watching the city's elite football team games on television.

Motivation to participate in the project

Female 1 summarised two important motives for participation in the project: the comprehensive health check that was offered the participants as well as a desire to get started with regular exercise that may be continued after the end of the project. Female 2 signed up for the project as it seemed exciting and because it would be nice to workout with colleagues. Female 3 wanted to get in regular training. Female 4 joined the project because she thought it was exciting to get her physical capabilities tested. Female 5 did also mention that the physical tests were a motivating factor for participation. Furthermore, she emphasised the social aspect of exercising together with colleagues and doing something together on another arena as an additional factor. Although football was not the most preferred intervention group, she was determined to give it a try, but at the same time determined to quit if it turned out that the participation caused bodily stress that could influence her working day.

Experience of participation

Female 1 highlighted the incredible fun of being a part of the football group and that the exercise is much more exhaustive in comparison to strength training that she had most experience with the recent years. With regard to the aerobic component of playing football, she also claimed that the activity is much easier to practice compared to running on a treadmill or running out in the woods. Asking about what makes playing football fun, she replied that it feels that time goes faster because you get so involved in following the ball, and the interaction with your teammates, as well as the opponents. She also emphasised that the atmosphere between the participants was very good with no disagreement, and that everyone seemed to take care of each other and tried to avoid hurting each other. In addition to experiencing the same enjoyment in participating in the football group after 12 weeks, she also perceived an improvement in both her own technical skills as well as cooperation between players of the teams. Moreover, she experienced the teamwork, the competition and the cheering associated with playing football as positive aspects of participating. Although she felt exhausted towards the end of every single training session (which she highly acknowledged), she had a lot of fun participating in the football exercise, and stated that the game makes you feel a little bit free. She also highlighted the positive effect from the intervention in view of expanded social meeting points at the hospital during working hours, where employees who did not previously know each other now have something common to talk about when they meet in the elevator or in the corridor. Female 2 stated during the first training week that she was sweating from the workout, but did not feel breathless, and thought the pulse had to be higher if you were supposed to get exhausted. After 12 weeks she emphasised that participation in the football group was associated with positive social relationships and happiness with lots of laughter. What makes it fun is that you are in constant activity with relatively high intensity and that you do not have such a high level of skill creates many fun situations. Furthermore, she acknowledges that she has improved her skills over these 12 weeks, but it still does not make her a football player (laughs). Furthermore, she says that the participation has been better than expected because of many lovely ladies that she did not know from before, and whom she now frequently stops and talks to in the corridors at work. Female 3 finds that the football activity has created a talking point at work where people who previously did not know each other now stop when they meet in the corridors to talk about the football exercise. Despite being skeptical and reluctant the first week of the intervention, female 4 experienced that as a group they had a lot of fun during the actual football activity. After 12 weeks, she realised that this skepticism disappeared due to feeling more confident and tougher facing the ball, and experienced that the football exercise changed from being unpredictable to becoming a more structured activity where all participants were more equal in terms of skills. She also claimed that at this point she was feeling more exhausted from football exercise compared to in the beginning because she had gradually become more active, i.e. running more during the game. Additionally, she felt an improvement in her physical capacity, not necessarily during playing football, but when she was out walking in the forest and/or during swimming. She also highlighted the social community that had been established, and the important influence this group affiliation had on the improvements they had achieved regarding interaction and overview when playing football. Furthermore, the pain she had in her knee disappeared. Because female 5 felt that everyone else had much better skills than her, she was satisfied that the exercise was organised by others. At the start, she found playing difficult with having to learn rules and thinking while taking part in the game, and also expressed that she felt it was mentally tough because she was constantly worried about hard balls that could hit her in the face. In spite of the fact that the balls used were of the kind of inner ball dressed with a soft surface, she stated at this point that the ball could be dangerous. In the start she also expressed that she did not run so much because she was nervous about bumping into the others. After 12 weeks, she highlighted the great fun it was to participate in the football group and that during the period she had managed to move boundaries by daring more than before and having the ability to push oneself harder. In addition, she found it less strenuous to climb the stairs up to the 8th floor at work, and that she needed less sleep during the daytime compared to before, and concludes that there has been an improvement in physical capacity. As a result of her experience of coping with the football activity itself through passing and shooting skills, she now was very satisfied being part of the football group, and emphasised that these new relationships appeared during the working day when participants randomly met in the elevator or in the corridors at the hospital.

Organisation and degree of compliance

Female 1 pointed out that it was very good with the close follow-up that was performed during the first 12 weeks. Female 2 claimed that football was an excellent form of exercise to perform indoors during winter time, but should be organised outdoors in the summer months to motivate her for further participation. With regard to the 4.00 p.m. session, she claimed that this could be challenging to accomplish over time because it assumes good will from colleagues who can take over assignments in the last half hour of the working day, whereas female 3 believed that the time of exercise made it difficult for participants with young children in kindergarten. Female 4 expressed that she occasionally found it difficult to find motivation to go to football exercise three times a week throughout the project period, but that this feeling disappeared as soon as she entered the gymnastic hall and met with the other participants, and that after the sessions she felt very excited and did not regret going to training. Female 5 emphasised the opportunity for both morning and afternoon exercises as very positive, as some of the participants were working shift work and the extra times gave them the opportunity to sustain their training frequency through the intervention period. In addition, she felt it was positive that newcomer exercises were carried out due to her lack of skills in the beginning.

After the 40-week intervention period ended in October 2011 and up to today, 10–12 of the original participants have maintained 1–2 weekly football sessions, and reveal that football exercise provides a certain level of compliance among target groups with little to no previous experience with football. In addition to the regular training these persons have in common, they are also regularly gathered for social events such as ahead of summer and Christmas holidays where they have dinner and drinks together, and substantiate the aforementioned impact of football activity on social relations.

References

Ahlstrom, L., Grimby-Ekman, A., Hagberg, M., & Dellve, L. (2010). The work ability index and single-item question: Associations with sick leave, symptoms, and health-a prospective study of women on long-term sick leave. *Scandinavian Journal of Work, Environment and Health*, *36*(5), 404–412.

Andersen, L., Christensen, K., Holtermann, A., Poulsen, O., Sjogaard, G., Pedersen, M., & Hansen, E. (2010). Effect of physical exercise interventions on musculoskeletal pain in all body regions among office workers: A one-year randomized controlled trial. *Manual Therapy*, *15*(1), 100–104.

Andersen, L. L., Kjaer, M., Sogaard, K., Hansen, L., Kryger, A. I., & Sjogaard, G. (2008). Effect of two contrasting types of physical exercise on chronic neck muscle pain. *Arthritis and Rheumatism*, *59*(1), 84–91. doi:10.1002/art.23256

Arvidson, E., Borjesson, M., Ahlborg, G., Jr., Lindegard, A., & Jonsdottir, I. H. (2013). The level of leisure time physical activity is associated with work ability-a cross sectional and prospective study of health care workers. *BMC Public Health*, *13*, 855. doi:10.1186/1471-2458-13-855

Barene, S., Krustrup, P., Brekke, O.-L., & Holtermann, A. (2014b). Soccer and Zumba as health-promoting activities among female hospital employees: A 40-weeks cluster randomised intervention study. *Journal of Sports Sciences*, *32*(16), 1539–1549.

Barene, S., Krustrup, P., Jackman, S. R., Brekke, O. L., & Holtermann, A. (2014a). Do soccer and Zumba exercise improve fitness and indicators of health among female hospital employees? A 12-week RCT. *Scandinavian Journal of Medicine and Science in Sports*, *24*(6), 990–999.

Blair, S. N., & Church, T. S. (2004). The fitness, obesity, and health equation: Is physical activity the common denominator? *JAMA: The Journal of the American Medical Association*, *292*(10), 1232–1234. Retrieved from www.ncbi.nlm.nih.gov/pubmed/15353537 http://jama.jamanetwork.com/data/Journals/JAMA/4943/JED40054.pdf. doi:10.1001/jama.292.10.1232

Borg, G. (1970). Perceived exertion as an indicator of somatic stress. *Scandinavian Journal of Rehabilitation Medicine*, *2*, 92–98.

Calbet, J. A., Dorado, C., Diaz-Herrera, P., & Rodriguez-Rodriguez, L. P. (2001). High femoral bone mineral content and density in male football (soccer) players. *Medicine and Science in Sports and Exercise*, *33*(10), 1682–1687.

Capodaglio, P., Castelnuovo, G., Brunani, A., Vismara, L., Villa, V., & Maria Capodaglio, E. (2010). Functional limitations and occupational issues in obesity: A review. *International Journal of Occupational Safety and Ergonomics*, *16*(4), 507–523.

Chalabaev, A., Sarrazin, P., Fontayne, P., Boiché, J., & Clément-Guillotin, C. (2013). The influence of sex stereotypes and gender roles on participation and performance in sport and exercise: Review and future directions. *Psychology of Sport and Exercise*, *14*(2), 136–144. doi:10.1016/j.psychsport.2012.10.005

Christensen, J. R., Faber, A., Ekner, D., Overgaard, K., Holtermann, A., & Sogaard, K. (2011). Diet, physical exercise and cognitive behavioral training as a combined workplace based intervention to reduce body weight and increase physical capacity in health care workers: A randomized controlled trial. *BMC Public Health*, *11*, 671. Retrieved from www.ncbi.nlm.nih.gov/pubmed/21871113. doi:10.1186/1471-2458-11-671

Church, T. S., Thomas, D. M., Tudor-Locke, C., Katzmarzyk, P. T., Earnest, C. P., Rodarte, R. Q., . . . Bouchard, C. (2011). Trends over 5 decades in U.S. occupation-related physical activity and their associations with obesity. *PloS One*, *6*(5), e19657. https://doi.org/10.1371/journal.pone.0019657

Coulomb-Cabagno, G., Rascle, O., & Souchon, N. (2005). Players' gender and male referees' decisions about aggression in French soccer: A preliminary study. *Sex Roles*, *52*(7–8), 547–553.

Creighton, D. L., Morgan, A. L., Boardley, D., & Brolinson, P. G. (2001). Weight-bearing exercise and markers of bone turnover in female athletes. *Journal of Applied Physiology*, *90*(2), 565–570.

Daltroy, L. H., Iversen, M. D., Larson, M. G., Lew, R., Wright, E., Ryan, J., . . . Liang, M. H. (1997). A controlled trial of an educational program to prevent low back injuries. *New England Journal of Medicine*, *337*(5), 322–328.

Deng, H. W., Xu, F. H., Davies, K. M., Heaney, R., & Recker, R. R. (2002). Differences in bone mineral density, bone mineral content, and bone areal size in fracturing and non-fracturing women, and their interrelationships at the spine and hip. *Journal of Bone and Mineral Metabolism*, *20*(6), 358–366. doi:10.1007/s007740200052

Ding, D., Lawson, K. D., Kolbe-Alexander, T. L., Finkelstein, E. A., Katzmarzyk, P. T., Van Mechelen, W., . . . Committee, L. P. A. S. E. (2016). The economic burden of physical inactivity: A global analysis of major non-communicable diseases. *the Lancet*, *388*(10051), 1311–1324.

Dirlewanger, M., Di Vetta, V., Giusti, V., Schneiter, P., Jequier, E., & Tappy, L. (1999). Effect of moderate physical activity on plasma leptin concentration in humans. *European Journal of Applied Physiology and Occupational Physiology*, *79*(4), 331–335.

Dunning, E. (1999). *Sport matters: Sociological studies of sport, violence, and civilization*. London and New York: Routledge.

Ellingson, L. D., Colbert, L. H., & Cook, D. B. (2012). Physical activity is related to pain sensitivity in healthy women. *Medicine and Science in Sports and Exercise*, *44*(7), 1401–1406. doi:10.1249/MSS.0b013e318248f648

Fredricks, J. A., & Eccles, J. S. (2005). Family socialization, gender, and sport motivation and involvement. *Journal of Sport & Exercise Psychology*, *27*(1), 3–31. doi:10.1123/jsep.27.1.3

Goetzel, R. Z., & Ozminkowski, R. J. (2008). The health and cost benefits of work site health-promotion programs. *Annual Review of Public Health*, *29*, 303–323. doi:10.1146/annurev.publhealth.29.020907.090930

Gormley, S. E., Swain, D. P., High, R., Spina, R. J., Dowling, E. A., Kotipalli, U. S., & Gandrakota, R. (2008). Effect of intensity of aerobic training on VO_2 max. *Medicine and Science in Sports and Exercise*, *40*(7), 1336–1343.

Gram, B., Holtermann, A., Sogaard, K., & Sjogaard, G. (2012). Effect of individualized worksite exercise training on aerobic capacity and muscle strength among construction workers: A randomized controlled intervention study. *Scandinavian Journal of Work, Environment and Health*, *38*(5), 467–475. Retrieved from www.ncbi.nlm.nih.gov/pubmed/22057836. doi:10.5271/sjweh.3260

Han, T. S., Richmond, P., Avenell, A., & Lean, M. E. (1997). Waist circumference reduction and cardiovascular benefits during weight loss in women. *International Journal of Obesity and Related Metabolic Disorders*, *21*(2), 127–134. Retrieved from www.ncbi.nlm.nih.gov/pubmed/9043967.

Hardin, M., Simpson, S., Whiteside, E., & Garris, K. (2007). The gender war in US sport: Winners and losers in news coverage of Title IX. *Mass Communication & Society*, *10*(2), 211–233.

Helge, E. W., Aagaard, P., Jakobsen, M. D., Sundstrup, E., Randers, M. B., Karlsson, M. K., & Krustrup, P. (2010). Recreational football training decreases risk factors for bone fractures in untrained premenopausal women. *Scandinavian Journal of Medicine and Science in Sports*, *20*(Suppl 1), 31–39.

Henriksen, P., Rayce, S., Melkevik, O., Due, P., & Holstein, B. (2016). Social background, bullying, and physical inactivity: National study of 11-to 15-year-olds. *Scandinavian Journal of Medicine and Science in Sports*, *26*(10), 1249–1255.

Hermann, J. M., & Vollmeyer, R. (2016). "Girls should cook, rather than kick!": Female soccer players under stereotype threat. *Psychology of Sport and Exercise*, *26*, 94–101. doi:10.1016/j.psychsport.2016.06.010

Hively, K., & El-Alayli, A. (2014). "You throw like a girl:" The effect of stereotype threat on women's athletic performance and gender stereotypes. *Psychology of Sport and Exercise*, *15*(1), 48–55. doi:10.1016/j.psychsport.2013.09.001

Holtermann, A., Jorgensen, M. B., Gram, B., Christensen, J. R., Faber, A., Overgaard, K., . . . Sogaard, K. (2010). Worksite interventions for preventing physical deterioration among employees in job-groups with high physical work demands: Background, design and conceptual model of FINALE. *BMC Public Health*, *10*, 120. doi:10.1186/1471-2458-10-120

Horneij, E., Hemborg, B., Jensen, I., & Ekdahl, C. (2001). No significant differences between intervention programmes on neck, shoulder and low back pain: A prospective randomized study among home-care personnel. *Journal of Rehabilitation Medicine*, *33*(4), 170–176.

Ilmarinen, J. (2007). The work ability index (WAI). *Occupational Medicine*, *57*(2), 160–160.

Jackman, S. R., Scott, S., Randers, M. B., Orntoft, C., Blackwell, J., Zar, A., . . . Krustrup, P. (2013). Musculoskeletal health profile for elite female footballers versus untrained young women before and after 16 weeks of football training. *Journal of Sports Sciences*, *31*(13), 1468–1474. doi:10.1080/02640414.2013.796066

Johnsen, N., Toftager, M., Melkevik, O., Holstein, B., & Rasmussen, M. (2017). Trends in social inequality in physical inactivity among Danish adolescents 1991–2014. *SSM-Population Health*, *3*, 534–538.

Kivimäki, M., Virtanen, M., Kawachi, I., Nyberg, S. T., Alfredsson, L., Batty, G. D., . . . Burr, H. (2015). Long working hours, socioeconomic status, and the risk of incident type 2 diabetes: A meta-analysis of published and unpublished data from 222 120 individuals. *The Lancet Diabetes & Endocrinology*, *3*(1), 27–34.

Krustrup, P., Aagaard, P., Nybo, L., Petersen, J., Mohr, M., & Bangsbo, J. (2010). Recreational football as a health promoting activity: A topical review. *Scandinavian Journal of Medicine and Science in Sports*, *20*(Suppl 1), 1–13. Retrieved from www.ncbi.nlm.nih.gov/pubmed/20210908. doi:10.1111/j.1600-0838.2010.01108.x

Krustrup, P., Hansen, P. R., Andersen, L. J., Jakobsen, M. D., Sundstrup, E., Randers, M. B., . . . Bangsbo, J. (2010). Long-term musculoskeletal and cardiac health effects of recreational football and running for premenopausal women. *Scandinavian Journal of Medicine and Science in Sports*, *20*(Suppl 1), 58–71. doi:10.1111/j.1600-0838.2010.01111.x

Krustrup, P., Hansen, P. R., Randers, M. B., Nybo, L., Martone, D., Andersen, L. J., . . . Bangsbo, J. (2010). Beneficial effects of recreational football on the cardiovascular risk profile in untrained premenopausal women. *Scandinavian Journal of Medicine and Science in Sports*, *20*(Suppl 1), 40–49. doi:10.1111/j.1600-0838.2010.01110.x

Krustrup, P., Nielsen, J. J., Krustrup, B. R., Christensen, J. F., Pedersen, H., Randers, M. B., . . . Bangsbo, J. (2009). Recreational soccer is an effective health-promoting activity for untrained men. *British Journal of Sports Medicine*, *43*(11), 825–831. doi:10.1136/bjsm.2008.053124

Kuorinka, I., Jonsson, B., Kilbom, A., Vinterberg, H., Biering-Sorensen, F., Andersson, G., & Jorgensen, K. (1987). Standardised Nordic questionnaires for the analysis of musculoskeletal symptoms. *Applied Ergonomics*, *18*(3), 233–237.

Lahelma, E., Martikainen, P., Laaksonen, M., & Aittomäki, A. (2004). Pathways between socioeconomic determinants of health. *Journal of Epidemiology and Community Health*, *58*(4), 327–332.

Lee, I. M., Shiroma, E. J., Lobelo, F., Puska, P., Blair, S. N., & Katzmarzyk, P. T. (2012). Effect of physical inactivity on major non-communicable diseases worldwide: An analysis of burden of disease and life expectancy. *Lancet*, *380*(9838), 219–229. doi:10.1016/s0140-6736(12)61031-9

Lenneis, V. (2016). *The life, work and recreational physical activity of female cleaners*. Department of Nutrition, Exercise and Sports, Faculty of Science, University of Copenhagen, Denmark.

Love, R., Adams, J., van Sluijs, E., Foster, C., & Humphreys, D. (2018). A cumulative meta-analysis of the effects of individual physical activity interventions targeting healthy adults. *Obesity Reviews*, *19*(8), 1164–1172.

Malik, S. H., Blake, H., & Suggs, L. S. (2014). A systematic review of workplace health promotion interventions for increasing physical activity. *British Journal of Health Psychology*, *19*(1), 149–180. doi:10.1111/bjhp.12052

Marmot, M., & Bell, R. (2012). Fair society, healthy lives. *Public Health, 126*(Suppl 1), S4–10. doi:10.1016/j.puhe.2012.05.014

Mujika, I. (1998). The influence of training characteristics and tapering on the adaptation in highly trained individuals: A review. *International Journal of Sports Medicine, 19*(7), 439–446.

Nielsen, G., Wikman, J. M., Jensen, C. J., Schmidt, J. F., Gliemann, L., & Andersen, T. R. (2014). Health promotion: The impact of beliefs of health benefits, social relations and enjoyment on exercise continuation. *Scandinavian Journal of Medicine and Science in Sports, 24*(S1), 66–75.

OECD. (2019). Working age population (indicator). OECD Publishing. https://doi.org/10.1787/d339918b-en.

Ortega, E., Garcia, J. J., Bote, M. E., Martin-Cordero, L., Escalante, Y., Saavedra, J. M., . . . Giraldo, E. (2009). Exercise in fibromyalgia and related inflammatory disorders: Known effects and unknown chances. *Exercise Immunology Review, 15*, 42–65.

Pedersen, M. T., Andersen, C. H., Zebis, M. K., Sjogaard, G., & Andersen, L. L. (2013). Implementation of specific strength training among industrial laboratory technicians: Long-term effects on back, neck and upper extremity pain. *BMC Musculoskeletal Disorders, 14*, 287. doi:10.1186/1471-2474-14-287

Premkumar, M., Sable, T., Dhanwal, D., & Dewan, R. (2013). Vitamin D homeostasis, bone mineral metabolism, and seasonal affective disorder during 1 year of Antarctic residence. *Arch Osteoporos, 8*(1–2), 129. doi:10.1007/s11657-013-0129-0

Proper, K. I., Koning, M., van der Beek, A. J., Hildebrandt, V. H., Bosscher, R. J., & van Mechelen, W. (2003). The effectiveness of worksite physical activity programs on physical activity, physical fitness, and health. *Clinical Journal of Sport Medicine, 13*(2), 106–117.

Randers, M. B., Nielsen, J. J., Krustrup, B. R., Sundstrup, E., Jakobsen, M. D., Nybo, L., . . . Krustrup, P. (2010). Positive performance and health effects of a football training program over 12 weeks can be maintained over a 1-year period with reduced training frequency. *Scandinavian Journal of Medicine and Science in Sports, 20*(Suppl 1), 80–89. Retrieved from www.ncbi.nlm.nih.gov/pubmed/20210904. doi:10.1111/j.1600-0838.2010.01091.x

Randers, M. B., Nybo, L., Petersen, J., Nielsen, J. J., Christiansen, L., Bendiksen, M., . . . Krustrup, P. (2010). Activity profile and physiological response to football training for untrained males and females, elderly and youngsters: Influence of the number of players. *Scandinavian Journal of Medicine and Science in Sports, 20*(Suppl 1), 14–23. Retrieved from www.ncbi.nlm.nih.gov/pubmed/20149143. doi:10.1111/j.1600-0838.2010.01069.x

Rongen, A., Robroek, S. J., van Lenthe, F. J., & Burdorf, A. (2013). Workplace health promotion: A meta-analysis of effectiveness. *American Journal of Preventive Medicine, 44*(4), 406–415. doi:10.1016/j.amepre.2012.12.007

Schmidt, H. C. (2016). Women's sports coverage remains largely marginalized. *Newspaper Research Journal, 37*(3), 275–298.

Schulz, K., Altman, D., & Moher, D. (2011). CONSORT 2010 statement: Updated guidelines for reporting parallel group randomised trials. *International Journal of Surgery (London, England), 9*(8), 672–677. doi:10.1016/j.ijsu.2011.09.004

Slater, A., & Tiggemann, M. (2011). Gender differences in adolescent sport participation, teasing, self-objectification and body image concerns. *Journal of Adolescence, 34*(3), 455–463. doi:10.1016/j.adolescence.2010.06.007

Sogaard, K., Blangsted, A. K., Nielsen, P. K., Hansen, L., Andersen, L. L., Vedsted, P., & Sjogaard, G. (2012). Changed activation, oxygenation, and pain response of chronically painful muscles to repetitive work after training interventions: A randomized controlled trial. *European Journal of Applied Physiology*, *112*(1), 173–181. doi:10.1007/s00421-011-1964-6

Sorensen, G., Landsbergis, P., Hammer, L., Amick, B. C., Linnan, L., Yancey, A., . . . Pratt, C. (2011). Preventing chronic disease in the workplace: A workshop report and recommendations. *American Journal of Public Health*, *101*(S1), S196–S207. Retrieved from http://dx.doi.org/10.2105/AJPH.2010.300075

Strijk, J. E. P., Proper, K. I. P., van Mechelen, W. P., & van der Beek, A. J. P. (2013). Effectiveness of a worksite lifestyle intervention on vitality, work engagement, productivity, and sick leave: Results of a randomized controlled trial. *Scandinavian Journal of Work, Environment and Health*, *39*(1), 66–75.

Strohacker, K., Wing, R. R., & McCaffery, J. M. (2013). Contributions of body mass index and exercise habits on inflammatory markers: A cohort study of middle-aged adults living in the USA. *BMJ Open*, *3*(5). doi:10.1136/bmjopen-2013-002623

Strom, V., Knardahl, S., Stanghelle, J. K., & Roe, C. (2009). Pain induced by a single simulated office-work session: Time course and association with muscle blood flux and muscle activity. *European Journal of Pain (London, England)*, *13*(8), 843–852. doi:10.1016/j.ejpain.2008.11.003

Sumanen, H., Lahelma, E., Pietiläinen, O., & Rahkonen, O. (2017). The magnitude of occupational class differences in sickness absence: 15-year trends among young and middle-aged municipal employees. *International Journal of Environmental Research and Public Health*, *14*(6), 625. Retrieved from www.mdpi.com/1660-4601/14/6/625.

Sundstrup, E., Jakobsen, M. D., Brandt, M., Jay, K., Persson, R., Aagaard, P., & Andersen, L. L. (2014). Workplace strength training prevents deterioration of work ability among workers with chronic pain and work disability: A randomized controlled trial. *Scandinavian Journal of Work, Environment and Health*, 244–251.

Tolonen, A., Rahkonen, O., & Lahti, J. (2017). Leisure-time physical activity and direct cost of short-term sickness absence among Finnish municipal employees. *Archives of Environmental & Occupational Health*, *72*(2), 93–98. Retrieved from https://doi.org/10.1080/19338244.2016.1160863

Toomingas, A., Mathiassen, S. E., & Tornqvist, E. W. (2016). *Occupational physiology*. Florida, USA: CRC Press.

Turner, C. H., & Robling, A. G. (2003). Designing exercise regimens to increase bone strength. *Exercise and Sport Sciences Reviews*, *31*(1), 45–50.

UEFA. (2017). Women's football across the national associations 2016/17. Retrieved from www.uefa.com/MultimediaFiles/Download/OfficialDocument/uefaorg/Women'sfootball/02/43/13/56/2431356_DOWNLOAD.pdf

Vainionpaa, A., Korpelainen, R., Vihriala, E., Rinta-Paavola, A., Leppaluoto, J., & Jamsa, T. (2006). Intensity of exercise is associated with bone density change in premenopausal women. *Osteoporosis International*, *17*(3), 455–463. Retrieved from www.ncbi.nlm.nih.gov/pubmed/16404492. doi:10.1007/s00198-005–0005-x

Waddell, G., & Burton, A. K. (2006). *Is work good for your health and well-being?* London, England: The Stationery Office.

WHO. (2008). Preventing noncommunicable diseases in the workplace through diet and physical activity: WHO/World Economic Forum report of a joint event. Geneva: WHO Press. Retrieved from https://apps.who.int/iris/bitstream/handle/10665/43825/9789241596329_eng.pdf?sequence=1&isAllowed=y

Wikman, J. M., Nistrup, A., Vorup, J., Pedersen, M. T., Melchor, P. S., Bangsbo, J., & Pfister, G. (2017, July 10). The effect of floorball training on health status, psychological health and social capital in older men. *AIMS Public Health*, *4*(4), 364–382. doi:10.3934/publichealth.2017.4.364. eCollection 2017.

Woitge, H. W., Friedmann, B., Suttner, S., Farahmand, I., Muller, M., Schmidt-Gayk, H., . . . Seibel, M. J. (1998). Changes in bone turnover induced by aerobic and anaerobic exercise in young males. *Journal of Bone and Mineral Research*, *13*(12), 1797–1804. doi:10.1359/jbmr.1998.13.12.1797

Yadav, A., Kataria, M. A., Saini, V., & Yadav, A. (2013). Role of leptin and adiponectin in insulin resistance. *Clinica Chimica Acta*, *417*, 80–84.

Ylinen, J., Takala, E. P., Nykanen, M., Hakkinen, A., Malkia, E., Pohjolainen, T., . . . Airaksinen, O. (2003). Active neck muscle training in the treatment of chronic neck pain in women: A randomized controlled trial. *JAMA*, *289*(19), 2509–2516. doi:10.1001/jama.289.19.2509

Ylinen, J. J., Hakkinen, A. H., Takala, E. P., Nykanen, M. J., Kautiainen, H. J., Malkia, E. A., . . . Airaksinen, O. V. (2006). Effects of neck muscle training in women with chronic neck pain: One-year follow-up study. *Journal of Strength and Conditioning Research*, *20*(1), 6–13. doi:10.1519/r-17274.1

Yu, W., Yu, I. T., Wang, X., Li, Z., Wan, S., Qiu, H., . . . Sun, T. (2013). Effectiveness of participatory training for prevention of musculoskeletal disorders: A randomized controlled trial. *International Archives of Occupational and Environmental Health*, *86*(4), 431–440. doi:10.1007/s00420-012-0775-3

Chapter 11

The implementation of Football Fitness

Søren Bennike, Laila Ottesen, Kenneth Grønlund Rasmussen, Birgitte Rejkjær Krustrup and Julie Midtgaard

1 Introduction

Exercise has well-documented health effects (Lee et al. 2012) and playing football can arguably play a role in improving health (Oja et al. 2015; Milanović et al. 2015, 2018). However, to get people involved and adhere long-term, the activities need to be motivating, easily accessible, and of similar importance to be organised in a form which is possible to realise (and sustain!) in a real-life setting. This is done by football associations all around the world, where the latest FIFA Big Count survey suggests that 270 million people worldwide are registered as football club members (FIFA 2006) indicating a very successful organisational form.

We have recently seen an increasing focus on football as prevention and adjunct to medical treatment (see e.g. Krustrup et al. 2010a, 2010b; Bangsbo et al. 2014; Bruun et al. 2014; Krustrup et al. 2018), explicitly emphasised with the publication of this book. This will arguably result in the development of 'football for health' initiatives, holding the potential to attract and activate participants which in many cases are unfamiliar to the game. It is very plausible that the organisation of these will require a different form than 'traditional' association football which holds a rather strong focus on skill development and competitive aspects. One example of a football for health initiative is Football Fitness (FF), of which a purposefully selected issue of the implementation process is under scrutiny in this chapter. The implementation process is highly important as the potential of health improvement related to football for health initiatives remain unfulfilled if participants are not playing due to an unsuccessful implementation.

Henderson (2009) notes that sport management literature has previously focused primarily on sport as spectatorship or entertainment, and not as an opportunity to promote participation in active behavior, which in turn can lead to better health. Moreover Ooms et al. (2015) highlight that little research has focused on understanding the implementation context of organised sports in relation to implementing health-enhancing physical activity, such as the initiative of FF and other football for health activities. Similarly, Finch and Donaldson (2010) emphasise that there has been increasing recognition of the need for research within real-world intervention contexts of community sport. As argued by the authors,

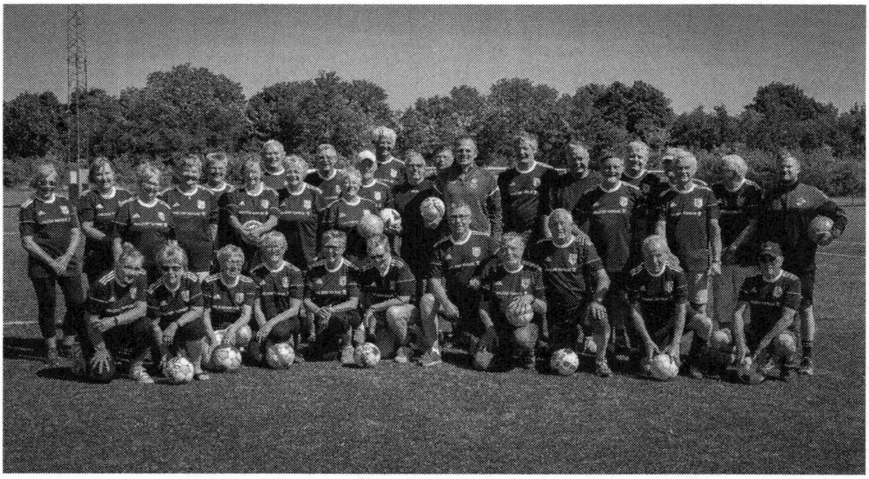

Photo 11.1 Football Fitness is for all age groups and experience levels. 75 women and men aged 60–90 are playing year-round in Frederikssund IK in Denmark.

if interventions are not widely adopted and sustained, it is unlikely that they will have a public health impact. A few studies point to challenges that are critical to the implementation of centrally developed health-related sporting activities in organised sport, such as the willingness and ability of grassroots sports clubs (see e.g. Skille 2008; Casey et al. 2009; Harris, Mori and Collins 2009; Skille 2009; May, Harris and Collins 2013; Kokko 2014; Ooms et al. 2015).

Building on institutional and implementational theory (Lipsky 1980; O'Toole and Montjoy 1984; Campbell 2004; Sydow, Schreyögg and Koch 2005; Winter 2012; May 2012; O'Toole 2012; Meyers and Nielsen 2012; Scott 2014), Bennike, Ottesen and other scholars have explored the initiative of FF and the implementation process (Krustrup and Ottesen 2014; Bennike, Wikman and Ottesen 2014a, 2014b; Bennike 2016; Bennike and Ottesen 2016; Ottesen, Bennike and Thing 2017; Bennike, Thing, and Ottesen 2018). These publications will frame the following, hoping to inspire students, researchers, practitioners and policy makers within the fields of recreational sport and health policy, as we believe that the organised recreational sports setting, such as association-based football, will experience increasing attention in sport for health initiatives.

2 Purposefully selected issues for understanding Football Fitness

In 2010, a working group of the Danish Football Association (DFA) provided a proposal to the DFA board with the purpose of launching the FF initiative. The proposal was greatly inspired by studies highlighting the potential of recreational small-sided football as a beneficial activity for improving cardiovascular and metabolic health effects (Krustrup et al. 2010a, 2010b) and accumulating social capital contributing positively to adherence (Ottesen, Jeppesen and Krustrup 2010). At the same time, FF stands as a reaction to a changing landscape of recreational sport (Bennike, Thing and Ottesen 2018), where public funding for sport is being questioned (MCD 2014) and a growing number of adults are active outside sport clubs in more flexible, health-oriented and often commercial organised activities (Pilgaard and Rask 2016). In addition, the Danish organised sports setting is being increasingly promoted as a setting for complementary treatment/exercise-based rehabilitation, secondary prevention and health promotion (Ottesen and Jacobsen 2011; Ibsen and Eichberg 2012; Danish Government 2014; Bennike 2016). In relation to FF, this has resulted in several partnerships between the DFA, grassroots clubs, municipalities and non-governmental organisations. Current examples are 'FF for rehabilitation' (Guldborgsund 2018), 'FF ABC'[1] (DCSa 2018) and 'FC Prostate®,' (DCSb 2018), all building on the framework of FF. Concerning FC Prostate®, a FF initiative targeting men diagnosed with prostate cancer, a specific educational program for non-professional coaches has been developed (Bjerre et al. 2018) supporting implementation and dissemination. This is in line with a more general and broader FF instructors educational program (FFI 2018). Both are incorporated in the educational system of the DFA. At this very moment, the DFA is planning the development of 'Football for the Heart', in which a similar education for volunteers who wish to organise FF in the context of cardiac rehabilitation is incorporated.

In the project proposal for FF (DFA 2010a) it is stated that the purpose of FF is to: 'Promote football as a health-beneficial activity', 'create an interest in football for fitness and exercise', and 'support football clubs in creating more flexibility in relation to adult players, primarily over the age of 25'.

Moreover, it is stated that if FF succeeds:

> we can expect very great gains in membership, with the associated membership fee income for the football clubs. On the other hand, if we fail in this, we can expect to see much greater competition from other providers of football as exercise on the Danish market in the future.

In a press release (DFA 2010b) of same year it is stated that key factors of FF are: 'A focus on health and enjoyment', 'a reduced membership fee compared to regular club members', 'no league tournament participation' and 'the possibility for clubs to present the concept in a local way and adapt to the participations'.

Overall, two aspects are very different from the organisation and working procedures of football normally conducted by the DFA and clubs (Bennike, Wikman and Ottesen 2014a). Firstly, it is an activity which is centrally developed and expected to be operationalised regionally and realised locally in a divisional organisational system, which is of particular interest in the following analysis. Secondly, it is an activity where a focus on competition is explicitly toned down and tactical and technical skills do not take highest priority. A local FF organiser explains (Bennike, Wikman and Ottesen 2014a): 'The less you know about football, the better you match our target group. The worse you are at football, the better you match our target group'.

The fact that FF teams do not engage in a league structure means that it can be adapted to local needs in terms of target group, activities, rules and the number of players. In relation to this follows the possibility of a more flexible format than traditional recreational football. A Football Development Officer (FDO) states (Bennike, Thing and Ottesen 2018):

> It is a concept that fits in with a lot of target groups and can be managed in many different ways. Some teams do ordinary fitness exercises, and some just play football. Others mix and match from activities that they are fond of. It is up to the clubs.

A FF administrator puts it this way (Ottesen, Bennike and Thing 2017):

> It is football when people have time for it . . . It is not compulsory in the same way as traditional football, it's not about training twice a week with a match at the weekend, it's more flexible in that way.

Together with the fact that FF, as mentioned previously, brings potential cross-sectoral partnerships, these differences represents a distinct break with the organisation of the 'traditional' understanding of association football (Bennike 2016; Bennike, Thing and Ottesen 2018), bringing potential fruitful perspectives, though also implementational challenges. In relation to this, it is important to add that Denmark does not have an established (and often commercial) 5-a-side culture with an emphasis on casual recreational participation that you might see elsewhere.

3 The implementation of Football Fitness

The following will focus on the implementation process of FF, based on theories related to public policy and administration. In the above, FF has been introduced as an initiative reacting to a changing socioeconomic environment influencing recreational football. It is being developed to renew the game of football – to create more flexibility, to emphasise the fun and social dimensions of the game, and to bring to the fore the healthy benefits of the game. To do so, it will need to challenge and influence the traditional understanding of football and the culture of the clubs and participants involved in FF as the target group. The implementation of FF is like the implementation of a policy enacted and implemented to influence the behaviour of civic institutions and citizens.

According to Winter (2012), implementation is a highly diverse process most often taking place in very different settings with many aspects and variables. This is also the case with the implementation of FF, as will unfold in the following. Winter (2012, 271) concludes that no general implementation theory exists, and he therefore advocates for a focus on partial rather than general implementation theories. In the following we have purposefully selected to focus on *interorganisational implementation behavior* (O'Toole and Montjoy 1984; O'Toole 2012), which has proven to be of crucial importance to the success of FF (Bennike and Ottesen 2016; Bennike 2016).

3.1 The influence of interorganisational implementation behavior

Three actors holding different implementational responsibilities are involved within the implementation creating three levels. These are displayed in Table 11.1 and is defined as the 'central DFA', the 'regional football county unions' (FCUs) and the 'local football clubs'. When two or more organisations are involved in the implementation *interorganisational implementation behavior (IIB)* will occur and influence the implementation (O'Toole and Montjoy 1984; O'Toole 2012). Of great importance to the understanding of IIB, three theoretical aspects are highlighted.

Firstly, do the actors responsible for implementation cooperate? And if so, how do they depend on each other? As illustrated in Table 11.1, each actor holds different implementational responsibilities, which are 'design and continuous adaptation of FF', 'operationalisation of FF' and 'realisation of FF'. At the same time, there is no linkage between the central and the local level, given that the cooperation between the DFA, a FCU and a club can be defined as a *sequentially interdependent chain* (Thompson 1967). This means that A proposes a program, including new routines for B, and so forth. In this sequentially interdependent chain, the working output of A becomes the working input of B, and so forth, highlighted by the arrows also displayed in Table 11.1. Thus, the process of implementation can be defined by two links of cooperation beginning with the cooperation

Table 11.1 Different implementation characteristics of the implementation levels

	Implementation task	*Interests*
Central level DFA	Design and continuous adaptation of FF ⇩	The game of football nationally Strong political voice
Regional level 6 FCUs	Operationalisation of FF ⇩	The game of football regionally Support member clubs Administer regional league tournaments
Local level +1600 Clubs	Realisation of FF	The game of football locally Daily running of club

between the DFA and a FCU, followed by the cooperation between a FCU and a club. Secondly, and of great importance to understanding the links of cooperation, O'Toole and Montjoy (1984) and O'Toole (2012) highlight the influence of the *interests* of the actors involved and the *form of cooperation*. These two aspects are closely related.

Regarding the interests of the DFA, their mission (DFA 2018) is to promote and develop Danish football – from a leisure activity to elite level, which gives the work of the DFA national interests. The DFA receives state funding under the Act of Allocation (Udlodningsloven 2015), and seems keenly aware of its position, e.g. in relation to contributing to national health-programmes (DFA 2018). This means that the central DFA works to advocate for football in a political perspective and is a strong voice in the political agenda. An illustrative case (on addition to the development of FF!) is the present national strategy of the DFA to contract 'welfare-alliances' with municipalities with the mission to make football contribute to the solution of social challenges, including health. In this case, it is providing football with an explicit social role related to the overall DFA vision of being *part of something bigger* (DFA 2018).

The FCUs define themselves as interest organisations of the clubs in their region (see e.g. FCU Zealand 2018a, 2018b). They are especially involved in regional leisure and children's football activities, whereas the DFA oversees the game at a higher level, including national team activity. The FCUs are taking care of tournament structures, referees, bookings and so on, making tournament administration and income their biggest responsibilities (Bennike et al. in review), as the clubs pay tournament fees. Moreover, they receive financial resources due to the membership of the DFA. Nevertheless, they are independent legal units working rather autonomously, holding regional variation to promote and develop football with regional interests (see e.g. FCU Zealand 2018a, 2018b). Other than finances from the DFA and tournament administration, they receive membership fees from the subscriptions of regional member clubs and fees for running coaching, refereeing and club management courses.

Regarding the interests of the club, a survey shows that the focus is mainly on activities for children and young ones, and the primary objective is to create a sense of social community for their members (Bennike, Wikman and Ottesen 2014b). Notwithstanding these characteristics, clubs function with local variation, as they are managed relatively autonomously, relying on their respective members, culture and structure to conduct the activities they feel are most suitable for them. Regarding the implementation of FF, this becomes very important, as they, in contrast to the FCU, can decline or accept to realise the initiative. The funding for clubs is provided by the municipalities in the form of rooms/halls/fields for sport, and on a member basis for members under the age of 25 in accordance with the Act of Enlightenment (Folkeoplysningsloven 2011). Moreover, membership fees and activities organised by volunteers represent the main income (Ibsen and Seippel 2010).

O'Toole (2012, 296) highlights three different forms of cooperation, strongly related to interests. One form is *authority*, where B cooperates with A because B feels it is an obligation. The cooperation derives from a sense of duty, so to speak. Based on the above, it is obvious that authority is not a thriving force due to strong levels of autonomy. Here, a group of FDOs are discussing the implementation (Bennike and Ottesen 2016):

KASPER: It is the way that the DFA is organised, which becomes a road block. The DFA is the big central, but it (FF) needs to be sold locally, which is two different accounts and two different legal units, and it causes bickering. Just because the big top organisation thinks this is fun, it is not necessary the case out there.

SVEND: The FCUs is self-governing in many ways. They belong to the DFA, and they do want to cooperate. But there is some power which is not clear. And we (as FDOs) sense this.

A second form of cooperation is *common interests*, which relates strongly to what is going to be implemented and how the content of the new initiative fits with the overall interests presented above. In this form, B cooperates with A because B feels that doing so would also serve B's interests. The cooperation exists because each participant values the goal of the new initiative. Both the DFA and the FCU want the game of football to maintain its strong position in Denmark and in each region. However, they do not seem to agree on how to accomplish this interest. Two FCU administrators state (Bennike and Ottesen 2016):

CHARLOTTE: I believe that this is a classic example on how we forget to listen (. . .). We have already asked the clubs, what their challenges are. We (the DFA) would like more members, the clubs are screaming for more coaches and more volunteers (. . .) Put in another way, we could have spent some of the funding's (for FF) differently.

JOHN: First of all, and I believe that this is the crucial challenge, the concept has its source in the DFA. Not in the clubs. I mean no matter how you put it; it is about getting more members overall in the DFA. We have made investigations in our clubs, showing that member attraction is not a main priority. They have other aspects they feel is more important. So, you have a mismatch between the desire of the DFA and the needs of the clubs.

These statements reveal two interesting aspects. Firstly, the FCUs understanding of FF is that it is designed to attract members, which is not the sole objective of FF. This understanding is logical though, as the DFA has set certain success criteria based on the number of FF participants. This is how the FCU is evaluated as an operational actor. They are asked to deliver results in terms of how many new FF clubs they establish. Two possible conclusions are that the DFA has not been successful in explaining the concept or that the FCUs have misunderstood it. Regardless, the FCU seems skeptical about FF, and a lack of common interest exists. Secondly, the FCUs refer to the clubs as 'our clubs'. This emphasises that the main interest of the FCUs is to support the clubs of their region of responsibility, in whatever seems to be the club's interests, which leads to another interesting aspect; in the view of the FCUs, a strong interest of the clubs is to attract more volunteers. This is not untrue, though it is not the only interest and the reason why clubs might be interested in FF is influenced by several local factors, such as the surrounding society and the club's culture (Bennike 2016). Moreover, if a club decides to implement FF, it will be directed by interest; otherwise FF would not have been initiated in the first place, as no club is forced to realise FF. If we look closer at how FF fits with the interests of the clubs, in a one-size-fits-all perspective, the reason FCU administrators believe that clubs are not interested in FF becomes clear. FF is designed to accommodate new target groups above 25 years of age, among others, which does not fit with the main interests of the clubs already stated, namely to carry out activities for children and young people and create a sense of social community for their existing members. As already stated, it would be wrong to apply the same yardstick to all clubs, but on the face of it, there is a mismatch between the characteristics of FF and the interests of (many) clubs.

The third form of cooperation is *exchange*, where B cooperates with A because B receives something in return other than achieving the goal. Regarding the implementation of FF, the DFA introduces the concept to the FCU, while financial resources follow, marked for the work of FF administrators and FDOs. Moreover, the DFA provides incitements for clubs to start. Initially, this was a starting kit, including a small amount of funding and equipment for the FCUs to deliver to a club willing to initiate FF. In addition, clubs who initiated FF had the possibility of buying a multi-court from the DFA with a discount of DKK 70,000 (approx. €9,400). Though based on this example, the DFA is, in practice, exchanging funds for the time spent on FF by the FCU as operators, and offering resources and an offer to be passed on from the FCU to the club as realiser of the initiative.

To sum up, authority is very limited in both links of cooperation, whereas common interests are more complex to analyse, as the interest is present in the central level, lacking in the regional level and present in the local level if they accept to work with the initiative. From this, one can argue that exchange is the strongest with both links of cooperation when it comes to putting the implementation process into action, as the FCU is paid to work with the implementation and the club receives a starting kit. O'Toole and Montjoy (1984, 492) state that if the actors experience common interest in the new program or have immensely strong authority, this might be enough to produce an effective implementation. But in the absence or sparsity of both common interest and authority, there is likely to be very little coordinated effort unless the necessary exchange is provided. The question to be asked is, if the exchange in this case is strong enough to work as a significant driver. Given that the starting kit and the significant discount on a new court comes from the DFA, it might be argued that the central level is exchanging with the local level, while the regional level serves as an intermediary with no gain. An important point mentioned, not yet elaborated on, is the fact that funding for the different levels comes from different cash flows. The DFA and the clubs do, to some extent, experience pressure from their surroundings being funded by the state and members, respectively. This is not the case for the FCUs, which are funded by clubs and the DFA. The regional level exists in a space bordering the central and local levels, but not the surrounding society (at least not to the same extent as the DFA and clubs). FF is designed to meet the changes in sporting activity patterns of individuals, funding for sport and the social role of organised sport, but the surroundings of the FCUs (the DFA and clubs) do not change at the same pace. This means that the regional level does not gain directly from FF, which limits motivation and interest in working with the implementation. Moreover, the main job of the FCU is to administer tournaments, which are not a feature of FF. So, by providing FF, they might feel they are undermining their existence.

According to Bennike and Ottesen (2016), and the experiences of the co-authors of this chapter connecting on different levels to the implementation of FF, the challenge of cooperation between implementational actors comes as no surprise. Next step is to consider how to reduce these challenges. Following the theory of IIB, we need to pay attention to the form of cooperation (authority, common interest and exchange) and try to adjust these. In that regard, we take the perspective that it is not possible to change the implementational system as being sequential and interdependent, nor possible to change the institutions involved. To change this 'setup' would be a complex, troublesome process, but necessary to optimise the implementation process. If it is in the common interest to optimise the implementation process, it is necessary to adjust the FF concept to fit with the interest of all implementation levels or to convince all that the concept is important and necessary. This is especially needed at the regional level. If we also take the view that it is not possible to change the concept, then exchange is the last form of cooperation to adjust. In this case, it is necessary to optimise the trade-off so that all implementation levels are satisfied. This, again, is especially needed at the regional level.

4. From news to everyday use

'*From news to everyday use*' (Guldbrandsson 2008) is a literature review on the implementation of health-enhancing initiatives in the health care sector. While the context is different from voluntarily organised football clubs, the conclusions can enrich a discussion of perspectives for future consideration for football for health initiatives (Bennike 2016). In the review, several traits are highlighted as critical to a successful implementation. New initiatives, such as FF, must respectively bring visible benefits and be in line with the norms, values and working methods of the organisations implementing it. Moreover, it should be easy to use and adaptable to the needs of the recipient. In the case of FF, and following the analysis presented above, these traits are predominantly present in the central and local level of implementation.

Regarding the DFA, they are, as mentioned previously, concerned with their political position and their ability to work strategically in that regard, of which FF is providing a clear message of how football can tackle health-related issues of huge important to the state and municipalities. In a study by Casey, Payne and Eime (2012) it is highlighted how big sporting organisations (800+ member clubs), such as the DFA, have high abilities and the capacity to work with health policy-related issues. In comparison, and although the FCUs member clubs are included in the DFA, smaller organisations, such as the regional FCUs, have less ability and capacity. This is an implementational challenge not to be overlooked – namely the cooperation of a central (DFA) and a regional (FCU) organisation, in which the all-important function of the latter is to administrate tournaments, not to build strong relations to health-related organisations. This structure or work-sharing agreement is a well-oiled machine for conducting tournaments and promoting the traditional understanding of the game. But it is not a machine which is very well oiled regarding the promotion of initiatives such as FF.

Regarding the clubs, it is important to highlight that they can adopt FF in a form which is suitable to them and their target group. Based on four cases, Bennike (2016) shows how the local organisation of FF relates strongly to the existing norms, values and working procedures of the organising club responsible for realisation. If the club does not feel it fits with existing norms, values and working procedures, they can close the team or simply decide not to work with it in the first place, which is the case of many clubs. From the same cases, Bennike (2016) points to the fact that the clubs are experiencing visible benefits from FF. A club chairmen states (Bennike 2016):

> FF (for women) has changed the club from an absolutely laddish atmosphere to a respectably place. It has created a new behavior. The male chauvinistic atmosphere, which me myself is a part of has heavily calmed down – all for the better. . . . This FF-team have put our club on the map. We can show the municipality that we are more than playing tournaments.

Moreover Bennike, Wikman and Ottesen (2014a) show, based on a questionnaire survey, that many of the clubs that offer FF find that it enhances club life, social activities and parental environment. These outcomes are in line with the clubs' overall focus, as already mentioned, on children and young people and on providing a social community for members. What does not appeal to the clubs at first glance, remembering that FF is targeting participants over the age of 25 and most often being new to the club, may produce the exact result that the clubs identify as their main purpose.

As shown, the success of initiatives like FF are dependent of the final actor. In this case, the football clubs serve as grassroots implementers. Firstly, if no clubs are willing to organise FF you will have no activity, and secondly, the activities are realised as organised by the clubs. This opens an important discussion when promoting FF among clinical populations, which often brings additional implementational actors neglected in the previous analysis. From this perspective, it is of pivotal importance to implementation to establish stable and formal infrastructures and cooperation across health sectors to secure recruitment of participants, including the potential consecutive referral of patients from either hospitals or municipality health care centers. Moreover, the implementation of FF as a complementary treatment and/or rehabilitation strategy requires proactive solutions to challenges related to sustainable economic models and clinical responsibility. Such new models and policies are usually contingent on solid evidence (including cost-effectiveness analyses) of the health effects. However, to date, football intervention studies in clinical populations (i.e. type 2 diabetes, prostate cancer, mild hypertension) are characterised by relatively small sample sizes ($n < 100$) and interventions delivered by trained physiologists in ideal settings (Milanović et al. 2018), and thus with little generalisability to the real-life sport clubs setting, which FF is part of. This is characterised by limited or unstable resources including involvement of volunteers and collection of member fees. As such, evidence of the health benefits of FF when implemented in the existing structure is still limited, and further research examining the effectiveness of FF in relation to improvement of clinically relevant outcomes in different patient groups is highly warranted. Also, further research into barriers and facilitators related to the referral of clinical populations, including experiences and attitudes of health professionals, policy makers and volunteers, are needed to guide and promote long-term sustainability.

In the article entitled 'Where is the implementation in sport policy and programme analysis? The English Football Association's Charter Standard as an illustration' (O'Gorman, 2011, 86), the author states that there are numerous studies that in essence touch upon implementation, yet most fail to explicitly address it and do not consider theories of implementation evident in social and political science. Our analysis presented is an exception. In line with O'Gorman and building on Ooms et al.'s (2015) request for more research seeking to understand the implementation context, we advocate for a stronger focus on gaining knowledge about the possibility of realising evidence-based football for health concepts in real-life settings, such as locally organised non-profit, state-funded football clubs. If this is not the case, great expectations from a central level will most likely be dashed on a local level. Why this does not seem to be the case with FF, now holding approx. 380 clubs (of +1600) and 500 teams targeting different groups of participants, is the fact that it is adaptable to the clubs securing interest. On that note, we argue for strong awareness regarding how the content (including expected outcomes!) of a given initiative match the organisational context in which it is to be implemented. Currently, FF is spreading to the Faroe Islands, Norway and Sweden, and we encourage scholars of different disciplines to explicitly focus on the realisation and implementation process of these or other football for health initiatives.

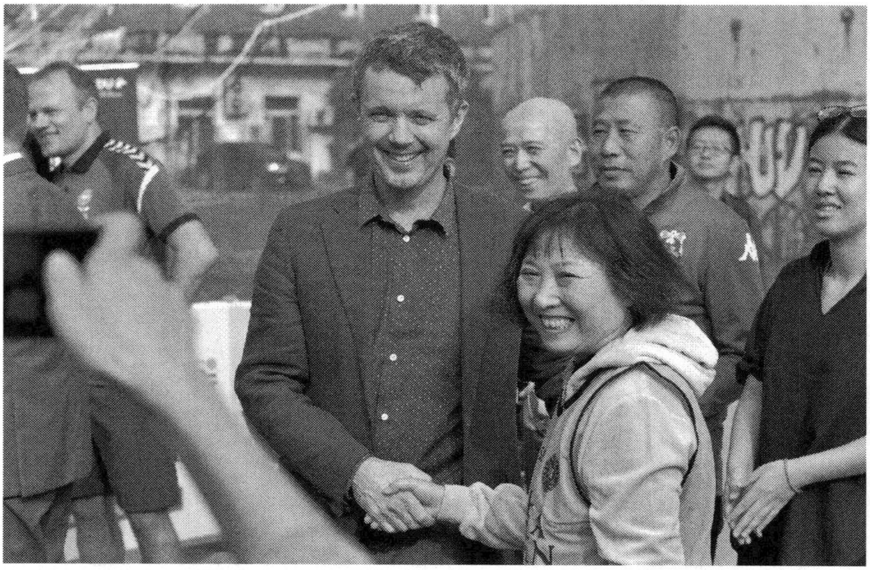

Photo 11.2 Football Fitness is currently being promoted in many countries, including China. His Royal Highness Crown Prince Frederik of Denmark is shaking hands with one of the Football Fitness players during the Beijing Design Week, September 2018.

Source: Photo Credit: The Royal Danish Embassy in Beijing.

Note

1 Football Fitness After Breast Cancer.

References

Bangsbo, J., A. Junge, J. Dvorak and P. Krustrup. 2014. Executive summary: Football for health prevention and treatment of non-communicable diseases across the lifespan through football. *Scandinavian Journal of Medicine & Science in Sports*. 24 (Suppl. 1):147–150.

Bennike, S. 2016. *Fodbold Fitness – Implementeringen af en ny fodboldkultur* [Football Fitness: The implementation of a new football culture]. PhD-Monograph. University of Copenhagen, Faculty of Science, Department of Nutrition, Exercise and Sports. Frederiksberg C.

Bennike, S. and L. Ottesen. 2016. How does interorganisational implementation behaviour challenge the success of Football Fitness? *European Journal for Sport and Society, Special Issue: Sport Organisations in Europe-Changes and Challenges*. 13 (1):19–37.

Bennike, S., R. Storm, J.M. Wikman and L. Ottesen (in review). The Organisation of Club Football in Denmark: A Contemporary Profile.

Bennike, S., L.F. Thing and L. Ottesen. 2018. Health through state supported voluntary sport clubs. In *Sport and Health: Exploring the Current State of Play*, edited by D. Parnel and P. Krustrup, 111–131. Abingdon, UK: Routledge.

Bennike, S., J.M. Wikman and L. Ottesen. 2014a. Football Fitness: A new version of football? A concept for adult players in Danish football clubs. *Scandinavian Journal of Medicine and Science in Sports*. 24 (Suppl. 1):138–146.

Bennike, S., J.M. Wikman and L. Ottesen. 2014b. *Fodbold Fitness – Implementeringsstudie. 2013* [Football Fitness: Implementation study, 2013]. Center For Holdspil og Sundhed. Institut for Idræt og Ernæring. Københavns Universitet.

Bjerre, E.D., M. Leth, N.M. Hammer and J. Midtgaard. 2018. Development of an educational program for non-professional soccer coaches in charge of community-based soccer in men with prostate cancer: A qualitative study. *Sports Medicine Open*. 4(1):31.

Bruun, D.M., E. Bjerre, P. Krustrup, K. Brasso, C. Johansen, M. Rørth and J. Midtgaard. 2014. Community-based recreational football: A novel approach to promote physical activity and quality of life in prostate cancer survivors. *International Journal Environmental Research and Public Health*. May 26;11(6):5567–5585.

Campbell, J.L. 2004. *Institutional Change and Globalization*. Woodstock, Oxfordshire: Princeton University Press.

Casey, M.M., W.R. Payne, S.J. Brown and R.M. Eime. 2009. Engaging community sport and recreation organisations in population health interventions: Factors affecting the formation, implementation, and institutionalization of partnerships efforts. *Annals of Leisure Research*. 12:129–147. DOI: 10.1080/11745398.2009.9686815.

Casey, M.M., W.R. Payne, and R.M. Eime. 2012. Organisational readiness and capacity building strategies of sporting organisations to promote health. *Sport Management Review*. Feb. 2012;15(1), 109–124.

Danish Government. 2014. Et sundere liv for alle – Nationale mål for danskernes sundhed de næste 10 år. [A healthier life for all: National goals for the health of the Danes in the coming 10 years]. Sum.dk. København.

DCSa (Danish Cancer Society). 2018. www.cancer.dk/nyheder/fodbold-fitness-skal-styrke-kvinder-efter-brystkraeft/. Visited 4.10.2018.

DCSb (Danish Cancer Society). 2018. www.cancer.dk/nyheder/fc-prostata-fodbold-sparkes-i-gang-over-hele-landet/+https://fcprostata.dk/. Visited 4.10.2018.

DFA (Danish Football Association). 2010a. Fodbold Fitness (motionsfodbold) [Football Fitness (exercise football)]. (internal document).

DFA (Danish Football Association). 2010b. Fodbold som fitness [Football as Fitness]. Press Release December.

DFA (Danish Football Association). 2018. DBU's værdigrundlag. [DFA values]. www.dbu.dk/oevrigt_indhold/om_dbu/dbus_strategi/vaerdigrundlag. Visited 4.10.2018.

FCU Zealand. 2018a. Ide- og strategigrundlag. [Idea and strategy basis]. www.dbusjaelland.dk/oevrigt_indhold/om-dbu-sjaelland/dbu_sjaellands_idegrundlag. Visited 4.10. 2018.

FCU Zealand. 2018b. DBU Sjællands love. [DBU Zealand love]. www.dbusjaelland.dk/oevrigt_indhold/om-dbu-sjaelland/dbusjaellands_love#%C2%A7%201%20Navn%20og%20form%C3%A5l. Visited 4.10.2018.

FFI (Football Fitness Instructors manuals). 2018. www.bevaegdigforlivet.dk/media/2690/26815_bdfl_fodboldfitness_kursist_a4-haefte_tryk.pdf+www.bevaegdigforlivet.dk/media/2691/26815_bdfl_fodboldfitness_oevelse_a4-haefte_tryk.pdf. Visited 4.10.2018.

FIFA (Fédération Internationale de Football Association). 2006. www.fifa.com/mm/document/fifafacts/bcoffsurv/bigcount.statspackage_7024.pdf. Visited 4.10.2018.

Finch, C.F. and A. Donaldson. 2010. A sports setting matrix for understanding the implementation context for community sport. *British Journal of Sports Medicine*. 44(13):973–978.

Folkeoplysningsloven. 2011. Bekendtgørelse af lov om støtte til folkeoplysende voksenundervisning, frivilligt folkeoplysende foreningsarbejde og daghøjskoler samt Folkeuniversitet (folkeoplysningsloven). [Act on support for adult education, Voluntary Association work and day high schools and University Extension (General Education Act)]. Kulturministeriet. LBK nr. 854 af 11/07/2011.

Guldborgsund. 2018. www.guldborgsund.dk/da/Borger/SUNDHED_OG_SYGDOM/Genoptraening/Fodbold_fitness.aspx. Visited 4.10.2018.

Guldbrandsson, K. (2008): *From news to everyday use – The difficult art of implementation.* Swedish National Institute of Public Health, Östersund R 2008:09.

Harris, S., K. Mori and M. Collins. 2009. Great expectations: Voluntary sports clubs and their role in delivering national policy for English sport. *Voluntas*. 20:405–423. DOI: 10.1070/s11266-009-9095-y.

Henderson, K.A. 2009. A paradox of sport management and physical activity interventions. *Sport Management Review*. 12:57–65.

Ibsen, B. and H. Eichberg. 2012. Dansk idrætspolitik – mellem frivillighed og statslig styring [Danish sport for all policy: Between voluntarism and governmental control]. In *Idrætspolitik i komparativ belysning – national og international*, edited by H. Eichberg, 147–209. Odense: Syddansk Universitetsforlag.

Ibsen, B. and Ø. Seippel. 2010. Voluntary organized sport in Denmark and Norway. *Sport in Society: Cultures, Commerce, Media, Politics*. 13(4):593–608.

Kokko, S. 2014. Guidelines for youth sports clubs to develop, implement, and assess health promotion within its activities. *Health Promotion Practice*. 15:373–382. DOI: 10.1177/1524839913513900.

Krustrup, B.R. and L. Ottesen. 2014. *Fodbold Fitness – Pilotstudie* [Football Fitness pilotstudy] Udarbejdet i 2011. Center For Holdspil og Sundhed. Institut for Idræt og Ernæring. Københavns Universitet.

Krustrup, P., P. Aagaard, L. Nybo, J. Petersen, M. Mohr and J. Bangsbo. 2010a. Recreational football as a health promoting activity: A topical review. *Scandinavian Journal of Medicine & Science in Sports*. 20 (Suppl. 1):1–13.

Krustrup, P., J. Dvorak, A. Junge and J. Bangsbo. 2010b. Executive summary: The health and fitness benefits of regular participation in small-sided football games. *Scandinavian Journal of Medicine & Science in Sports*. 20 (Suppl. 1):132–135.

Krustrup, P., C.A. Williams, M. Mohr, P.R. Hansen, E.W. Helge, A.-M. Elbe, M. de Sousa, et al. 2018. Editorial: The "Football is medicine" platform: Scientific evidence, large-scale implementation of evidence-based concepts and future perspectives. *Scandinavian Journal of Medicine & Science in Sports*. 28(Suppl. 1):3–7.

Lee, I.M., E.J. Shiroma, F. Lobelo, P. Puska, S.N. Blair and P.T. Katzmarkzyk. 2012. The lancet physical activity series working group: Effect of physical inactivity on major non-communicable diseases worldwide: An analysis of burden of disease and life expectancy. *Lancet*. 380(9838):19–229.

Lipsky, M. 1980. *Street Level Bureaucracy: Dilemmas of the Individual in Public Service*. New York: Russel Sage Foundation.

May, P.J. 2012. Policy design and implementation. In *The Sage handbook of public administration* (2nd ed.), edited by B.G. Peters and J. Pierre, 279–291. Thousand Oaks, CA: Sage Publication.

May, T., S. Harris and M. Collins. 2013. Implementing community sport policy: Understanding the variety of voluntary club types and their attitudes to policy. *International Journal of Sport Policy and Politics*. 5:397–419. DOI: 10.1080/19406940.2012.735688.

MCD (Ministry of Culture Denmark). 2014. *Udredning af idrættens økonomi og struktur. Analyse*. Af: Kulturministeriet, Idrættens analyseinstitut og KPMG. http://kum.dk/uploads/tx_templavoila/Udredning%20af%20idrattens%20okonomi%20og%20struktur,%20Analyse%201.pdf. Visited 4.10.2018.

Meyers, M.K. and V.L. Nielsen. 2012. Street-level bureaucrats and the implementation of public policy. In *The Sage handbook of public administration* (2nd ed.), edited by B.G. Peters and J. Pierre, 305–318. Thousand Oaks, CA: Sage Publication.

Milanović, Z., S. Pantelić, N. Čović, G. Sporis and P. Krustrup. 2015. Is recreational soccer effective for improving VO2max a systematic review and meta-analysis. *Sports Medicine*. 45:1339–1353.

Milanović, Z., S. Pantelić, N. Čović, G. Sporis, M. Mohr and P. Krustrup. 2018. Broad-spectrum physical fitness benefits of recreational football: A systematic review and meta-analysis. *British Journal of Sports Medicine*. 2018:1–14.

O'Gorman, J. 2011. Where is the implementation in spot policy programme analysis? The English Football Association's Charter Standard as an illustration. *International Journal of Sport Policy and Politics*. 3(1):85–108.

Oja, P., S. Titze, S. Kokko, U.M. Kujala, A. Heinonen, P. Kelly, P. Kaski and C. Foster. 2015. Health benefits of different sport disciplines for adults: Systematic review of observational and intervention studies with meta-analysis. *British Journal of Sports Medicine*. 49:434–440.

Ooms, L., C. Veenhof, N.S. Veldhoven and D.H. de Bakker. 2015. Sporting programs for inactive population groups: Factors influencing implementation in the organized sports setting. *BMS Sports Science, Medicine, and Rehabilitation*. 7:1–14. DOI: 10.1186/s13102-015-0007-8.

O'Toole, L.J., Jr. 2012. Interorganizational relations and policy implementation. In *The Sage handbook of public administration* (2nd ed.), edited by B.G. Peters and J. Pierre, 292–304. Thousand Oaks, CA: Sage Publication.

O'Toole, LJ., Jr. and R.S. Montjoy. 1984. Interorganizational policy implementation: A theoretical perspective. *Public Administration Review*. 44:491–503. London.

Ottesen, L., S. Bennike and L.F. Thing 2017. The emergence of the Danish Football Fitness concept. *Proceedings of the 8th World Congress on Science and Football*. Copenhagen.

Ottesen, L. and Jacobsen, P.J. 2011. Idræt og velfærdspolitik – Indledning. *Forum for Idræt. Idræt og velfærdspolitik*, January.

Ottesen, L., R.S. Jeppesen and B.R. Krustrup. 2010. The development of social capital through football and running: Studying an intervention program for inactive women. *Scandinavian Journal of Medicine & Science in Sports*. 20:118–131.

Pilgaard, M. and S. Rask. 2016. *Danskernes motions-og sportsvaner 2016*. [Sports participation in Denmark 2016]. København: Idrættens Analyseinstitut.

Scott, W.R. 2014. *Institutions and Organizations: Ideas, Interests, and Identities* (4th ed.). Thousand Oaks, CA: Sage Publications.

Skille, E. 2008. Understanding sport clubs as sport policy implementers: A theoretical framework for the analysis of the implementation of central sport policy through local and voluntary sport organizations. *International Review for the Sociology of Sport*. 43:181–200. DOI: 10.1177/1012690208096035.

Skille, E. 2009. State sport policy and voluntary sport clubs: The case of the Norwegian sports city programme as social policy. *European Sport Management Quarterly*. 9:63–79. DOI: 10.1080/16184740802461736.

Sydow, J., G. Schreyögg and J. Koch 2005. Organizational paths: Path dependency and beyond. *21st. EGOS Colloquium*, June 30–July 2, Berlin, Germany.

Thompson, J.D. 1967. *Organizations in Action*. New York: McGraw-Hill.
Udlodningsloven. 2015. Bekendtgørelse af lov om udlodning af overskud fra lotteri samt heste-og hundevæddemål udlodningsloven) [Act on distribution of profits from lotteries, horse racing and dog racing (distribution law)]. LBK nr. 115 af 1/01/2015.
Winter, S.C. 2012. Implementation. In *The Sage handbook of public administration* (2nd ed.), edited by B.G. Peters and J. Pierre, 254–318. Thousand Oaks, CA: Sage Publication.

Chapter 12

Injury prevention in football

The 11+ programme

Mario Bizzini, Oliver Faude and Jiri Dvorak

12.1 Introduction

Football is the most popular sport worldwide, and is played competitively on amateur or recreational level by almost 300 million people. While football can be considered a healthy leisure activity, football, as a contact team sport, entails also a certain risk of injury. The medical treatment of football-related injuries can have a significant socio-economic impact in terms of related healthcare costs (Bizzini, Junge, and Dvorak 2013).

In 1994, FIFA realised their responsibility towards player's health and safety, and founded the FIFA – Medical Assessment and Research Centre (F-MARC) in order to create and disseminate scientific knowledge on various medical topics in football, to reduce football injuries and thus, to promote football as a health enhancing leisure activity (Dvorak 2009). This chapter presents the theoretical background, development, scientific evaluation, implementation and dissemination strategies of injury prevention programmes (The 11 and later The 11+), under the leadership of F-MARC (1994–2016), in order to provide a role model of how an international sports governing body can make its sport safer.

12.2 Development of injury prevention programmes

The first scientific study on injury prevention in football was published in 1983 (Ekstrand, Gillquist, and Liljedahl 1983). Over the next 20 years, only a few authors reported studies on prevention of football injuries. In 2000, F-MARC conducted its first study on the prevention of football injuries in male Swiss youth teams, showing 21% fewer injuries in the intervention compared to the control group (Junge et al. 2002). The interventions were focused on improving the structure and content of the training by educating and supervising the coaches and players. The prevention program included general interventions such as improvement of warm-up, regular cool-down, taping of unstable ankles, adequate rehabilitation, promotion of the spirit of fair play and 10 sets of exercises designed to improve coordination, stability of ankle and knee, flexibility and strength of trunk, hip and leg muscles. Based on the experiences with this pilot study and in cooperation with international experts, F-MARC developed in 2003 a simple injury prevention programme for amateur football players called 'The 11'.

The 11 comprises 10 evidence-based or best-practice exercises (core stability, balance, dynamic stabilisation and eccentric hamstring strength) and the promotion of Fair Play. The programme was designed to reduce the most common football injuries (ankle and knee sprains, hamstring and groin strains). It can be completed in 10 to 15 minutes and requires no equipment other than a ball. The 11 was implemented in two countrywide campaigns (Switzerland and New Zealand) in cooperation with the national accident insurance companies and the national football associations (Bizzini, Junge, and Dvorak 2013).

In Switzerland, the implementation of The 11 and its effects on the injury rates were evaluated by an independent research institute. Four years after the launch of the programme, teams that included The 11 as a part of their warm-up had 11.5% fewer match injuries and 25.3% fewer training injuries than team that warmed-up as usual (Junge et al. 2011). In New Zealand, the implementation of The 11 resulted in a 8.2 dollars of return of investment (per invested dollar) for the national accident insurance company after seven years (Bizzini, Junge, and Dvorak 2013).

In two controlled randomised studies (RCTs) on The 11, only small effects were found in terms of injury prevention in male and female players. Compliance issues and exercise dosage were discussed as the main points of concern (Bizzini, Junge, and Dvorak 2013). Based on experiences with The 11, 'PEP' (Prevent Injury and Enhance Performance programme) (Gilchrist et al. 2008) and other exercised-based programmes to prevent football injuries, an advanced version ('The 11+') were developed in 2006 together with the OSTRC and the Santa Monica Orthopaedic and Sports Medicine Research Foundation. The 11+ is a complete warm-up programme with running exercises in the beginning and at the end to activate the cardiovascular system, and specific preventive exercises focussing on core and leg strength, balance and agility, each of three levels of increasing difficulty (to providing variation and progression). It takes about 20 to 25 minutes to be completed, and requires a minimum of equipment (a set of cones, and balls) (http://fifamedicinediploma.com/courses/injury-prevention/). The 11+ should replace the usual warm-up few times a week (Bizzini, Junge, and Dvorak 2013). As from 2007, different research groups worldwide evaluated the preventive and performance effects of this basic prevention programme (Bizzini and Dvorak 2015; Al Attar et al. 2016; Thorborg et al. 2017).

12.3 Evidence of injury prevention for 11+ in female and male players

The efficacy of The 11+ was first proven in young female players, which was similar for PEP, a non-contact ACL prevention programme. A significant reduction (up to 50%) of injuries was found in young female players in large RCTs when the warm-up exercises were performed at least twice a week (Soligard et al. 2008; Steffen, Meeuwisse et al. 2013). In both studies the role of compliance was documented, showing a further reduction of injury risk in those players with higher adherence to the programme. Recently, a similar impact of The 11+ was reported in two RCTs involving male players (Owoeye et al. 2014; Silvers-Granelli et al. 2015). Owoeye et al. (2014) found a lower (ca. 40%) incidence of injuries in young Nigerian male players who conducted The 11+ exercises, and Silvers-Granelli et al. (2015) reported similar results in American male NCAA Division I-II players – when performing the programme regularly (2–3 ×/week). These four RCTs impressively showed how a basic injury prevention programme, with proper players' compliance, significantly reduces injuries both in female and male amateur football. Recent systematic reviews on structured neuromuscular warm-up programmes underline the evidence behind the preventive effects of The 11+ in youth amateur football (Bizzini and Dvorak 2015; Al Attar et al. 2016; Thorborg et al. 2017). A recent systematic review and meta-analysis concluded that The 11+ has a substantial injury-preventing effect by reducing football injuries in recreational/ subelite football by 39% (Thorborg et al. 2017).

12.4 The 11+ Kids

In other age groups, especially in children (below 14 years of age), there is a paucity of research in injuries and their prevention (Rossler et al. 2014). A systematic review analysed the epidemiology of football injuries in children and adolescents as a foundation for preventive strategies in children playing football (Faude, Rossler, and Junge 2013). The results of this review served as a basis for developing an adapted '11+ Kids' programme.

This preliminary programme was pilot tested with regard to feasibility and neuromuscular training adaptations (Rossler et al. 2016). The results of this pilot study were used to further adapt the programme which was finally evaluated with regard to its efficacy in reducing injuries in children´s football in a large multi-national cluster randomised controlled trial, including nearly 4,000 children of 7 to 13 years of age in four European countries (Rossler, Junge, et al. 2018). Injury incidence was reduced by nearly 50% in the intervention group which conducted 11+ Kids as a warm-up compared to a control group which performed their routine warm-up (Rossler, Junge, et al. 2018). Likely more important is the observation that nearly three quarters of all severe injuries (i.e. a lay-off time of more than four weeks) could be prevented (Beaudouin et al. 2018). The compliance analysis showed that one 11+ Kids session per week relevantly reduced injury risk. Two sessions per week, however, resulted in a near maximal efficacy with additional sessions not relevantly increasing the effect. A cost-effectiveness analysis of these data revealed that the 11+ Kids programme reduced the healthcare costs by more than 50% compared with a usual warm-up (Rossler, Verhagen, et al. 2018).

12.5 The referees

The match officials are an important but often unrecognised part of football. In modern football, referees (especially at elite level) are exposed to considerable

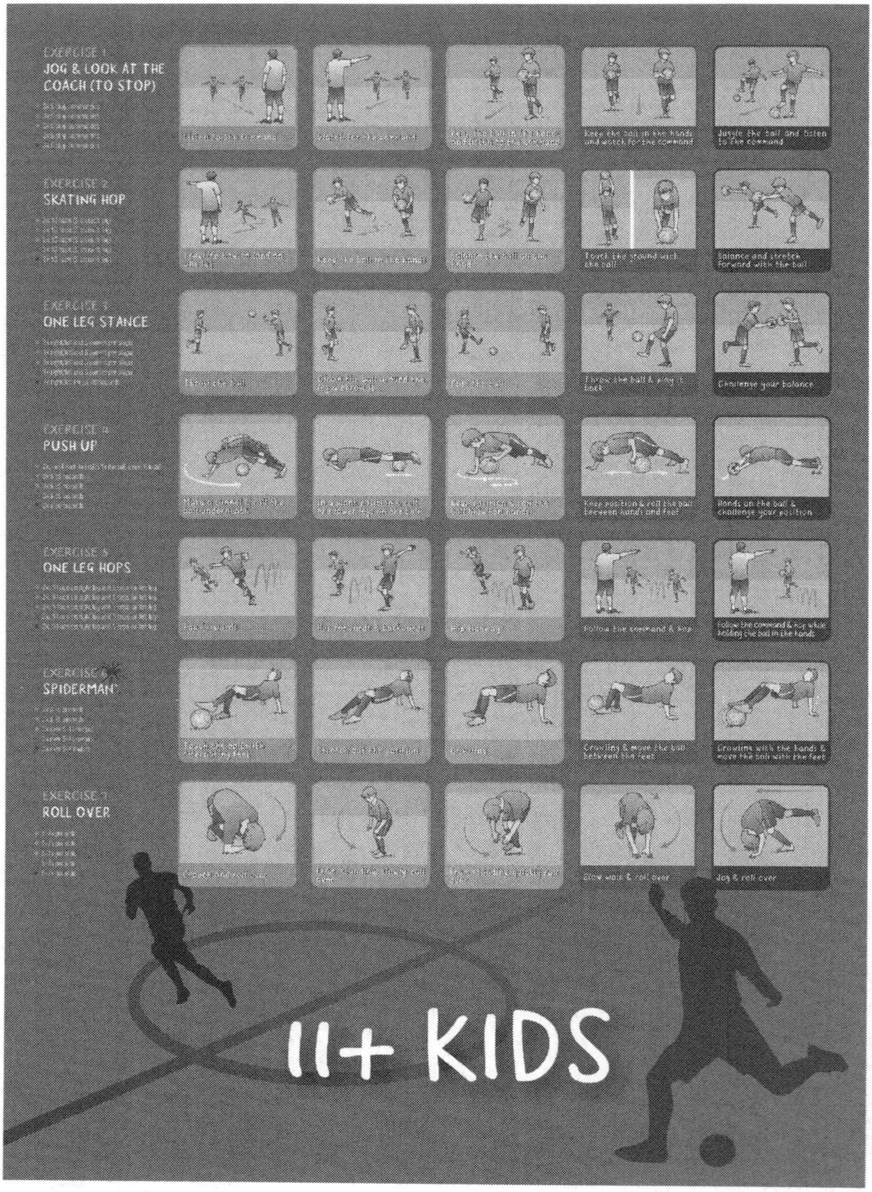
EXERCISE 1
JOG & LOOK AT THE COACH (TO STOP)
Keep the ball in the hands and watch for the command
Juggle the ball and listen to the command
EXERCISE 2
SKATING HOP
Balance and stretch forward with the ball
EXERCISE 3
ONE LEG STANCE
Challenge your balance
EXERCISE 4
PUSH UP
Keep position & roll the ball between hands and feet
Hands on the ball & challenge your position
EXERCISE 5
ONE LEG HOPS
Follow the command & hop
Follow the command & hop while holding the ball in the hands
EXERCISE 6
SPIDERMAN
Crawling & move the ball between the feet
Crawling with the hands & move the ball with the feet
EXERCISE 7
ROLL OVER
Slow walk & roll over
Jog & roll over
11+ KIDS

Figure 12.1 11+ KIDS poster (with permission of C. von Grebel and M. Bizzini, Zürich, Switzerland).

amounts of match and training loads. While several (but to a lesser extent than in players) studies have addressed different aspects of performance and training, the associated injury risk in referees has been investigated recently. Based on the their specific injury profile and on the success of 11+, an '11+ Referee' injury prevention programme for referees and assistant referees has been developed and pilot tested (Weston et al. 2012). The programme is being distributed worldwide (since 2013) within FIFA Refereeing courses, and can be accessed online (http://fifamedicinediploma.com/courses/referee/).

12.6 Performance and warm-up effects of the 11+

'What are the performance benefits of such exercises?' is one of the most common questions by football coaches when exposed to a so-called 'injury prevention programme'. Various studies have investigated the performance effects of the 11+ in male and female players. An RCT found significantly better neuromuscular control (quicker stabilisation time of lower extremity and core) in Italian amateur male players after nine weeks of the 11+ practice (Impellizzeri et al. 2013). Others (Steffen, Emery, et al. 2013) showed significant better functional balance in Canadian young female players performing the 11+ during a season in another RCT. Further studies found improved knee strength ratios, static/dynamic balance and agility skills in Asian male players after performing the 11+ warm-up for an average time of two months. A pre-post study in Italian male amateur players showed how 11+ induces similar physiological responses as other published warm-ups (Bizzini et al. 2013). Recently, two studies showed how 11+ exercises can trigger core and hip musculature activation, therefore improving neuromuscular control (Figure 12.1). Other studies have found positive performance enhancement effects of the 11+ in male futsal players (Bizzini et al. 2013).

A recent systematic review and meta-analysis reported beneficial adaptations in various neuromuscular performance markers, e.g. balance/stability measures, leg power and isokinetic hamstring and quadriceps strength as well as hamstring-to-quadriceps ratio, but also in sprint abilities and sport-specific skills as a result of multimodal injury prevention programmes (Faude et al. 2017). Similarly, there is evidence that injury prevention programmes focusing on core stability, leg strength, dynamic balance/stability and eccentric hamstrings strength improve potential biomechanical risk factors for lower-limb ligament and muscle injuries (Lopes et al. 2018; Pappas et al. 2015; Ribeiro-Alvares et al. 2018). These improvements in neuromuscular and biomechanical parameters substantiate the preventive efficacy of exercise-based injury prevention programmes.

While epidemiological data are available in professional football, almost no prevention studies in elite-level players have been published so far. Recent published surveys on the preventative strategies in premier league clubs and national teams showed that most of the rated preventive exercises were components of the 11+ programme (McCall et al. 2014; McCall et al. 2015). Although evidence on injury prevention in professional adult players is limited, it seems likely that the basics of exercise-based injury prevention may also work in elite players and the regular implementation in the training process can be recommended. According to the particular needs of elite players and the circumstances in the professional setting, adaptations and refinements on an individual basis might be indicated.

12.7 Development of an implementation strategy

From the beginning of F-MARC activities in injury prevention, the coach – especially at lower levels – was identified as the key instigator in performing injury prevention programmes with her/his players. The successful countrywide campaign in Switzerland was the first example demonstrating how a basic injury prevention programme can be disseminated and implemented at a large scale in amateur football through coaching education (Junge et al. 2011). For the countrywide campaign in Switzerland, The 11 was integrated in the coach education of the Swiss Football Association (Schweizerischer Fussballverband, SFV) using a 'teach the teacher' strategy or 'cascade approach'. All instructor coaches of the SFV were educated by sports physical therapists on how to deliver the programme to the coaches in their licensing or refresher courses. During a period of three years, 5000 licensed amateur coaches were subsequently instructed on performing The 11 with their teams and received the information material (Junge et al. 2011). The same strategy was used in New Zealand, where The 11 was implemented as part of the 'SoccerSmart Program'. In Belgium, the introduction of the 11+ (via coaching courses by the National Football Federation), together with other preventive policies (i.e. no matches if weather conditions are bad) have led to an overall reduction of football-related injuries (Bizzini and Dvorak 2015).

An RCT evaluating different delivery methods of the 11+ found that a preseason coaching workshop was more effective than unsupervised delivery, additional on-field supervision in terms of adherence and even reduced injury risk in teams performing the injury prevention programme (Steffen, Meeuwisse, et al. 2013). Delivery strategies should be further tailored to coaches and players, as other factors (knowledge, beliefs, experience) may also influence their behaviour towards endorsing injury prevention programmes.

The 11+ is best taught to coaches in a workshop that includes theoretical background knowledge and practical demonstration of the exercises. After raising the coach's motivation and awareness of injury prevention, the exercises should be briefly explained and demonstrated. It is helpful to select a participant to perform the exercise, while the instructor highlights the correct execution of the exercises. The participants should then perform the exercises and be corrected by the instructor(s). The participants should get 'a feeling' for the exercises and appreciate the challenges behind each exercise. In the second half of the workshop, each of the participants should teach at least one of the exercises to the group and get feedback on this from the instructor (Bizzini, Junge, and Dvorak 2013).

12.8 Worldwide dissemination of the 11+

In 2009, FIFA started the dissemination of the programme in its 209 Member Associations (MAs). Based on the experience with the countrywide implementation in Switzerland and New Zealand, a guideline on how to implement the The 11+ injury prevention programme at a large scale in amateur football was developed. The implementation was conducted either in close cooperation with MAs or via FIFA Coaching Instructor courses. F-MARC supported the MAs in the preparation of the educational material in the local language and the workshops for the first group of instructors in initiating the cascade training (Bizzini, Junge, and Dvorak 2013). Various important national Football Associations (such as Germany, Brazil, Italy and Japan) integrated The 11+ in their basic coaching curriculum or their physical training/education curriculum. Despite implementation problems, other countries followed these role models, and in general, the interest towards injury prevention in football has increased over the years (Bizzini, Junge, and Dvorak 2013).

12.9 Implementation challenges

While the scientific evidence has proven that 11+ can prevent football injuries, its implementation in the field (as for other injury prevention programmes) remains a challenging task. FIFA has included the programme in all official coaching courses, and presented this concept of prevention at several occasions on all continents. Despite numerous promotional activities in more than 80 countries and three FIFA Medical Conferences (Zürich 2009; Budapest 2012; Zürich 2015), so far the 11+ has been endorsed by only 20 MAs (about 10% of all MAs) of FIFA (Bizzini and Dvorak 2015). Current and past World Cup Champions such as Germany, Brazil and Japan (Women's World Cup) symbolise that the (political) willingness at MA executive levels is crucial in order to strongly support the message of prevention. Therefore, the firm commitment by a MA to realise a given implementation plan, allocating persons and resources for the 11+ 'project' is fundamental. The example by the DFB in Germany, as outlined above, shows that this is also feasible in a large country. Furthermore, implementation strategies at various levels, as illustrated by the RE-AIM Sports Setting Matrix (Finch and Donaldson 2010) and implementation drivers are needed to plan programme adoption, implementation and sustainability.

12.10 Conclusion

Since the introduction of the 11+, research studies and implementation campaigns with this programme have been conducted in four continents (Europe, North America, Africa and Asia). Substantial scientific evidence supports the dissemination and implementation of the 11+ as a basic injury prevention programme in amateur football. Although important results have been achieved, a lot of work remains to be done, especially in prioritising 'injury prevention' in the overall enhancement of the health of football players within the MA's responsibilities. The two countrywide campaigns in Switzerland and New Zealand represent successful examples of injury prevention in amateur football: not only the incidence of football injuries can be reduced, but the health-related costs can also be impressively diminished.

References

Al Attar, W. S., N. Soomro, E. Pappas, P. J. Sinclair, and R. H. Sanders. 2016. "How Effective are F-MARC Injury Prevention Programs for Soccer Players? A Systematic Review and Meta-Analysis." *Sports Medicine* 46 (2):205–217. doi: 10.1007/s40279-015-0404-x.

Beaudouin, F., R. Rossler, K. Aus der Funten, M. Bizzini, J. Chomiak, E. Verhagen, A. Junge, J. Dvorak, E. Lichtenstein, T. Meyer, and O. Faude. 2018. "Effects of the '11+ Kids' injury prevention programme on severe injuries in children's football: A secondary analysis of data from a multicentre cluster-randomised controlled trial." *British Journal of Sports Medicine*. doi: 10.1136/bjsports-2018–099062.

Bizzini, M., and J. Dvorak. 2015. "FIFA 11+: An effective programme to prevent football injuries in various player groups worldwide-a narrative review." *British Journal of Sports Medicine* 49 (9):577–579. doi: 10.1136/bjsports-2015-094765.

Bizzini, M., F. M. Impellizzeri, J. Dvorak, L. Bortolan, F. Schena, R. Modena, and A. Junge. 2013. "Physiological and performance responses to the 'FIFA 11+' (part 1): Is it an appropriate warm-up?" *Journal of Sports Sciences* 31 (13):1481–1490. doi: 10.1080/02640414.2013.802922.

Bizzini, M., A. Junge, and J. Dvorak. 2013. "Implementation of the FIFA 11+ football warm up program: How to approach and convince the Football associations to invest in prevention." *British Journal of Sports Medicine* 47 (12):803–806. doi: 10.1136/bjsports-2012-092124.

Dvorak, J. 2009. "Give Hippocrates a jersey: Promoting health through football/sport." *British Journal of Sports Medicine* 43 (5):317–322. doi: 10.1136/bjsm.2009.059618.

Ekstrand, J., J. Gillquist, and S. O. Liljedahl. 1983. "Prevention of soccer injuries: Supervision by doctor and physiotherapist." *American Journal of Sports Medicine* 11 (3):116–20. doi: 10.1177/036354658301100302.

Faude, O., R. Rossler, and A. Junge. 2013. "Football injuries in children and adolescent players: Are there clues for prevention?" *Sports Medicine* 43 (9):819–837. doi: 10.1007/s40279-013-0061-x.

Faude, O., R. Rossler, E. J. Petushek, R. Roth, L. Zahner, and L. Donath. 2017. "Neuromuscular adaptations to multimodal injury prevention programs in youth sports: A systematic review with meta-analysis of randomized controlled trials." *Frontiers in Physiology* 8:791. doi: 10.3389/fphys.2017.00791.

Finch, C. F., and A. Donaldson. 2010. "A sports setting matrix for understanding the implementation context for community sport." *British Journal of Sports Medicine* 44 (13):973–978. doi: 10.1136/bjsm.2008.056069.

Gilchrist, J., B. R. Mandelbaum, H. Melancon, G. W. Ryan, H. J. Silvers, L. Y. Griffin, D. S. Watanabe, R. W. Dick, and J. Dvorak. 2008. "A randomized controlled trial to prevent noncontact anterior cruciate ligament injury in female collegiate soccer players." *American Journal of Sports Medicine* 36 (8):1476–1483. doi: 10.1177/0363546508318188.

Impellizzeri, F. M., M. Bizzini, J. Dvorak, B. Pellegrini, F. Schena, and A. Junge. 2013. "Physiological and performance responses to the FIFA 11+ (part 2): A randomised controlled trial on the training effects." *Journal of Sports Sciences* 31 (13):1491–1502. doi: 10.1080/02640414.2013.802926.

Junge, A., M. Lamprecht, H. Stamm, H. Hasler, M. Bizzini, M. Tschopp, H. Reuter, H. Wyss, C. Chilvers, and J. Dvorak. 2011. "Countrywide campaign to prevent soccer injuries in Swiss amateur players." *American Journal of Sports Medicine* 39 (1):57–63. doi: 10.1177/0363546510377424.

Junge, A., D. Rosch, L. Peterson, T. Graf-Baumann, and J. Dvorak. 2002. "Prevention of soccer injuries: A prospective intervention study in youth amateur players." *American Journal of Sports Medicine* 30 (5):652–659. doi: 10.1177/03635465020300050401.

Lopes, T. J. A., M. Simic, G. D. Myer, K. R. Ford, T. E. Hewett, and E. Pappas. 2018. "The effects of injury prevention programs on the biomechanics of landing tasks: A systematic review with meta-analysis." *American Journal of Sports Medicine* 46 (6):1492–1499. doi: 10.1177/0363546517716930.

McCall, A., C. Carling, M. Nedelec, M. Davison, F. Le Gall, S. Berthoin, and G. Dupont. 2014. "Risk factors, testing and preventative strategies for non-contact injuries in professional football: Current perceptions and practices of 44 teams from various premier leagues." *British Journal of Sports Medicine* 48 (18):1352–1357. doi: 10.1136/bjsports-2014-093439.

McCall, A., M. Davison, T. E. Andersen, I. Beasley, M. Bizzini, G. Dupont, R. Duffield, C. Carling, and J. Dvorak. 2015. "Injury prevention strategies at the FIFA 2014 World Cup: Perceptions and practices of the physicians from the 32 participating national teams." *British Journal of Sports Medicine* 49 (9):603–608. doi: 10.1136/bjsports-2015-094747.

Owoeye, O. B., S. R. Akinbo, B. A. Tella, and O. A. Olawale. 2014. "Efficacy of the FIFA 11+ warm-up programme in male youth football: A cluster randomised controlled trial." *Journal of Sports Science and Medicine* 13 (2):321–328.

Pappas, E., E. J. Nightingale, M. Simic, K. R. Ford, T. E. Hewett, and G. D. Myer. 2015. "Do exercises used in injury prevention programmes modify cutting task biomechanics? A systematic review with meta-analysis." *British Journal of Sports Medicine* 49 (10):673–680. doi: 10.1136/bjsports-2014-093796.

Ribeiro-Alvares, J. B., V. B. Marques, M. A. Vaz, and B. M. Baroni. 2018. "Four weeks of nordic hamstring exercise reduce muscle injury risk factors in young adults." *Journal of Strength and Conditioning Research* 32 (5):1254–1262. doi: 10.1519/JSC.0000000000001975.

Rossler, R., L. Donath, M. Bizzini, and O. Faude. 2016. "A new injury prevention programme for children's football: FIFA 11+ Kids-can improve motor performance: A cluster-randomised controlled trial." *Journal of Sports Sciences* 34 (6):549–556. doi: 10.1080/02640414.2015.1099715.

Rossler, R., L. Donath, E. Verhagen, A. Junge, T. Schweizer, and O. Faude. 2014. "Exercise-based injury prevention in child and adolescent sport: A systematic review and meta-analysis." *Sports Medicine* 44 (12):1733–1748. doi: 10.1007/s40279-014-0234-2.

Rossler, R., A. Junge, M. Bizzini, E. Verhagen, J. Chomiak, K. Aus der Funten, T. Meyer, J. Dvorak, E. Lichtenstein, F. Beaudouin, and O. Faude. 2018. "A multinational cluster randomised controlled trial to assess the efficacy of '11+ Kids': A warm-up programme to prevent injuries in children's football." *Sports Medicine* 48 (6):1493–1504. doi: 10.1007/s40279-017-0834-8.

Rossler, R., E. Verhagen, N. Rommers, J. Dvorak, A. Junge, E. Lichtenstein, L. Donath, and O. Faude. 2018. "Comparison of the '11+ Kids' injury prevention programme and a regular warmup in children's football (soccer): A cost effectiveness analysis." *British Journal of Sports Medicine*. doi: 10.1136/bjsports-2018-099395.

Silvers-Granelli, H., B. Mandelbaum, O. Adeniji, S. Insler, M. Bizzini, R. Pohlig, A. Junge, L. Snyder-Mackler, and J. Dvorak. 2015. "Efficacy of the FIFA 11+ injury prevention program in the collegiate male soccer player." *American Journal of Sports Medicine* 43 (11):2628–2637. doi: 10.1177/0363546515602009.

Soligard, T., G. Myklebust, K. Steffen, I. Holme, H. Silvers, M. Bizzini, A. Junge, J. Dvorak, R. Bahr, and T. E. Andersen. 2008. "Comprehensive warm-up programme to prevent injuries in young female footballers: Cluster randomised controlled trial." *British Medical Journal* 337:a2469. doi: 10.1136/bmj.a2469.

Steffen, K., C. A. Emery, M. Romiti, J. Kang, M. Bizzini, J. Dvorak, C. F. Finch, and W. H. Meeuwisse. 2013. "High adherence to a neuromuscular injury prevention programme (FIFA 11+) improves functional balance and reduces injury risk in Canadian youth female football players: A cluster randomised trial." *British Journal of Sports Medicine* 47 (12):794–802. doi: 10.1136/bjsports-2012-091886.

Steffen, K., W. H. Meeuwisse, M. Romiti, J. Kang, C. McKay, M. Bizzini, J. Dvorak, C. Finch, G. Myklebust, and C. A. Emery. 2013. "Evaluation of how different implementation strategies of an injury prevention programme (FIFA 11+) impact team adherence and injury risk in Canadian female youth football players: A cluster-randomised trial." *British Journal of Sports Medicine* 47 (8):480–487. doi: 10.1136/bjsports-2012-091887.

Thorborg, K., K. K. Krommes, E. Esteve, M. B. Clausen, E. M. Bartels, and M. S. Rathleff. 2017. "Effect of specific exercise-based football injury prevention programmes on the overall injury rate in football: A systematic review and meta-analysis of the FIFA 11 and 11+ programmes." *British Journal of Sports Medicine* 51 (7):562–571. doi: 10.1136/bjsports-2016-097066.

Weston, M., C. Castagna, F. M. Impellizzeri, M. Bizzini, A. M. Williams, and W. Gregson. 2012. "Science and medicine applied to soccer refereeing: An update." *Sports Medicine* 42 (7):615–631. doi: 10.2165/11632360-000000000-00000.

Chapter 13

Watching Football as Medicine

Promoting health at the football stadium

Keith D. Parry, Emma S. George, Jess Richards and Andy Stevens

Introduction – Stadium-based health

French Neo-Marxist sociologist Jean-Marie Brohm (1978) claimed that the Olympic Games acts as an 'opiate' for the people, keeping them enthralled and pacified. He went on to argue that the televising of sports events allows the ruling class to reduce the population to 'a servile mass' in a move that is eerily similar to the use of 'bread and circuses' to appease and distract the citizens of Ancient Rome. Although such a view may sound alarmist, spectator sport is contradictory and is indeed based on large numbers of the population passively engaging in mass entertainment. The majority of those involved in the sporting spectacle are largely inactive and sedentary, watching a minority expend energy and effort for their amusement. Therefore, watching sport may be detrimental to the health of 'the people' when their sedentary behaviour is considered in combination with the poor food options provided at venues and the highly stressful nature of sport fandom (Parry 2012). It may be unsurprising that watching sport has been previously linked to a variety of health impacts, including an increased risk of acute cardiovascular events (Čulić 2011; Olsen et al. 2015; Onozuka & Hagihara 2018).

Citizens of many nations are now, more than ever, spending copious amounts of time 'enthralled' by watching sport on television and live at venues. Perhaps as a result of this obsession with watching sport, in the United Kingdom, only 65% of men and 60% of women aged 16 and over met the recommended aerobic guidelines (Sport England 2018), with 21% of men and 25% of women in England classified as inactive (NHS Digital 2018). As previously documented (Parry et al. 2018), rates of sport participation are far lower than rates of sport spectatorship, both in terms of watching sport at a stadium or from home via the media. Indeed, watching sport is one of the most popular leisure choices in many countries, but the prolonged periods of sedentary behaviour that are associated with modern sport consumption can have a detrimental impact on health (Grøntved & Hu 2011). Physical activity and sedentary behaviour guidelines have been established in many countries with the aim of minimising both the amount of time that populations are spending in front of screens and overall sedentary behaviour (see, for example, Department of Health 2017). Therefore, to avoid a modern passive population that is appeased by 'pies and football' it is important that health promotion is encouraged with regard to fans attending live sport, specifically through the provision of healthier eating options and physical activity initiatives, and with a particular focus on young people to encourage lifelong healthy lifestyles. Moves aimed at encouraging stadia to adopt healthy initiatives that benefit fans and staff alike, such as the introduction of a meat-free menu by Forest Green Rovers (as will be discussed later), are gaining increasing scholarly attention including a special edition in the journal *Sport and Society* focusing on the concept of Healthy Stadia, which are defined as:

> those which promote the health of visitors, fans, players, employees and the surrounding community . . . places where people can go to have a positive healthy experience playing or watching sport.
>
> (Philpott & Seymour 2011, 69).

This chapter will assess the potential that *watching* football holds for health promotion. We commence by critically examining the state of stadium food and highlight recent moves towards healthier eating. We will then discuss a number of evidence-based programmes that encourage football fans to be more physically active and the potential that stadium design holds for increasing physical activity. After acknowledging the challenges that stadium-based health promotion activities are faced with, we will provide an instructive case study on Forest Green Rovers, the world's first vegan football club. We finish by detailing the way forward for health promotion through football stadia.

Healthy eating at stadia

> The game day activities many fans relish are undoubtedly unhealthy . . . poor eating and drinking habits may extend beyond game day.
>
> (Woods 2012, 1)

The consumption of food and drink plays an important role in the stadium experience (Parry, Hall & Baxter 2017), but, as indicated in the above quote, football stadia are not associated with healthy eating. Excessive alcohol consumption and unhealthy fast food have been equated to what Ireland and Watkins (2010) termed the 'football fan diet'. In their study of fast food sold at an unidentified Premier League football club, they explored how attending football matches was a 'release' for football fans from their everyday life where fans typically engaged in indulgent behaviour. This indulgence has been encouraged by the presence of all-you-can-eat food promotions by teams such as the Detroit Tigers and the Los Angeles Dodgers in Major League Baseball, which only added an extra US$15–20 onto the price of a ticket. In 2010 19 of the 30 teams in the league offered such a package (Paulas 2011).

An ethnographic study on the match day experiences of Everton Football Club fans found that consuming fast food also had symbolic meanings attached to it. Meanings tied to particular types of food were reflective of and attached to match day memories, experiences and traditions (Richards 2016). For example, the smell of fast food and the sizzling sounds of burgers outside of the football stadium remains tied to what Gaffney and Bale (2004, 33) have described as 'sensing the stadium'. The smells that fans experience en route to and once inside a stadium evoke responses that familiarise them with sport. Smells, like familiar landmarks, anchor fans spatially within a sports stadium, evoking feelings of routine, comfort and familiarity. Whilst eating at home symbolises intimacy and family, eating while watching a sports match symbolises festivity, excitement, and builds atmosphere for the upcoming fixture – encouraging excessive eating.

However, studies by Ireland and Watkins (2010, 684) and Parry, Hall and Baxter (2017, 210) also highlight the dissatisfaction that fans feel with the choice and quality of the food on offer with comments such as 'awful', 'atrocious', 'terrible food choices (no fresh/healthy food at all)' and 'exorbitant prices' used to describe the typical offerings. Worryingly, some fans go to great lengths to avoid purchasing food and beverage once inside the stadium. These lengths reportedly involve binge eating on food and beverages *before* they enter a venue (Martin & O'Neill 2010, 14). These practices are contrary to healthy eating guidelines that encourage smaller, balanced and regular meals (National Health and Medical Research Council 2013).

In the absence of a clear definition of healthy eating options, we turn to discussions such as those offered by the World Health Organisation (WHO), who identify the high levels of fat, sugars and cholesterol in unhealthy foods (WHO 2015). Stadium food has typically been high in levels of saturated fat and sugar (Philpott & Seymour 2011), similar to the offerings found in fast food restaurants (Sukalakamala, Sukalakamala & Young 2013) and would thus be considered unhealthy. Furthermore, European stadia have frequently been situated in less affluent areas, with a high density of low-quality housing. The inhabitants of these neighbourhoods are often accustomed to eating fast food-style offerings as they typically either have poorer health literacy (being unaware of the health implications of their food choices), or are happy to eat offerings that are less healthy and of lower quality as they are cheaper (Drygas et al. 2013). Yet even those fans who have a better understanding of the implications of food choices may also eat unhealthily at sports matches. Indeed, it has been reported that some fans see football matches as 'a place for an occasional unhealthy pie' (Ireland & Watkins 2010, 685).

Whereas few stadia have, hitherto, had a healthy eating policy (Drygas et al. 2013), recent moves by the European Healthy Stadia Network have seen the 'implementation of robust, evidence-driven policies and practices' (European Healthy Stadia Network 2019) along with a series of guidance documents and toolkits to facilitate the development of stadia as health-promoting environments. In addition to issuing guidance on achieving a tobacco-free stadium and promoting active travel, they have developed a new benchmarking tool for healthy match-day catering, which is supported by the British Heart Foundation. Their 'Healthy Match Mark' focusses on the sale of healthier food options, food preparation and healthier cooking techniques, the control of portion size and condiments, the supply of healthier beverages, pricing and the promotion of healthier options.

Therefore, as evidenced through the growing Healthy Stadia agenda, it is possible to overcome the fractious relationship between sport and health promotion (McKenna et al. 2017) and use venues to promote and even encourage healthy lifestyles and choices. The aforementioned contradictory nature of spectator sport also opens up an important discussion around the social obligation of professional sporting bodies to encourage fans to be more active and not only to use sport as a lucrative spectacle for television. Furthermore, given that the location is crucial for delivering health interventions, particularly those aimed at men, stadia are uniquely placed to promote physical activity to some population groups.

Football Fans in training and other programmes

Men are a hard-to-reach population group for the promotion of healthy lifestyles (Department of Health and Ageing 2010; Pagoto et al. 2012). There are limited programmes designed specifically for men, however, evidence suggests that when gender-specific approaches are used to shape the development and delivery of health promotion programmes, men may be more likely to engage (Bottorff et al. 2015; George et al. 2012; Gray et al. 2013; Morgan et al. 2011).

Sporting organisations, and professional football clubs in particular, are perfectly positioned to deliver important health and social messages and researchers are increasingly using sport as a vehicle for health promotion (Cade et al. 2017; Hunt et al. 2014; Lewis, Reeves & Roberts 2017; Pringle 2009). The Football Fans in Training (FFIT) programme (Hunt et al. 2014; Gray et al. 2013) demonstrates the potential for professional sporting organisations to engage with their fans in a way that truly contributes to the health and wellbeing of the community. This 12-week programme, developed in collaboration between the Scottish Professional Football League Trust and the University of Glasgow, involved gender-sensitised group-based education and physical activity sessions and was delivered across 13 Scottish professional football clubs (Hunt et al. 2014). Significantly, this intervention was staged at the clubs' home stadia, capitalising on the importance of the stadium to fans. The programme successfully recruited male football fans with a body mass index of 28kg/m^2 or over who were aged between 35 and 65 years. FFIT was delivered by Scottish Premier League Community Coaches according to a defined protocol and educations sessions focused on topics relating to weight management, including increasing physical activity and improving dietary intake. The intervention also comprised an incremental walking programme, where men were encouraged to monitor their daily step counts using pedometers (Gray et al. 2013).

Results from a two-group, pragmatic randomised controlled trial with 747 participants (Hunt et al. 2014) demonstrated a significant treatment effect for absolute weight and percentage weight loss ($p < 0.0001$), after adjusting for club and weight at baseline. Significant treatment effects were also observed for waist circumference, body mass index, body fat percentage and blood pressure, demonstrating that a gender-sensitised weight loss intervention could be effectively delivered at the stadia of professional football clubs (Hunt et al. 2014).

This innovative approach to men's health and recruitment capitalises on sport fandom and uses the inherently masculine context of a football stadium to deliver health messages. The effectiveness of FFIT has led to the development of an additional football-based programme in Europe (Wyke et al. 2019), and spin-off programmes in rugby union in New Zealand (Maddison et al. 2019), rugby league (see below) and Australian Rules football in Australia (Quested et al. 2018) and ice hockey in Canada (Caperchione et al. 2017; Petrella et al. 2017).

The EuroFIT randomised controlled trial recruited 1,113 overweight men aged 30–65 years with a body mass index of 27 kg/m^2 or above across 15 professional football clubs in England, the Netherlands, Norway and Portugal (Wyke et al. 2019). EuroFIT extended FFIT by incorporating an app (MatchFIT), physical activity and a sedentary behaviour monitoring device (SitFIT) to encourage participants to self-monitor their activity. Weekly education sessions targeted physical activity, sedentary time and diet, and were delivered by trained coaches at club facilities or their 'iconic' stadia (Wyke et al. 2019). At 12 months, significant between-group differences favouring the intervention were observed for outcomes including steps/day, dietary intake, weight, wellbeing and self-esteem.

Both FFIT and EuroFIT provide evidence to support the use of football club facilities and stadia to promote weight management, physical activity, sedentary time and diet in middle-aged men. Due to its success, and the demand from women, FFIT is now also available to female football fans (http://spfltrust.org.uk/ffit/) and the programme is delivered as a sustainable, community engagement initiative through the Scottish Premier Football League Trust. Sustainability and transferability should be key goals for any health promotion initiative, so to see this level of engagement beyond the scope of a contained, rigorous randomised controlled trial is promising. This framework could be utilised in a number of professional sporting contexts and tailored to meet the needs of local communities.

In New Zealand, Maddison and colleagues (2019) tailored the FFIT programme to be delivered at the grounds of professional rugby union clubs in Auckland and Dunedin (RUFIT-NZ). Overweight men aged 25–65 years were recruited for a pilot study testing the feasibility of the tailored programme. Significant treatment effects were observed for body weight, waist circumference, blood pressure and cardiorespiratory fitness, suggesting that the FFIT programme could be successfully tailored for the New Zealand population.

The FFIT programme has also been replicated in Australia, with the AussieFIT programme being delivered in Western Australia through professional Australian Rules football clubs in the elite Australian Football League (AFL) at either the clubs' playing or training facility (Quested et al., 2018). Outcome data are not yet available, but the results from the EuroFIT and RUFIT-NZ programmes are promising, and it is anticipated that the AussieFIT programme will show similar results. There is also a range of excellent programmes being delivered through professional football clubs for which formal outcome data are not yet available or are not being collected. For example, the Western Bulldogs AFL club based in Melbourne, Australia also deliver a 10-week FFIT-inspired programme called Sons of the West (http://sonsofthewest.org.au/). The free programme delivers education sessions and activities to promote physical activity, nutrition and mental health. Although the effectiveness of the programme has not been formally evaluated, anecdotal evidence suggests this programme is successfully engaging the local community and improving health outcomes.

In the National Rugby League, the Canterbury-Bankstown Bulldogs deliver the Active Breed men's health initiative (https://activebreed.thebulldogs.com.au//home). This 12-week programme engages male rugby league football fans in the Greater Sydney region and involves weekly education and physical activity sessions within the club's inner sanctum and training facility, Belmore Sports Ground – a stadium that hosted Bulldogs' games from 1936 until 1998. This programme is also inspired by FFIT, but was developed in partnership with sport, health and community partners. The education component of the programme focuses on physical activity, nutrition, health service engagement, mental health and violence prevention. Participants engage in tailored activity sessions including gym-based workouts in the same gym used by the players and touch football games. Active Breed is embedded within the club and incorporates visits from club coaches, current and former players, and health experts.

The professional football context is a powerful drawcard for fans, and this should be harnessed for the continued promotion of health and wellbeing. However, it is also worth considering the potential that stadia have for increasing physical activity levels of spectators at regular games in addition to during interventions.

Stadium design and fan activity levels at games

The MatchFIT app is not the only example of the potential that mobile technology holds for stadia-based health initiatives. Indeed, as is detailed in this volume (see Chapter 14), the Fan Fit app has been used to both track activity levels and create an active fan community in a variety of sports clubs. Global Positioning System (GPS)-enabled devices, such as smartphones and smartwatches, can be used to provide visual overviews and tracking data of research participants en route to specific sport locations (Andrew 2013; Gong et al. 2014; Rasmussen 2013). Indeed, wearable technology has been used since the 1990s to track trip data, and gained popularity because of the improvement in the accuracy of GPS technology. In fact, the first attempts to validate a commercially available GPS device (the GPS45 Garmin) for the measurement of human movement was published in 1997 (Schutz & Chambaz 1997).

Although wearable devices have been used to explore skill development and/or health and wellbeing implications of professional athletes, their potential to track sports fans' movement, engagement and physical exertion has only recently been explored. There is much potential for the use of these devices as a substantial amount of empirical data can be generated from a study incorporating wearable technology into the research design. An additional benefit of utilising this technology is that the data collection process is completely normalised and operates 'innocently and efficiently' to limit field distortion (Jones, Marshall & Denison 2016), primarily because wearable technology enables users to access information naturally in their own environment rather than forcing them to enter into a digital world (York & Pendharkar 2004). The psychological benefits of being a sports fan have been extensively researched (Bransombe & Wann 1991; Wann 2006), but going to a sports match may also have additional physical health benefits not yet explored within research and academic literature. Despite people becoming increasingly aware of their wellbeing and the state of their bodies, with body sensor networks embedded into garments to track bodily data in order to sustain healthier lives (Uğur 2013), the physical benefits of attending sports matches remains under-researched.

Sports fan-related research is increasingly identifying that the match day experience entails much more than just attending the stadium and involves visiting particular locations (often routinely) while travelling to watch live sport (Richards & Parry 2019). Gaffney (2008) identifies that stadia function as sites and symbols of social memory, representation and meaning for sports fans, with match day travel yielding particular significance. Travel in this way both consolidates and strengthens fan identity, with fans either sharing modes of transport (train/car), or meeting at a particular venue and walking together to the match. Historically, the routes walked by fans from public transport links or through densely packed housing to the stadium have involved at least moderate degrees of physical activity. However, while the (often extraordinary) lengths that fans travel by car to attend matches is frequently documented, the distances that fans walk to games and the associated levels of physical activity have been ignored. Recent technological advancement has provided researchers with the tools to collect, analyse and integrate micro-level data on an individual's location, time and intensity of activity in space (Yin 2013). For example, a recent study by Murray et al. (2017) on the social and physical benefits of watching golf found that spectators of the 2016 Paul Lawrie Matchplay tournament walked a mean of 11,589 steps, with 82.9% of the 339 spectators surveyed reaching their recommended daily step count. Additionally, they note the physical, social and mental health benefits of walking the course.

We are currently conducting a pilot study exploring the use of wearable technology to understand how sports fans interact with stadia during sports matches, as well as assessing any health benefits of match day travel. The project aims to provide a more holistic account of sports fans' routes to stadia and explore an alternative narrative of match day related to health. Preliminary findings suggest that attending a live sporting fixture involves more physical activity and physical movement than first anticipated – and certainly more than fans who watch matches on television. Initial data collection took place at a number of venues in Sydney, Australia. Within the Australian context, the ticket to a sporting fixture generally includes the cost of public transportation and, for this reason, most participants travelled by train to their chosen sporting match. Our findings suggest that travelling to the match, regardless of the mode of transportation and even without engaging in active travel measures, involves not inconsiderable levels of physical activity. Fans that took public transport had a higher rate of physical activity (mostly due to walking to and from a train station), but even those who drove still had substantially higher levels of physical activity than fans watching it on television, as most car parks are situated at least a reasonable walk from the stadium. Indeed, the shortest distance travelled by participants when attending a stadium was 1.5kms.

Tracked levels of physical activity varied depending on the design of the stadium and the type of sporting event being watched. Those stadia that allow fans to move around during games, such as oval-shaped cricket grounds, provided greater opportunities for physical activity during games and resulted in greater distances covered by participants. Rectangular football stadia, where fans are typically allocated seats in particular sections and often segregated from either opposition fans or exclusive corporate facilities, result in lower levels of physical activity. Indoor arena sports, such as basketball and netball, offer high levels of entertainment during breaks in play (and which involve shorter match-time), resulting in a greater tendency for spectators to remain sedentary and hence lower levels of activity. However, for sports that were longer in duration, such as cricket, there was an increase in the physical movement in and around the stadium.

As it is now recognised that prolonged bouts of sedentary behaviour should be broken up with physical activity in order to improve metabolic health (Healy et al. 2008), sporting organisations should not only consider the role that the design of stadia plays in health promotion, but also the activities that they provide during events to reduce the amount time that fans are seated. As an example, in North America, the San Diego Padres have for a number of years been incorporating physical activity breaks for spectators during their games (Yancey et al. 2009) as part of a holistic approach to health promotion that also includes competitively priced healthier food options.

Challenges to stadium-based approaches

Facilities and stadia have been identified as 'cultural landmarks to deliver health-related messages, interventions and projects' (Martin et al. 2016, 177). Yet using football stadia as health promotion sites is not without challenges. As an example, an initiative that aimed to create health awareness and motivate men to consider adopting and/or engaging in recommended health behaviours disseminated health messages both inside and outside an English football stadium, but found that 'only a small number of men engaged with health services at the stadium on match days' (Curran, Drust & Richardson 2014, 924). As noted, fans have regular match day routines that are grounded in tradition and meaning (Richards & Parry 2019). They are resistant to any interruptions to these routines and so, Curran, Drust and Richardson (2014, 929) have concluded that 'we cannot assume that male supporters will absorb health messages in and around all sport stadia on match days'. Health messages can also be hard to deliver when stadia are more often the home of 'unhealthy' messages.

In numerous countries, television advertising of products such as alcohol, gambling and fast food is now regulated; recognising the negative impact that these products can have, particularly on children. Similarly, the governing body of football in England, the English Football Association, has restricted the sponsorship of playing kits worn by teams consisting entirely of players under the age of 18 by any 'service or other activity which is considered by The [Football] Association as detrimental to the welfare, health or general interest of young persons' (The Football Association 2017, 6). They primarily identify alcohol and gambling as being 'detrimental' based on the fact that they are age-restricted products. However, Parry et al. (2018) note that the main sponsors of sport, particularly for mega events and venues are often fast food, fizzy drink, alcohol, gambling and (previously) tobacco companies. Moreover, even when venues limit their unhealthy sponsors, the clubs playing there may not follow suit. In an analysis of association football clubs in Australia, we found that the teams in the elite men's competition, the A-League had, on average, two unhealthy food or beverage companies amongst their main sponsors in 2018. In addition, the league itself has fast-food giant McDonald's as one of its 'official partners'. While the clubs were less likely to have official betting sponsors/partners, the league again has a major betting company as an official partner. The negative impact of (less healthy) food and beverage, betting and alcohol companies sponsoring sporting events has been identified (Carter et al. 2012; Garde & Rigby 2012; Sherriff, Griffiths & Daube 2010), and yet the lucrative deals offered by these profitable sponsors means that they continue to be appealing for venues and sports organisations. As a result, health-promoting policies regarding stadium food can be lost within the 'noise' generated by the proliferation of messages promoting unhealthy options. Until binding regulations or voluntary measures are introduced this situation may be difficult to change.

As has previously been argued (Parry et al. 2018), a football stadium (and sports stadia generally) is a specific environment that, like airports and concert venues, is physically sealed off from the outside world. It is an enclosed commercial domain that is designed in the context of a monopoly or oligopoly (depending on how many independent suppliers are contracted to service it) around offering food and beverages. The sale of these is often outsourced to a small number of licensed suppliers (Lee, Heere, & Chung 2013) who pass on the costs of supplying their necessarily limited offerings to sport fans. Under this model, food and beverages that are cheap to produce, and typically less healthy, are favoured due to their promise of larger returns than more expensive or more time-intensive healthy alternatives. Consequently, some teams and venues have little or no influence or control over the food and beverage on offer.

In rare instances, clubs that retain control over their stadium and catering offerings can move away from the accepted practices and the indulgent behaviour associated with modern football. One club, Forest Green Rovers, are challenging these norms, promoting sustainable practices and encouraging healthier eating and lifestyles. The following case study analyses this unique example.

Forest Green Rovers: 'the world's first vegan football club'

Forest Green Rovers Football Club were already unique when the 'village team on the top of a hill in the middle of nowhere' (Garry 2017) became the smallest club to be promoted to the Football League (FIFA 2018), the professional divisions of association football in England and Wales. The club's stadium, The New Lawn, is located in Nailsworth, Gloucestershire, which has a population of just 5,794 (Garry 2017) – smaller than the average attendance of many of the club's rivals in League Two (the lowest division in the Football League) and some in the National League. However, it has been their off-the-pitch strategy rather than the team's performance in the Football League that has won recognition from the likes of FIFA and the United Nations, as the organisation became the first vegetarian (Vegetarian Living n.d.), and then the first the vegan (BBC 2015) football club in the world.

Rovers were founded in 1889 and have had modest success as a non-league club in local and regional leagues, with their most notable trophy being the 1982 FA Vase (Anderson 2017). In 2011, the club was acquired by Ecotricity (Ecotricity Group Limited 2011), a company owned by Dale Vince, who was appointed chairman of the club. Ecotricity is a provider of sustainable energy, transport and food services, which is based in the nearby town of Stroud, Gloucestershire. The club was acquired to provide a new channel for the company to promote sustainability projects (Forest Green Rovers 2018). Since then, Rovers have implemented a sustainability programme which has encompassed the club's food and drink services, with the club's environmental policy being 'to promote healthier food for our players, staff, visitors and fans' (Forest Green Rovers 2018, 4). The most prominent, and most contentious, part of the programme has been the introduction of a vegetarian and, subsequently, vegan menu in 2015 (see Figure 13.1). The meat-free policy was initially introduced for players 'for health and performance reasons' (Haynes 2011, 38) and subsequently to all staff and spectators 'as a good health initiative and also an environmental one' (Stuart 2017, 6).

As we will detail below, many were initially sceptical about the menu and the rationale behind it. However, a comprehensive systematic review and meta-analysis on observational studies of vegetarian and vegan diets (Dinu et al. 2017) found that a vegetarian diet was associated with a significantly lower risk of ischaemic heart disease incidence and mortality and cancer. A vegan diet was also associated with a significantly lower risk of cancer (Dinu et al. 2017).

Forest Green Rovers have generated worldwide publicity for their policy, although much of it has drawn on stereotyped perceptions of vegetarian and vegan menus being restricted to hummus (Haynes 2011, 38) and lentils (Daily

Mail 2011). Vince has been described as a 'hippy' (James 2017) and the club as 'eco-warriors' (Edwards 2018, 49). Reporting of the menus has been predominately negative: Meat products have been *banned* (Daily Mail 2011), while the vegan menu has been *imposed* (Haynes 2011, 38) on fans and players. The vegan menu has both been blamed for poor performances, typically in the sport pages of the tabloid newspapers (cf. Witcoop 2017), and for good performances, such when Rovers won promotion to the Football League, more often by broadsheets (cf. Burnton 2017).

The non-meat menus have received support from the club's own staff, players and fans, but less so from those from opposition teams. Importantly, the policy has been endorsed by Rovers' manager Mark Cooper and the players (Stuart 2017; Williams 2015), although they have had to address scepticism, misconceptions and suspicion. Staff had to overcome concern from players that a vegan diet was 'weird or wrong' (Caulkin 2017, 12) and there have been reports of players ignoring the policy, although Rovers maintain that it only applies at the club's facilities and events.

Some opposition clubs have – intentionally or otherwise – been antagonistic towards the meat-free menu. When Lincoln City played Rovers in November 2018, they placed an advertisement for a steak restaurant in the match programme next to a feature on Forest Green Rovers (Johnson 2018). The chairman of Carlisle United, Andrew Jenkins, described Rovers' policy as 'strange' (Scott 2018, 10) when his team visited The New Lawn in December 2017. He refused to even try any of the products: 'I couldn't pull myself together to sample the food on offer. I don't want to be sarcastic, but what would happen if, when vegetarians came to our club, all we could offer was an all-meat menu?' (Scott 2018, 10). However, Carlisle United did then offer a vegan option on their menus when they hosted Rovers later in the season (Bawden 2019).

There is generally more acceptance of the unique menu on offer at The New Lawn from Rovers' own supporters and neutral spectators than there is from opposition fans. Complaints are more likely to be from away fans, although some are open-minded and even anticipate the new products on offer, with a few visitors changing their opinions about vegetarian and vegan products. The menu is frequently debated on the *FGR Forum* message board, which is available on the club's website (Forest Green Rovers n.d.). Threads relating to food and drink are more prominent than on comparable forums of other clubs. There are a variety of opinions, but overall the forum indicates that there is a lot of support for many aspects of the club's sustainability programme. The opinions of other visitors to The New Lawn, however, are much more divisive. Reviews of the matchday experience on the *Football Ground Guide* and *TripAdvisor* websites cover a range of issues, but comments on the club's food and drink service are common. It is evident that many first-time visitors are sceptical about the menu, although some change their minds as a consequence of attending a match at The New Lawn. More notable is that the fan experience is, again, adversely affected by perceptions of the poor-quality products and particularly by perceived low quality of facilities and customer service.

2010	Ecotricity acquires Forest Green Rovers.
2011	Rovers remove red meat products such as burgers and sausages from the menu at The New Lawn, although free-range and sustainable poultry and fish continue to be served.
2015	Introduce a vegetarian menu to become first vegetarian football club in the United Kingdom.
2015	The meat-free brand Quorn become a club sponsor.
2015	Introduce a vegan menu to become the first vegan football club in the world.
2016	Club is named "Menu of the Year" at the 2016 Sports and Leisure Catering Awards.
2017	Rovers' Creamy Vegan Pie is highly commended in the Vegetarian Pie category at the 2017 British Pie Awards.
2017	Win the National League play-off final at Wembley Stadium to gain promotion to Football League for the first time.
2017	Menu registered with The Vegan Society's Vegan Trademark.
2019	Rovers' Sweet Potato, Spinach & Chickpea Curry Pie wins silver in the Vegan Pie category and, along with the Q Pie, is awarded bronze in the Sports Pie category at the 2019 British Pie Awards.

Figure 13.1 Timeline of Forest Green Rovers' food journey.

The sustainability strategy of Forest Green Rovers, and specifically the introduction of vegetarian and vegan menus, has received a significant and mixed response from the media and from the staff, players and fans of the club and its opponents. There has been scepticism from the media (Oliver 2017), but Rover's non-meat policy has generated publicity that the club and its sponsors would likely have not otherwise received. The club claims that all staff, including the manager and players, support the policy, although various news outlets reported that a delivery of chicken and fish and chips was made to the team bus after a match in November 2018 (Hughes 2018). There have also been 'misconceptions' and 'suspicion' (Caulkin 2017, 12) from other club owners and 'a lot of animosity' (Garry 2017) from opposition fans.

The club has been constrained by the size and quality of its facilities (Forest Green Rovers 2019), but have plans for a larger stadium with new and enhanced facilities (Forest Green Rover no date). Whether a meat-free menu or even more healthy products can be introduced by larger clubs, perhaps even in Premier League, or at other sports and events, is more questionable (Gordon 2017).

Future directions

The development of the European Healthy Stadia Network and its subsequent guidance and toolkits has provided the impetus for practitioners and academics to push for healthier practices at football stadia. The Healthy Match Mark, in particular, is an important step towards healthier eating options at stadia as this index-based benchmarking tool assesses catering practices at an organisational level. However, it is also important that fans are provided with greater information on nutrient values at the point of sale to allow informed decisions on food choices to be made. These measures should, surely, be a minimum requirement for any venues that are constructed or run via public funding. Yet such moves will not be met without resistance as fans are reluctant to break from the tradition practices and match day routines detailed above.

This chapter has also detailed the potential that wearable technology can play in providing a greater understanding of the activity levels of sport spectators. With further research in this area it will be possible to understand the degree to which infrastructure and stadium design influence activity levels on the way to/from and during games. The use of wearable technology will also facilitate the evaluation of in-stadia physical activity interventions, providing insight into the efficacy of this form of health intervention. During a period when some venues are struggling to attract spectators to games, data on the levels of physical activity that are associated with watching sports matches at stadia may provide an additional incentive for sports fans and spectators to 'get off the couch' and go to a game. A holistic approach to healthy stadia (including active travel, stadium design, healthy eating and physical activity activations) can, therefore, become a key component of *Watching* Football as Medicine.

However, for these approaches to be successful, the continued presence of advertising of unhealthy products and services at sports stadia must be challenged. Given that there are often restrictions on the advertising of these products on television, it may also be time to restrict this advertising at sports venues and of sporting organisations. The resistance to such a move is likely to come from clubs and sporting organisations, as these sponsors make significant financial contributions so that they can associate their products with the healthy lifestyle associated with professional sport.

References

Anderson, John. 2017. *Sky Sports Football Yearbook 2017–2018*. 48th ed. London: Headline Publishing Group.

Andrew, Adrienne, Kevin Eustice, & Andy Hickl. 2013. "Using Location lifelogs to Make Meaning of Food and Physical Activity." Paper presented at the International Conference on Pervasive Computer Technologies for Healthcare and Workshops, Venice, May 5–8.

Bawden, Tom. 2019. "Why Forest Green Rovers could be the greenest sports club in the world." *i News*, January 1. https://inews.co.uk/news/environment/why-forest-green-rovers-could-be-the-greenest-sports-club-in-the-world/.

BBC. 2015. "Football club goes vegan in 'world first'." *BBC*, October 31. www.bbc.co.uk/news/uk-england-gloucestershire-34680213.

Bottorff, Joan L., Cherisse L. Seaton, Steve T. Johnson, Cristina M. Caperchione, John L. Oliffe, Kimberly More, Haleema Jaffer-Hirji, & Sherri M. Tillotson. 2015. "An updated review of interventions that include promotion of physical activity for adult men." *Sports Medicine* 45 (6): 775–800.

Branscombe, Nyla & Wann. 1991. "The positive social and self-concept consequences of sports team identification." *Journal of Sport & Social Issues* 15 (2): 115–127. doi: 10.1177/019372359101500202.

Brohm, Jean-Marie. 1978. *A Prison of Measured Time*. London: Pluto Press.

Burnton, Simon. 2017. "Forest Green hope Dale Vince's eco vision brings promotion from National League." *The Observer*, May 13.

Cade, Daniel, Kathryn Curran, Andy Fuller, Jenny Hacker, Clive Knight, Simon Lansley, Daniel Parnell, & Matthew Philpott. 2017. "Perspectives from those involved in healthy stadia." *Sport in Society* 20 (2): 187–201.

Caperchione, Cristina M., Joan L. Bottorff, John L. Oliffe, Steven T. Johnson, Kate Hunt, Paul Sharp, Kayla M. Fitzpatrick, Ryley Price, Larry S. Goldenberg. 2017. "The HAT TRICK programme for improving physical activity, healthy eating and connectedness among overweight, inactive men: Study protocol of a pragmatic feasibility trial." *BMJ Open* 7 (9): e016940.

Carter, Mary-Ann, Richard Edwards, Louise Signal, & Janet Hoek. 2012. "Availability and marketing of food and beverages to children through sports settings: A systematic review." *Public Health Nutrition* 15 (8): 1373–1379.

Caulkin, George. 2017. "Club where meat is off the menu and the pitch is fed seaweed: Forest Green Rovers head in to their first League season on a mission to change attitudes, says George Caulkin." *The Times*, July 29.

Čulić, Viktor. 2011. "Football matches and acute cardiac events: Potential effects of a complex psychosocial phenomenon on cardiovascular health." *International Journal of Epidemiology* 40 (5): 1422–1425.

Curran, Kathryn, Barry Drust, & Dave Richardson. 2014. "'I just want to watch the match': A practitioner's reflective account of men's health themed match day events at an English Premier League football club." *Soccer & Society* 15 (6): 919–933.

Daily Mail. 2011. "Who ate all the lentils? Vegan football boss bans matchday meat pies and burgers." *Daily Mail*, February 11.

Department of Health. 2017. "Australia's physical activity and sedentary behaviour guidelines." *Australian Government Department of Health*. www.health.gov.au/internet/main/publishing.nsf/Content/health-pubhlth-strateg-phys-act-guidelines.

Department of Health and Ageing. 2010. "National male health policy: Building on the strengths of Australian males." Edited by Department of Health and Ageing Canberra.

Dinu, Monica, Rosanna Abbate, Gian Franco Gensini, Alessandro Casini, & Francesco Sofi. 2017. "Vegetarian, vegan diets and multiple health outcomes: A systematic review with meta-analysis of observational studies." *Critical Reviews in Food Science and Nutrition* 57 (17): 3640–3649.

Drygas, Wojciech, Joanna Ruszkowska, Matthew Philpott, Olav Björkström, Mike Parker, Robin Ireland, Federico Roncarolo, & Maria Tenconi. 2013. "Good practices and health policy analysis in European sports stadia: Results from the 'Healthy Stadia' project." *Health Promotion International* 28 (2): 157–165. doi: 10.1093/heapro/dar088.

Ecotricity Group Limited. 2011. "Directors' report and financial statements." Stroud, Gloucestershire: Ecotricity Group.

Edwards, Richard B. 2018. "Vegans to be cheerful: Forest green: Football's eco-warriors." *The People*, November 18.

European Healthy Stadia Network. 2019. "Policy guidance for stadia" Accessed March 20, 2019. https://healthystadia.eu/policy-guidance-for-stadia/.

FIFA. 2018. "The village club earning UN honours and global acclaim." Accessed October, 29, 2018. www.fifa.com/sustainability/news/y=2018/m=10/news=the-village-club-earning-un-honours-and-global-acclaim.html.

Football Association. 2017. *A Guide to the FA Kit and Advertising Regulations Season 2017–18.* London: The Football Association.

Football Ground Guide. n.d. "Forest Green Rovers: The New Lawn." Accessed March 25, 2019. www.footballgroundguide.com/leagues/england/league-two/forest-green-rovers-the-new-lawn.html.

Forest Green Rovers. 2018. "FGR footprint report 2018." Nailsworth, Gloucestershire: Forest Green Rovers.

Forest Green Rovers. 2019. "NEWS: Work begins on new bar." Accessed February 21, 2019. www.fgr.co.uk/news/february-2019/news-work-begins-on-new-bar.

Forest Green Rovers. n.d. "FGR forum." Accessed March 25, 2019. http://forum.fgrfc.net/.

Gaffney, Christopher. 2008. *Temples of the Earthbound Gods: The Stadiums of Rio de Janeiro and Buenos Aires.* Austin: University of Texas Press.

Gaffney, Christopher & John Bale. 2004. "Sensing the stadium." In *Sites of Sport: Space, Place, Experience*, edited by Patricia Vertinsky & John Bale, 25–38. London: Routledge.

Garde, Amandine & Neville Rigby. 2012. "Going for gold: Should responsible governments raise the bar on sponsorship of the Olympic Games and other sporting events by food and beverage companies?" *Communications Law* 17 (2): 42–49.

Garry, Tom. 2017. "Forest Green Rovers: The village team that reached the English Football League." *BBC*, May 15. www.bbc.co.uk/sport/football/39923153.

George, Emma S., Gregory S. Kolt, Mitch J. Duncan, Cristina M. Caperchione, W. Kerry Mummery, Corneel Vandelanotte, Pennie Taylor, & Manny Noakes. 2012. "A review of the effectiveness of physical activity interventions for adult males." *Sports Medicine* 42 (4): 281–300. doi: 10.2165/11597220-000000000-00000.

Gong, Lie, Takayuki Morikawa, Toshiyuki Yamamoto, & Hitomo Sata. 2014. "Deriving personal trip data from GPS data: A literature review on the existing methodologies." *Procedia- Social and Behavioural Sciences* 138: 557–565. doi: 10.1016/j.sbspro.2014.07.239.

Gordon, Dan. (2017) "HUNGER GAMES." *Stadia*, March 2017.

Gray, Cindy M., Kate Hunt, Nanette Mutrie, Annie S. Anderson, Jim Leishman, Lindsay Dalgarno, & Sally Wyke. 2013. "Football Fans in training: The development and optimization of an intervention delivered through professional sports clubs to help men lose weight, become more active and adopt healthier eating habits." *BMC Public Health* 13 (1): 232.

Grøntved, Anders & Frank B. Hu. 2011. "Television viewing and risk of type 2 diabetes, cardiovascular disease, and all-cause mortality." *The Journal of the American Medical Association* 305 (23): 2448–2455. doi: 10.1001/jama.2011.812.

Haynes, Natalie. 2011. "If you're going to impose your ethical choices, go the whole hog." *The Independent*, February 12.

Healy, Genevive, David Dunstan, Jo Salmon, Ester Cerin, Jonathan Shaw, Paul Zimmet, & Neville Owen. 2008. "Breaks in sedentary time: Beneficial associations with metabolic risk." *Diabetes Care* 31 (4): 661–666.

Hughes, Janet. 2018. "'My car was full of fish and chips': Taxi driver's surprise at taking huge order of chicken and fast food to 'vegan' club Forest Green after match." Accessed April 23, 2019. www.gloucestershirelive.co.uk/news/gloucester-news/my-car-full-fish-chips-2217567.

Hunt, Kate, Sally Wyke, Cindy M. Gray, Annie S. Anderson, Adrian Brady, Christopher Bunn, Peter T. Donnan, et al. 2014. "A gender-sensitised weight loss and healthy living programme for overweight and obese men delivered by Scottish Premier League football clubs (FFIT): A pragmatic randomised controlled trial." *The Lancet* 383 (9924): 1211–1221.

Ireland, Robin & Francine Watkins. 2010. "Football fans and food: A case study of a football club in the English Premier League." *Public Health Nutrition* 13 (5): 682–687.

James, Stuart. (2017). "Forest Green: The eco-friendly club with a robot mower and big ambitions." Accessed April 23, 2019. www.theguardian.com/football/2017/jul/31/forest-green-rovers-league-two.

Jones, Luke, Phil Marshall, and Jim Denison. 2016. "Health and well-being implications surrounding the use of wearable GPS devices in professional rugby league: A Foucauldian disciplinary analysis of the normalised use of a common surveillance aid." *Performance Enhancement & Health* 5: 38–46.

Johnson, Alan (*@AFootballWriter*). 2018. "@AFootballWriter twitter post." November 3, 11:31am. https://twitter.com/AFootballWriter.

Lee, Seunghwan, Bob Heere, & Kyu-soo Chung. 2013. "Which senses matter more? The impact of our senses on team identity and team loyalty." *Sport Marketing Quarterly* 22 (4): 203–213.

Lewis, Colin J., Matthew J. Reeves, & Simon J. Roberts. 2017. "Improving the physical and mental well-being of typically hard-to-reach men: An investigation of the impact of the *Active Rovers* project." *Sport in Society* 20 (2): 258–268.

Maddison, Ralph, Elaine Anne Hargreaves, Sally Wyke, Cindy M. Gray, Kate Hunt, Justin Ihirangi Heke, Stephen Kara, et al. 2019. "Rugby Fans in Training New Zealand (RUFIT-NZ): A pilot randomized controlled trial of a healthy lifestyle program for overweight men delivered through professional rugby clubs in New Zealand." *BMC Public Health* 19 (1): 166.

Martin, Angus, Simon Morgan, Daniel Parnell, Matthew Philpott, Andy Pringle, Michael Rigby, Andy Taylor, & Jon Topham. 2016. "A perspective from key stakeholders on football and health improvement." *Soccer & Society* 17 (2): 175–182.

Martin, David S. & Martin O'Neill. 2010. "Scale development and testing: A new measure of cognitive satisfaction in sports tourism." *Event Management* 14 (1): 1–15.

McKenna, Jim, Thomas Quarmby, Nicky Kime, Daniel Parnell, & Stephen Zwolinsky. 2017. "Lessons from the field for working in Healthy Stadia: Physical activity practitioners reflect on 'sport'." *Sport in Society* 20 (2): 316–324.

Morgan, Philip J., Janet M. Warren, David R. Lubans, Clare E. Collins, & Robin Callister. 2011. "Engaging men in weight loss: Experiences of men who participated in the male only SHED-IT pilot study." *Obesity Research & Clinical Practice* 5 (3): e239–e248.

Murray, Andrew, Kieren Turner, Daryll Archilbald, Chloe Schiphorst, Steffan Griffin, Hilary Scott, Roger Hawkes, et al. 2017. "An observational study of spectators' step counts and reasons for attending a professional golf tournament in Scotland." *BMJ Open Sport & Exercise Medicine* 3 (1): 1–7. doi: 10.1136/bmjsem-2017-000244.

National Health and Medical Research Council. 2013 "Australian dietary guidelines: Summary." Accessed February 23, 2019. www.nhmrc.gov.au/guidelines-publications/n55.

NHS Digital. 2018. "Statistics on obesity, physical activity and diet England: 2018." Accessed April 23, 2019. https://files.digital.nhs.uk/publication/0/0/obes-phys-acti-diet-eng-2018-rep.pdf.

Oliver, Brian. 2017. "A vegan diet helps them win: But are sports stars committed to the cause?" *The Observer*, July 30.

Olsen, Peter., John Elliott, Chris Frampton, & Paul Bradley. 2015. "Winning or losing does matter: Acute cardiac admissions in New Zealand during Rugby World Cup tournaments." *European Journal of Preventive Cardiology* 22 (10): 1254–1260.

Onozuka, Daisuke & Akihito Hagihara. 2018. "Out-of-hospital cardiac arrests during the Japanese professional baseball championship series." *American Journal of Cardiology* 121 (12): 1471–1476.

Pagoto, Sherry L., Kristin L. Schneider, Jessica L. Oleski, Juliana M. Luciani, Jamie S. Bodenlos, & Matt C. Whited. 2012. "Male inclusion in randomized controlled trials of lifestyle weight loss interventions." *Obesity* 20 (6): 1234–1239.

Parry, Keith D. 2012. "Game of two passions: A football fan's autoethnography." *Qualitative Research Journal* 12 (2): 238–250.

Parry, Keith D., Tim Hall, & Al Baxter. 2017. "Who ate all the pies? The importance of food in the Australian sporting experience." *Sport in Society* 20 (2): 202–218.

Parry, Keith D., David Rowe, Emma S. George, & Tim Hall. 2018. "Healthy sport consumption: Moving away from pies and beer." In *Sport and Health: Exploring the Current State of Play*, edited by Daniel Parnell, Kathryn Curran & Matthew Philpott. London: Routledge.

Paulas, Rick. 2011. "An MLB guide to all you can eat." Accessed October 7, 2019. https://www.espn.com/travel/news/story?id=6559938.

Petrella, Robert J., Dawn P. Gill, Guangyong Zou, Ashleigh De Cruz, Brendan Riggin, Cassandra Bartol, Karen Danylchuk, et al. 2017. "Hockey fans in training: A pilot pragmatic randomized controlled trial." *Medicine and Science in Sports and Exercise* 49 (12): 2506.

Philpott, Mathew & Russel Seymour. 2011. "The European healthy stadia network: Sports stadia, public health and sustainability." In *Sustainability and Sport*, edited by Jill Savery & Keith Gilbert. Champaign, IL: Common Ground.

Pringle, Alan. 2009. "The growing role of football as a vehicle for interventions in mental health care." *Journal of Psychiatric and Mental Health Nursing* 16 (6): 553–557.

Quested, Eleanor, Dominika Kwasnicka, Cecilie Thøgersen-Ntoumani, Daniel F. Gucciardi, Deborah A. Kerr, Kate Hunt, Suzanne Robinson, et al. 2018. "Protocol for a gender-sensitised weight loss and healthy living programme for overweight and obese men delivered in Australian football league settings (Aussie-FIT): A feasibility and pilot randomised controlled trial." *BMJ Open* 8 (10): e022663.

Rasmussen, Thomas, Jesper Ingvardson, Katrin Halldorsdottir, & Otto Neilssen. 2013. "Using Wearable GPS devices in travel surveys: A Case study in the Greater Copenhagen Area." Paper presented at the Proceedings from the Annual Transport Conference, Denmark, August 20–22.

Richards, Jessica. 2016. "Sports space: A conceptual model of Everton football club matchday fan movement." PhD diss., The University of Sydney, Sydney.

Richards, Jessica & Keith D. Parry. 2019. "Beers and blurred boundaries: The spatial and gendered organisation of pre-match venues for English football." *Fans International Review for the Sociology of Sport* 1–19. https://doi.org/10.1177/1012690219835487.

Schutz, Yves & A. Chambaz. 1997. "Could a satellite-based navigation system (GPS) be used to assess the physical activity of individuals on earth?" *European Journal of Clinical Nutrition* 51 (5): 338–339. www.ncbi.nlm.nih.gov/pubmed/9152686.

Scott, Charlie. 2018. "20 cup stories you may have missed." *The Times*, January 8.

Sherriff, Jill L., Denise Griffiths, & Mike Daube. 2010. "Cricket: Notching up runs for food and alcohol companies?" *Australian and New Zealand Journal of Public Health* 34 (1): 19–23.

Sport England. 2018. "Active lives adult survey: May 17/18 report." Accessed April 22, 2019. www.sportengland.org/media/13768/active-lives-adult-may-17-18-report.pdf.

Stuart, James. 2017. "Forest Green: The club with a robot mower, its own hostel and big ambition." *The Guardian*, July 31.

Sukalakamala, Piyavan, Sophitmanee Sukalakamala, & Pam Young. 2013. "An exploratory study of the concession preferences of generation Y consumers." *Journal of Foodservice Business Research* 16 (4): 378–390. doi: 10.1080/15378020.2013.824278.

Trip Advisor. n.d. "The new lawn stadium." Accessed March 25, 2019. www.tripadvisor.co.uk/Attraction_Review-g315974-d12863034-Reviews-The_New_Lawn_Stadium-Nailsworth_Stroud_Stroud_District_Cotswolds_England.html.

Uğur, Seçil. 2013. *Wearing Embodied Emotions A Practice Based Design Research on Wearable Technology*. Milan; New York: Springer.

Vegetarian Living. n.d. "Rovers' red card to meat." Accessed March 25, 2019. www.vegetarianliving.co.uk/interviews.php?do=view&article=55.

Wann, Daniel. 2006. "Understanding the positive social psychological benefits of sport team identification: The team identification: Social psychological health model." *Group Dynamics: Theory, Research, and Practice* 10 (4): 272–296. doi: 10.1037/1089-2699.10.4.272.

WHO (World Health Organisation). 2015. "Healthy diet". Accessed January 28, 2019. www.who.int/mediacentre/factsheets/fs394/en/.

Williams, Jack. 2015. "No more meat pies at soccer's greenest stadium." *New York Times*, April 6.

Witcoop, Darren. 2017. "Reality bites for the vegan trailblazers: Inside the EFL." *Daily Express*, December 22.

Woods, Lindsey. 2012. "Happily unhealthy: A case study of sports fans." *The Chronical: Columbia College Chicago*, April 30. https://columbiachronicle.com/f70b752b-5f65-5e66-8d2e-ce39d6335918.

Wyke, Sally, Christopher Bunn, Eivind Andersen, Marlene N. Silva, Femke Van Nassau, Paula McSkimming, Spyros Kolovos, et al. 2019. "The effect of a programme to improve men's sedentary time and physical activity: The European Fans in Training (EuroFIT) randomised controlled trial." *PLoS Medicine* 16 (2): e1002736.

Yancey, Antronette, David Winfield, Judi Larsen, Michele Anderson, Portia Jackson, Jeff Overton, Shawn Wilson, Allen Rossum, & Shiriki Kumanyika. 2009. "'Live, learn and play': Building strategic alliances between professional sports and public health." *Preventive Medicine* 49 (4): 322–325.

Yin, Robert. 2013. *Case Study Research: Design and Methods*. 5th ed. Thousand Oaks, CA: Sage Publications.

York, Judy & Parag Pendharkar. 2004. "Human: Computer interaction issues for mobile computing in a variable work context." *International Journal of Human-Computer Studies* 60 (5–6): 771–797. doi: 10.1016/j.ijhcs.2003.07.004.

Chapter 14

Smartphone fitness apps and football fans

A case study of Fan Fit

Alex Fenton, Anna M. Cooper-Ryan and Cristina M. Vasilica

Introduction

This chapter explores the current evidence base in relation to building a community of participation of supporters through a digital health smartphone application and resulting interactions. As part of this, we explore the relevant policy agenda, which is likely to impact football clubs in the digital era. Then, to help illustrate how fans can be engaged digitally, we present an example of how action research for a digital intervention project (called Fan Fit) has been implemented in the real world to benefit the physical activity of sports fans.

The massive global growth of smartphone apps, social media networks and increased Internet connectivity presents great opportunities for engaging fans. Lawrence and Crawford (2018) highlight that football fans are now hyper-digitalised. That is, they are always connected through websites and apps on their phones and other devices. Meanwhile, the market for digital fitness apps and devices continues to grow (Tu et al., 2018). This presents prevention opportunities for health issues such as heart disease, obesity and diabetes. Globally there is an increasing concern around the rise of non-communicable disease, with the Global Burden of Disease study finding that ischaemic heart disease was the leading cause of death globally in 2017, with stroke being the third most common (Institute for Health Metrics and Evaluation, 2018). In the United Kingdom (UK), The British Heart Foundation report in 2017 compiled a number of data sources finding that 39% of adults did not meet the government guidelines around physical activity and that on average men spend 78 days a year sitting. There was also much variation in activity levels across different regions (British Heart Foundation, 2017).

As well as with adults, obesity and sedentary lifestyles in young people is a growing societal problem (Mitchell et al., 2009; Tremblay et al., 2011; Saunders et al., 2014). These issues are particularly prevalent in towns and cities in the North of England (including Salford and Manchester) and in Scotland (British Heart Foundation, 2017). The increases in these non-communicable lifestyle issues, the interest in fitness app usage and the rise in smartphone ownership, have influenced the digital project outlined in this chapter.

Major manufacturers of hardware and software such as Google, Intel and Apple and the largest social media platforms are working to get ahead in the rise of mobile health (m-health). With the considerable growth of smartphones and apps, people are becoming more connected, and arguably more conscious about their own health and wellbeing. However, in areas such as weight management, there is a need for more collaborative ventures to develop effective evidence-based digital health projects. This presents a major opportunity for football clubs and for academic research to gain new insight into digital fitness for fans. Social media and fitness apps can be used to combine people's love of football, support interaction with fans and players, and to help fans become more aware of their own fitness and wellbeing through friendly competition.

Utilizing all opportunities to engage people in a healthier lifestyle is of growing importance to local and national governments and healthcare providers (such as the NHS and Public Health departments in the UK, and insurance companies in the US) in order to reduce operational strain and rising costs caused by unhealthy lifestyles and the associated health issues. On an international scale, Sweeney and Quimby (2012) highlighted the dangers and cost of global health and fitness issues, saying 'within the next ten years China, India, and the United Kingdom are projecting losses in national income of US$828 billion due to reduced economic productivity associated with chronic disease'. In the UK, in 2016–17, there were 617 thousand admissions to hospital where obesity was a factor with the majority of these people aged 35–64. When they were asked about their weight, 45% believed they were around the right weight and 45% said they were too heavy. This demonstrates that people can be unclear about obesity, which can also impact their engagement with support programmes (NHS Digital and National Statistics, 2018).

Many of the lifestyle non-communicable diseases have a variety of symptoms, which include high blood pressure and high blood cholesterol. These are often caused by smoking, weight gain, inactivity and poor diet. In the North-West of England, 27% of adults in 2012 were recorded as obese, which contributes to the much lower life expectancy found in the region (Public Health England, 2012). The picture is similar across Europe, where we face tough health challenges, such as the number one killer – heart disease – which is reported to cause almost twice as many fatalities as cancer across the continent (Townsend, Nichols, Scarborough, & Rayner, 2015). Throughout Europe, these premature deaths are closely linked to social inequality, particularly related to those who fall into lower income brackets and living in less privileged communities. An example can be found through the 'Scottish Effect' and the 'Glasgow Effect', where life expectancy is lower than the expected average in more deprived areas (Dahlgren and Whitehead, 2007).

Mobile devices and sports fans

The majority of sports clubs have embraced digital technologies including smartphones and apps at the board and fan level. Sports clubs at all levels are embracing smartphones by engaging their fans through platforms such as Twitter, Facebook, Instagram and YouTube (McCarthy et al., 2014). Larger sports clubs have marketing and communications departments and both large and small clubs are using social media to connect with their fans. Fans of clubs at all levels are utilising mobile devices and cameras to produce video and photos to feed into these social media platforms (Fenton and Helleu, 2019). Although the majority of clubs have at least a basic website and social media presence, clubs and fans at all levels are interested in how to effectively use social media, apps, the Internet of Things, video games and other technologies to further engage fans and connect with each other (Anagnostopoulos et al., 2018; Fenton, 2018).

Successful digital channels and apps have been found to increase fan engagement, the frequency of engagement and ultimately make the brand of a sports club better known (Fenton and Helleu, 2019). As such, digital media has an important role to play in building, promoting and maintaining a fan base. Understanding the benefits and challenges of digital media to engage fans is therefore crucial. The dual purpose of engagement and conversation through digital platforms and the growth in popularity of fitness apps has led to the creation of *Fan Fit* as a real-world research project which aims to support clubs with their corporate-social responsibility through digital fan engagement and wellbeing. Longer term this might produce outcomes for both fans and the clubs. The former are engaged in looking after their own health and wellbeing by reducing obesity and related diseases (Coughlin, 2016; Jee, 2017). Involving people within large networks (e.g. fans of a club), offering support and advice, and gaining the drive and additional resources that can help to motivate achievement of personal exercise goals.

There is considerable scope for research and development to understand the use of apps and virtual communities for the 'always on' generation of smartphone-owning fans, where data and the customer (fan) is central to the activity and often found to be wanting constant updates and engagement (Heinze et al., 2016). In order to do this successfully it is important to understand the needs and behaviours of fans and the ways they communicate online.

Sports policy and CSR

In sports, the concept of doing sport for good is widely adopted by the industry as part of corporate social responsibility (CSR) (Breitbarth et al., 2011). In a broader sense, CSR is a long-standing concept in that organisations are socially accountable to stakeholders and the public. CSR presents a variety of approaches and theories with a long history, evolving from the Paris Agreement and linking into the Sustainable Development Goals (SDG) which were adopted in 2016 (Garriga and Melé, 2004). As part of the SDGs, organisations are expected to contribute to the global determination to achieve the goals. As part of this, it could be said that the view held by football clubs that they have a responsibility to their communities of fans to encourage wellbeing, healthy living, exercise and research can feed into the SDGs. Implementation of CSR models within the football industry are widely adopted and discussed in literature (e.g. Breitbarth et al., 2011; Zeimers et al., 2019). However, as with many things, the challenges associated with implementation of CSR are associated with managerial alignment of strategies, conflict and access to resources which triggers inconsistent application of CSR (Anagnostopoulos and Shilbury, 2013).

The SDG of good health and wellbeing is prominent in the healthy stadia agenda, with the healthy stadia agenda (source) being concerned with promoting positive health behaviours through in-stadium healthier living choices, community initiatives and workforce development (source). In relation to population health, sports stadia enable access to large number of individuals, and often a chance to target hard-to-reach groups to tackle issues such as diet, nutrition, physical activity and other lifestyle behaviours (Ramshaw et al., 2013). The underpinning principle is that supportive social communities influence positive healthy behaviours. This also relates to adopting a 'settings approach' to public health 'bringing to bear public health resources on everyday sites of mass interaction' (Parnell et al., 2017). Specifically, utilizing sports club brands to promote health and fitness of fans.

Action research (AR) and CSR

One method that can support clubs to develop projects and help fan engagement is to undertake AR. AR began in the health sciences as a method to create practical and useful research in multiple iterations. It was popularised for use in the medical field by (Lewin, 1946) and in more recent times, AR has grown in prominence within the social sciences to support practical and insightful research. It has been utilised within the academic community to cross the gap that exists between academia and practice (Cavicchi et al., 2014). Although it has been used less in relation to healthy stadia, AR could provide a framework for the implementation of CSR within the football industry to address existing challenges and refine solutions to issues being tackled (e.g. supporting the health and wellbeing of fans). The underlying concept of AR is to undertake multiple iterations of a project/activity to support effective engagement/design and delivery (e.g. fan engagement activities and programme implementation) (Heinze et al., 2016). Each AR iteration involves planning, acting, observing and reflecting (as shown in the diagram below). AR typically uses a combination of researchers and practitioners of different fields and as part of the research and implementation to help combine different skill sets and build on community assets.

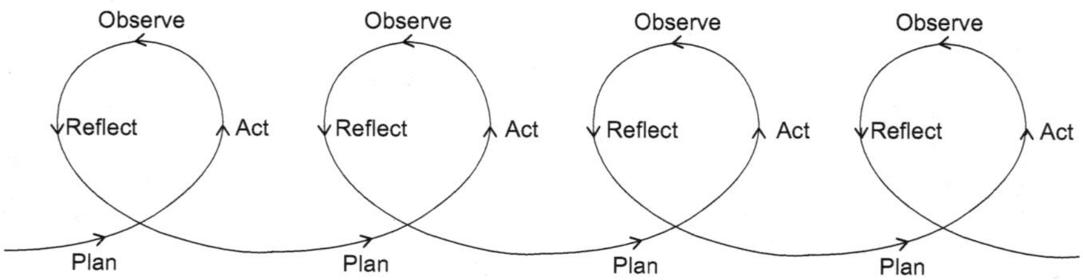

Figure 14.1 The AR cycle.
Source: Heinze et al., 2016.

Fan Fit case study

In the next part of this chapter we present a case study of Fan Fit as an example of how a smartphone application can be utilised by a sports club to support their fans' health and wellbeing, meet the healthy stadia agenda and CSR of sports clubs. The combination of the health issues outlined above, the rise of smartphones for fan interactions, the rise in health apps and increases everyday use of wearable technologies (such as fitness wristbands) sets the context for Fan Fit.

Fan Fit is a project based at the University of Salford, UK aimed at improving the fitness and wellbeing of fans through their engagement with technology. This project utilised the concept of AR in a number of ways, with underpinning research projects taking the form of multiple projects which engaged students as well as external partners. To ensure the evidence base of the app the research and design team was comprised of academics with backgrounds in information systems and health sciences, and students working across a range of topics including digital marketing, digital development, User Experience and business planning. We also worked with several external companies including app developers and User Experience experts, sports clubs and fans. Drawing on a range of expertise and backgrounds is crucial for tacking complicated situations such as lifestyle health issues, which often have complex behavioural influences and aetiologies. It also ensures that beyond the evidence base, there is engagement from those who participate in any ongoing development, participation in initial pilot research and evaluation of the app as it is developed and also used by professional clubs to support fan health and wellbeing. This builds on the knowledge that understanding the needs of a community and building on assets is more likely to lead to behaviour change, as well as the importance of doing research 'with' not 'on' people (Involve, 2019).

The project was initially named Footy Fit, but renamed to Fan Fit when it became apparent that the app might work effectively for other kinds of sports clubs. In 2018, a version of Fan Fit was created for Salford Red Devils Rugby league club, which provided the first implementation partnering with a professional sports club. A version for a Scottish football club is in development at the time of writing through a collaboration with the Healthier Lives Data Fund from the Scottish Government and Nesta.

Fan Fit began as an idea to engage football fans and raise awareness of fitness levels through their love of their favourite teams. The concept therefore was to combine fitness as gamification (game-like features) with social media information from their favourite club. Fan Fit has created a fitness app for people that may not traditionally use this kind of app or fitness wristbands.

The first version of the app created the basic ability to track walking and running, combined with football club social media feeds and video with live information embedded directly into it. It was designed to become an official app of a sports club, rebranded into the clubs colours so that it is recognisable as being part of a club's offering to their fans. Fan Fit includes the usual club app functions such as pulling in club news, fixtures, team and social media feeds. Furthermore, on a day-to-day basis, Fan Fit tracks movement in terms of steps and minutes, allowing fans to set their own daily minutes target and compete against other fans in leagues. The built-in leagues are split into:

1 Global – all-time highest number of steps since the app is launched
2 Monthly – highest steps from the start to the finish of a calendar month
3 Personal – allows fans to create their own mini league containing their own friends and others they want to compete against

The leagues are designed to create an active community, with more people choosing to walk on match days, and encouraging them through the app, which in turn can reinforce achievement and improve motivation. Working in partnership with a sports club means this can be done through physical prizes linked to the club (e.g. season tickets, shirts and fitness wristbands). For all users, digital badges (graphic designed icons) can also be earned for maintaining levels of fitness to encourage the maintenance of behaviour change through a process of reward and recognition.

This type of fan app provides a productive way in which fan groups can interact with each other, through sharing their achievements on the app and through social media such as Facebook and Twitter. For example, the people involved within a network (e.g. fans of a club) offer support, advice, and gain the drive and additional resources that can help to motivate achievement of personal exercise goals. Word of mouth and social media conversation about the app and the use of club-based and exercise-based competition between fans can help to reinforce their motivation.

Through the implementation of the app, we have observed increased social media engagement and interaction with the app. Through the app, clubs, researchers and potentially health professionals can learn about the walking/running habits of supporters over time. Fan Fit tracks and measures the number of steps and active minutes which are tracked automatically through the phone or a fitness wristband. This data can then in turn help clubs to support their fans and work with health providers to improve the health and wellbeing advice/support that is provided to supporters, which feeds into the Healthy Stadia agenda (Parnell et al., 2017). With Fan Fit to date, there were three key iterations (phases) of the AR cycle, which are outlined below and can be used as a guide for others in the future.

Phase 1 of the project began with formulating the original idea through working with football clubs and evaluating similar projects. To support this, a target audience survey was created which was augmented using qualitative data from participant observation and focus groups using an ethnographical approach (Atkinson, 2015). We used a netnography approach, which is a set of standards and guidelines for conducting participant observation online through social media (Kozinets, 2015). The gathering of this information allowed the initial app development to begin,

Table 14.1 Phases of AR undertaken within the case study

Phase 1	*Phase 2*	*Phase 3*
Plan – Initial idea to create a fitness app for a football club called Footy Fit	Plan – create rebranded instance of the app for Salford Red Devils Rugby club called 'Red Devils Fan Fit'	Plan – create rebranded version of Fan Fit app for Rangers FC called 'Fit Bears'
Act – secure internal funding and appoint app develop to develop a minimum viable product (MVP)	Act – secure internal funding, appoint student and then app development company to develop app Beta on Android and then iPhone	Act – secure external funding and develop new version with new features identified in phase 2
Observe – use of target audience survey, user experience testing, focus groups and Masters projects to gather data	Observe – use of focus groups, user experience testing, social network analysis and netnography	Observe – use of focus groups, analytics data and netnography
Reflect – shape future direction and roadmap of new features, rebrand to Fan Fit	Reflect – shape future direction and source external funding and new partners	Reflect – shape future direction for a potential fourth phase

after which focus groups and User Experience testing with university students was employed. This helped to refine the app and led to the development of a MVP (minimum viable product). At this stage, further focus groups with university staff and students were employed to develop the road map of features for the app. A larger survey with the general public in Manchester helped to determine the target audience and horizon scanning to identify barriers to adoption. Further, social network analysis designed to map out and analyse social media conversations provided a better understanding of the connections between developers, academics and research participants who are important to a project of this type of app. Finally, once there was a working prototype app, further focus groups and user experience testing were conducted to gain the views on the app by those it targets (e.g. sport club fans).

Target-audience survey

Working with masters students at the University of Salford, we formulated some initial survey questions to understand more about the audience for Fan Fit including:

- Demographic information
- How many people owned a smartphone or fitness wristband

- What sports people were interested in
- How comfortable they were in sharing their fitness scores with friends or publically
- If they would be interested in an app which combined news from their favourite club with fitness features

The structured survey aimed to gauge the market for an app such as Fan Fit. It also aimed to understand the factors that could hinder the adoption of Fan Fit within the UK, asking about potential barriers. Overall, the survey aimed to allow understanding of the possibilities of people using an app such as Fan Fit, their preferences and potential adoption figures. Our initial survey (n=123) found that the target audience surveyed was receptive to the use of a smartphone app designed to support improvements in physical activity.

Netnography

As outlined, a further method utilised was the adoption of a netnography approach of participant observation online (Kozinets, 2015) and blending of methods including interviews and social network analysis (Fenton and Procter, 2019). This allowed the team to interact with fans that were using the Fan Fit app to gather feedback as part of the AR cycle. Through this we were able to gain an insight into how the app was discussed on social media, for example:

> 'I've done 182 steps and 0 minutes of activity with #Fan Fit lol can tell it's my week off'
>
> 'Been on #Fan Fit for weeks. The competition starts now eh??
> I will be definitely involved in that! It will be great for all fans to get #Fan Fit'
>
> 'I'm at 226.432 steps and because of this iv lost 7lbs I'm very very competitive!'
>
> 'After the walking challenge last month, I actually felt confident enough today to manage my first run in 5 years since my knee injury only 1 1/4 miles but a start:-)'

One of the challenges found in initial testing is the engagement and downloading of the app by supporters and players. A challenge with a club app can be the buy-in from all aspects of clubs from management, communication teams, outreach teams and players.

App engagement

Having engagement from all aspects and players (which fans most want to engage with) can also support the adoption of an app. Of the fans that downloaded the app, 76.6% of users were male and 23.4% were female, which is similar to many clubs' fan population. There was also a range of ages of fans that downloaded the

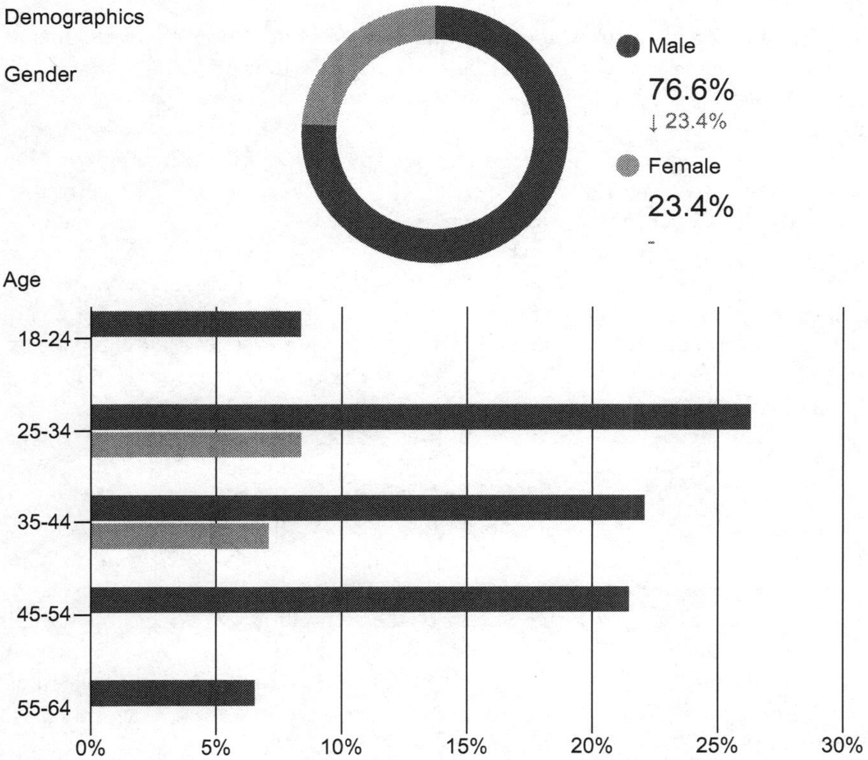

Figure 14.2 Demographic information derived from Red Devils Fan Fit app usage December 2018.

app from 18–64, with the most popular age being 25–44 years old, a key demographic for many health and wellbeing initiatives.

From this project there are a number of transferable lessons, which have been learned through the engagement. The Fan Fit team initially felt that engaging team players to also use the app would be motivating for fans. However, in the case study to date it was found that players were not able to use their phones or fitness wristbands for both practical and operational reasons. Although clubs do capture GPS movements of players, it was not possible to input this data directly into the app to allow them to be part of the competition this way. Going forward, apps of this nature need to establish a way to engage both the fans and the club's players and staff to allow the interaction and building of a larger community. Engaging players in this kind of activity in the future could let them act as ambassadors and influencers for use of the app and build social capital, and thus help increase fans motivation to exercise and remain healthy (Fenton, 2017).

Conclusion and recommendations

The monitoring and improvement of the health and fitness through digital means is a hot topic for practical research. This is in part due to its potential and versatility. In the light of CSR and the healthy stadia agenda, organisations are interested in a healthy workforce and customers, and are often supporting positive changes in the community. Meanwhile, health services are increasingly keen on prevention rather than cure, in part due to the economic conditions which are being experienced by many countries as well as increasing life expectancy. This means there is growing importance to maintain healthy lifestyles for longer. This has led to a need for more effective public health strategies across a variety of settings, so football, smartphones and research all have their part to play in addressing these health issues. Within the current political and social context, for example financial cuts, increased pressures on the NHS through staff shortage and increased numbers of people with chronic diseases, more effective community integrated solutions are necessary. Involving large communities of fans using digital solutions could trigger positive outcomes in that people are healthier with the potential to address some of the existing societal and political challenges.

In this chapter, we have explored the methodological approaches of AR in relation to a smartphone app to engage fans around fitness embedded into the digital community eco-system of their own club. According to evidence collected to date, it seems that the app is welcomed amongst the community of fans although there is a need to consider engagement challenges going forward. We believe that AR offers the correct methodological approach to actively change and improve initiatives, which may offer a potential solution to support and guide CSR initiatives (Zeimers et al., 2019).

Alongside engaging fans in relation to lifestyle behavior change, sports clubs are also increasingly engaged in campaigns around mental wellbeing. These offer development opportunities for smartphone apps, which can support a person physical as well as mental wellbeing. In relation to mental wellbeing, apps such as Headspace have attracted a great deal of attention as a way to use smartphone apps to improve mental health and wellbeing. Through taking an AR approach, which combines a passion for a sports club with physical health and mental wellbeing, there is the potential that sports club can have a greater impact in reaching and engaging harder to reach and wider groups to support the wellbeing agenda.

Furthermore, through initiatives such Fan Fit, general practitioners could prescribe social activities to support people's wellbeing by linking them with social activities such as football, as it is known that harder to reach groups can be reluctant to engage with traditional NHS prevention services (Bickerdike et al., 2017). As such, digital sports communities could offer attractive support environments and camaraderie both online and offline. The link amongst healthy stadia and social prescribing offer an interesting area of research in the wider field of Football as Medicine. On a regional and national level, funders should also be open to innovative projects and collaborations in order to support impact on a larger scale.

A challenge can be the crosscutting nature of projects in relation to digital, sports and health and wellbeing in relation to gaining funding.

An important aspect of the creation of any app is that it is designed with the user in mind. As such, we propose the use of AR and user-centred design to ensure that fans and those at the club are involved at all stages, and that robust evaluation is included in any design or use of these types of applications. This will also ensure that any app aligns with a clubs branding, principles, engagement strategies and the needs of fans to create behavioral change. Finally, there is a clear need for more research to investigate the use of AR as a process in implementing digital health projects within the football industry.

References

Anagnostopoulos, C., Parganas, P., Fenton, A. and Chadwick, S. (2018) Branding in pictures: Using instagram as a brand management tool in professional team sport organisations. *European Sport Management Quartely*, 18(4) pp. 1–46.

Anagnostopoulos, C. and Shilbury, D. (2013), Implementing corporate social responsibility in English football. *Sport, Business and Management: An International Journal*, 3(4) pp. 268–284.

Atkinson, P. (2015) *For Ethnography*. Sage. [Online] [Accessed on 19th November 2015] https://uk.sagepub.com/en-gb/eur/for-ethnography/book234711.

Bickerdike, L., Booth, A., Wilson, P. M., Farley, K. and Wright, K. (2017) Social prescribing: Less rhetoric and more reality: A systematic review of the evidence. *BMJ Open*, 7(4) p. e013384.

Breitbarth, T., Hovemann, G. and Walzel, S. (2011) Scoring strategy goals: Measuring corporate social responsibility in professional European football. *Thunderbird International Business Review*, 53(6) pp. 721–737.

British Heart Foundation (2017) *Physical Inactivity and Sedentary Behaviour Report 2017*.

Cavicchi, A., Santini, C. and Bailetti, L. (2014) Mind the "academician-practitioner" gap: An experience-based model in the food and beverage sector. *Qualitative Market Research: An International Journal*, 17(4) pp. 319–335.

Coughlin, S. S. (2016) The need for research-tested smartphone applications for promoting breastfeeding. *mHealth*, 2(5) p. 18.

Dahlgren, G. and Whitehead M. (2007). European strategies for tackling social inequities in health: Levelling up Part 2. Copenhagen, WHO Regional Office for Europe (Studies on social and economic determinants of population health, No. 3).

Fenton, A. (2017) *The Field Behind the Screen: Social Capital and the Social Media Communications of a Football Club Brand*. University of Salford, Salford, UK.

Fenton, A. (2018) Digital sport & fan engagement. *Alex Fenton Blog*. [Online] [Accessed on 26th March 2019] http://alexfenton.co.uk/digital-sport-for-fan-engagement/.

Fenton, A. and Helleu, B. (2019) Digital and social media. *In* Chadwick, S., Parnell, D., Widdop, P. and Anagnostopoulos, C. (eds.) *Routledge Handbook of Football Business and Management*. 1st ed., Routledge, Abingdon, UK.

Fenton, A. and Procter, C. (2019) Studying social media communities: Blending methods with netnography. *In Sage Research Methods Cases*. Sage, Thousand Oaks, CA.

Garriga, E. and Melé, D. (2004) Corporate social responsibility theories: Mapping the territory. *Journal of Business Ethics*, 53(1/2) pp. 51–71.

Heinze, A., Fletcher, G., Rashid, T. and Cruz, A. (2016) *Digital and Social Media Marketing: A Results Driven Approach*. Routledge, Abingdon, UK.

Institute for Health Metrics and Evaluation (IHME) (2018) *Findings from the Global Burden of Disease Study 2017*. Seattle, WA.

Involve (2019) *Involve: Supporting Public Involvement in NHS, Public Health and Social Care Research*. [Online] [Accessed on 2nd May 2019] www.invo.org.uk/.

Jee, H. (2017) Review of researches on smartphone applications for physical activity promotion in healthy adults. *Journal of Exercise Rehabilitation*, 13(1) pp. 3–11.

Kozinets, R. V. (2015) *Netnography Redefined*. Sage Publications, Thousand Oaks, CA.

Lawrence, S. and Crawford, G. (2018) *Digital Football Cultures: Fandom, Identities and Resistance*. Routledge, London.

Lewin, K. (1946) Action research and minority problems. *Journal of Social Issues*. John Wiley & Sons, Ltd (10.1111), 2(4) pp. 34–46.

McCarthy, J., Rowley, J., Ashworth, C. J. and Pioch, E. (2014) Managing brand presence through social media: The case of UK football clubs. *Internet Research*. Emerald Group Publishing Limited, 24(2) pp. 181–204.

Mitchell, J. A., Mattocks, C., Ness, A. R., Leary, S. D., Pate, R. R., Dowda, M., Blair, S. N. and Riddoch, C. (2009) 'Sedentary behaviour and obesity in a large cohort of children.' *Obesity (Silver Spring)*, 17(8) pp. 1596–1602.

NHS Digital and National Statistics (2018) *Statistics on Obesity, Physical Activity and Diet*. NHS Digital and National Statistics, England.

Parnell, D., Curran, K. and Philpott, M. (2017) 'Health stadia: A settings-based approach to health.' *In* Parnell, D. and Krustrup, P. (eds.) *Sport and Health: The Current State of Play*. 1st ed., Routledge, Abingdon, UK, pp. 238–250.

Public Health England (2012) *UK Health Profiles*. Public Health England.

Ramshaw, G., Gammon, S. and Huang, W.-J. (2013) Acquired pasts and the commodification of borrowed heritage: The case of the Bank of America Stadium tour. *Journal of Sport & Tourism*, 18(1) pp. 17–31.

Saunders, T. J., Chaput, J.-P. and Tremblay, M. S. (2014) Sedentary behaviour as an emerging risk factor for cardiometabolic diseases in children and youth. *Canadian Journal of Diabetes*, 38 pp. 53–61.

Sweeney, D. R. and Quimby, D. G. (2012) Exploring the physical health behavior differences between high and low identified sports fans. *The Sport Journal*, 15(1), pp. 1–12.

Townsend, N., Nichols, M., Scarborough, P. & Rayner, M. (2015) Cardiovascular disease in Europe – epidemiological update 2015, *European Heart Journal*, 36(40) pp. 2696–2705.

Tremblay, M. S., Leblanc, A. G., Kho, M. E., Saunders, T. J., Larouche, R., Colley, R. C., Goldfield, G. and Gorber, S. C. (2011) Systematic review of sedentary behaviour and health indicators in school-aged children and youth. *International Journal of Behavioral Nutrition and Physical Activity*, 8 p. 98.

Tu, R., Hsieh, P. and Feng, W. (2018) Walking for fun or for "likes"? The impacts of different gamification orientations of fitness apps on consumers' physical activities. *Sport Management Review*, In press, corrected proof.

Zeimers, G., Anagnostopoulos, C., Zintz, T. and Willem, A. (2019) Corporate social responsibility (CSR) in football. Exploring modes of CSR implementation. *In* Chadwick, S., Parnell, D., Widdop, P. and Anagnostopoulos, C. (eds.) *Routledge Handbook of Football Business and Management*. Routledge, Abingdon, UK.

Chapter 15

Football and mental health

Alan Pringle and Tim Carter

Introduction

In recent years there has been a growing interest in the use of football as a vehicle for mental health interventions. This has resulted in the development of a range of projects utilising football as a sport and football clubs as a venue for mental health work (Heun and Pringle 2018).

Friedrich and Mason (2017) observe that most of these mental health interventions seek to complement rather than replace 'standard' or conventional treatment, and many are underpinned by the 'recovery-based' philosophy that has become popular in mainstream psychiatric services. Rather than focusing on diagnosis and trying to identify and reduce symptoms, recovery approaches focus on identifying and a person's abilities, promoting hope and developing networks that help social inclusion (Repper and Perkins 2003; Slade 2009). Repper and Perkins (2003), in their defining text on Mental Health and Recovery, suggest that the challenge facing people with mental health problems is to retain, or rebuild, a meaningful and valued life, and, like everyone else, to grow and develop within and beyond the limits imposed by their cognitive and emotional difficulties. Recovery in their view is not about 'getting rid' of problems. It is about seeing people beyond their problems – their abilities, possibilities, interests and dreams – and recovering the social roles and relationships that give life value and meaning.

According to Spandler and McKeown. (2012), football is of great use in mental health interventions because it can act as a 'hook', facilitating an initial interest and providing a 'way in' to discuss mental health issues. This idea of a hook is reiterated by Pringle et al. (2014) when they identify that components of the club infrastructure, such as the ground or the badge, can be important for engaging fans and reaching them with information on interventions. This idea is reiterated by Curran et al. (2014) who suggest that the brand of professional football clubs has an important role in reaching, attracting and engaging participants in health improvement activities. As such, identifying with the club and the game can also help to overcome some of the stigma men can feel is associated with seeking help for mental health difficulties by focusing initially on the club or the game rather than the presenting problem.

The use of football as a vehicle for engaging people has partially been driven by the fact that a high proportion of those who engage heavily in playing or supporting football are men, and for mental health services, men are often regarded as what Sport England (2008) calls a 'Hard to Reach (HTR)' group. Men's reluctance to engage with services can be seen in their resulting poor health statistics for both physical health and mental health, and men have therefore been highlighted as a particular area of concern for health practitioners and professionals in various fields of healthcare. Curran et al. (2016) suggest that community-based, football-led health improvement programmes endorsed by professional football clubs appear well-positioned to connect with, and attract, men from these HTR populations. Henderson et al. (2014) observe that football is increasingly used to facilitate recovery in mental health services, often in partnership with football clubs, a partnership that is applauded by Curran et al. (2016) who feel that the role taken by professional football clubs and especially the clubs' health programmes is a 'huge success in both engaging and retaining their target audiences'. It must, however, be emphasised that this approach is not a panacea for delivering mental health intervention and has some associated problems and limitations.

Although football-based mental health interventions often have men as their target group, they are not exclusive in this area, and a range of interventions using football are delivered targeting women, school-age children and other parts of the community.

This chapter outlines some of the ways in which mental health care has utilised the game and venues associated with the game to build programmes and examines the way that healthcare providers such as the NHS, third sector organisations and football clubs themselves have begun to develop strategies to impact positively on mental health in their local communities. Some of the programmes developed involve playing football, (Darongkamas et al. 2011; McElroy et al. 2008) some involve watching football (Pringle 2009) and some involve using football venues as a base for interventions to take place (White et al. 2011; Nickell and Pringle 2011).

The Football League and Premier League in the United Kingdom have a historical commitment to highlighting mental health issues with examples including the inclusion of a football and mental health group in the 'Time to Change' programme that involved representatives from both leagues (Nickell and Pringle 2011) and the commitment to mental health issues by the English Football League who named the mental health charity organisation 'Mind' as their official charity partner for the 2018/19 football season. This promotion of mental health across the country meant that every club in the league had some form of mental health promotional activity during the season and an additional graphic joined to the players' names on the back of their shirts that represented the logo of Mind.

History

The use of sport and exercise is not a new phenomenon in mental health settings. Cherry and Munting (2005) describe how team games, initially cricket but later other games including football, were played in mental asylums in various parts of Britain from the mid-nineteenth century until the asylum system was dismantled in the move to 'care in the community'.

County provision of care for the 'mentally ill lunatics' became a compulsory requirement in 1845, with each county providing a large in-patient facility. The population then (around 5,000) grew to around 40,000 by 1880, and by 1939 it had risen to more than 130,000. This number remained roughly constant until improvements in treatments and medication began to reduce the numbers in the 1950s. The enactment of Care in the Community legislation closed the asylums throughout the 1980s and 1990s.

Although the game was very insular in nature, with matches mostly being either internally between staff and patients or between different asylums playing each other, the value of football was recognised as a way of engaging patients in activity and developing some measure of social inclusion. Brown (2013) observes that Victorian local newspapers included several accounts of outings where one asylum played another 'including one from Sussex Lunatic asylum that included pies, football and plenty of home brewed beer'.

More importantly, suggest Cherry and Munting (2005), staff and patients often played in the same team and this process broke down some of the barriers between patients and staff. They describe how one member of asylum staff speaking about his experiences of playing sport in the asylum in the 1950s soon realised that 'being mentally ill and sane, as far as I'm concerned, is just a narrow gap'. Through engaging in sport, patients became motivated and their keenness to improve their sports skills allowed nursing staff to coach them and secure their trust, providing an avenue for other forms of therapy.

The closure of large hospital units meant that people who would previously have been admitted to in-patient care were now looked after for the most part in either their own homes or in small units. For a period of time football more or less disappeared from the mental health landscape, but a resurgence in interest in how the worlds of football and mental health could work together took shape as the new century dawned. One of the main drivers in this process was not the NHS or the rapidly expanding private healthcare companies that delivered mental health care but the developing 'Football in the Community' network and the third sector.

Football in the community

Much of the mental health work carried out in or by football clubs is organised through the professional clubs in England's 'Football in the Community' (FitC) organisation. Parnell et al. (2013) describe how the national FitC scheme programme was launched in 1986 with the aim of building a greater link between clubs and their communities. Interestingly, the development of FitC organisations came at exactly the same time as the closure of the asylum system in the UK was taking place. These FitC schemes had an initial focus on traditional coaching schemes aimed mostly at children and young people, but over the years the community arm in several clubs has taken on a huge role in influencing health in local communities. Walters and Chadwick (2009) observe that many of these schemes have developed good working connections within their community and as these organisations have begun to carry out interventions that have no direct football connection. Many clubs have gone on to drop the word 'football' from their name, and are known by names such as Everton in the Community, Arsenal in the Community or Pompey in the Community.

Curran et al. (2014) observe that community programmes are now found in the majority of professional football clubs in England and are usually run as a separate entity to the football club, with many having their own staff and independent funding streams to finance their staff and their programmes. As an example of this, a study by Jenkins and James (2012) found that out of 23 clubs that had been involved in the Premier League only three of the clubs' community schemes were located within the organisational structure of the football club and managed directly by the club. Despite this financial, structural and strategic independence from the football club, the majority of schemes maintain association with the club in name and by using club logos.

While a geographical location is certainly of interest when considering community, Hoskin (2015) suggests that the real essence of community is more than a structured association through geographical location and that bonds are formed with football clubs by people often hundreds of miles from where they live. Skinner et al. (2008) observe this when they suggest that 'a sense of community arises out of the fundamental human need to create and maintain social bonds, to develop a sense of belonging and to further develop a self-identity'. For the purposes of mental health interventions, this is important because whilst a majority of participants in any programme may have allegiance to the club running a programme, a number will not. In the early groups of the 'It's a Goal!' programme run in Macclesfield Town, for example (Pringle and Sayers 2004), some participants were supporters of Liverpool and Manchester United, but it was the draw of football that was primarily engaging them rather than specific loyalty to one club. Similarly, when evaluating a programme run by Arsenal's community programme, Hoskin (2015) found people attending programmes who were fans of Arsenal's big rivals Tottenham Hotspur and Chelsea.

Using football clubs as a venue, using the language of football as a metaphor and using the playing of the game as a tool for engagement has meant that FitC organisations have had a huge impact on the mental health of their local communities by delivering a wide range of interventions aimed at all ages in the community. Some FitC organisations like Notts County FitC offer mental health programmes aimed at the whole age range in the community, from primary school age children right through to programmes aimed at people with dementia.

This is not to say that all successful interventions and programmes are run through FitC organisations, but, as they develop further and build stronger partnerships with organisations like their local NHS Trusts and universities, FitC organisations can be a pivotal player in the delivery of mental health interventions that use football as a vehicle for mental health improvement.

Playing football

Many of the mental health programmes run to support people with mental health problems involve playing the game. The pioneering work investigating the role of exercise on mental health was undertaken for the most part by William Morgan, who, in his early work found that fitness levels between psychiatric inpatients were lower than non-hospitalised controls (Morgan 1968). Since this pioneering work, numerous studies have documented the effect of exercise on various mental health disorders. Engaging in exercise can have positive benefits on mental wellbeing and psychological functioning in adults (Malcolm et al. 2013) and for children and young people (Lubans et al. 2012; Biddle and Asare 2011). Specifically it has been reported that engaging in exercise can lead to improvements in self-esteem and self-perception (Ekeland et al. 2004), mood (Peluso and Andrade 2005), sleep and insomnia (Bushman 2013; Carter et al. 2016) and psychological stress (Hamer et al. 2009)

In a Cochrane review, Gorczynski and Faulkner (2010) sought to determine the mental health effects of exercise/physical activity programmes for people with schizophrenia or schizophrenia-like illnesses. Although only a small number of trials were included, they tended to report significant improvement in numerous mental health outcomes for this population, such as reducing anxiety, reducing symptoms of the depression that can accompany schizophrenic presentations and increases in positive affect. Effects were also observed for positive and negative psychotic symptoms of the condition. Holley et al. (2011) similarly reviewed the influence of physical activity on the psychological wellbeing of people diagnosed with schizophrenia concluding that overall, physical activity has a beneficial effect. When evaluating a football programme specifically designed for people with schizophrenic-type conditions, Moloney and Rohde (2017) reported that the programme had a positive impact on the mental health of the participants and that football had helped them cope with their illness and provided hope that they could recover. Participants also described how 'participation in the programme provided a distraction from psychotic symptoms, led to improvements in concentration and alertness and improvements in self-esteem'.

Because the symptoms of schizophrenia often develop in late teens, just at the point where young people are taking exams or starting work or trying to build adult relationships, they are often not successful in developing the skills needed to achieve well in these areas. If someone is going to be good at football their skills are usually well developed before this age, so many players on mental health teams find football one area of their lives where they can succeed well and playing can often offer a degree of perceived social status and normalcy. Mason and Holt (2012) found that for participants in their study, the playing of football had been an important part of the participants' past lives, and as such, playing now offered a reconnection with a pre-illness identity. In particular, memories of football were strongly associated with enjoyment and a positive sense of self. Illness was often the reason they were no longer playing football and so playing again signified a return to health.

There is also some, albeit limited, evidence to suggest that exercise is effective at reducing post traumatic stress disorder (PTSD) symptoms (Diaz and Motta 2008).

The most extensively researched application of exercise within the field of mental health is in its potential for treating depression where the impact has been very positive (Brown et al. 2013; Hughes et al. 2013). In the most recent Cochrane review, Cooney et al. (2013) included 39 trials (2326 participants) that investigated the effect of exercise on depression and found a generally positive outcome when exercise was included as part of a treatment programme. Stanton and Happell (2014) conducted a systematic review of exercise interventions examining the effect of exercise interventions on the health of people hospitalised for treatment and overall, the studies examining the effect of exercise on depression reported a significant reduction in depression compared to control conditions.

There are a number of potential mechanisms that have been suggested to underpin the exercise depression relationship. Plausible reasons include neurobiological mechanisms that mediate changes in depressive symptoms and mood, and psychosocial mechanisms that result in improved mastery and elevations in self-efficacy. However, at present it seems as though we are not able to do more than speculate as to which mechanism, if any, may contribute to the observed effect reported in numerous trials over the years.

An important aspect to consider when evaluating a healthcare intervention is to determine how acceptable it is to the target population (Ayala and Elder 2011). Of all the different types of exercise available it is of interest how many interventions targeting primarily depression or psychosis in men focus primarily on using football as the method of exercise to engage people. It was of interest in the early days of the Nottinghamshire Healthcare Positive Goals league how often people (mostly men) participating in the process stated that they 'never did exercise' and 'didn't like exercise', but when offered football stated that they would happily play.

Examples of playing football have included The Positive Mental Attitude (PMA) Football League, a project developed by former professional footballer and coach Janette Hynes in London (Hynes 2008). Having run football sessions as part of her job as an occupational therapist for in-patients she found that on discharge, there was no similar option for the people who had participated. The evaluations of this league found that involvement in the programme helped people who participated in a range of ways, including increasing people's confidence and self-esteem by interacting with other people in the community. From its inception in 2005 the league developed in strength, winning a number of awards, and the PMA London League now functions as an organizing body for mental health football across the city, supporting the development of Community Football Clubs and coordinating and administrating PMA London Football competitions.

Similarly, the league that was developed in the North East of England by Grassroots Initiatives, a small, user-led, voluntary organisation, (originally known as the CSIP league) found improvements in the mental health of participants from the process. McEroy et al. (2008) describe findings from an evaluation carried out by the University of Nottingham involving 130 players in the league that concluded that players felt higher levels of self-esteem, that they were more positive about themselves and about their lives, and reported increases in confidence and a reduction in symptoms of mental health problems.

Across the UK in the intervening years, various leagues and one-off competitions have flourished and the involvement of service-user teams playing locally and moving further afield has become a regular feature of mental health care. Often these involve collaborative working within organisations such as the Positive Goals League in Nottinghamshire which receives funding from the Nottinghamshire NHS Trust but is run through a partnership between the Nottinghamshire FA and Notts County FitC.

Moving further afield, international football between service-user teams has become a regular feature for some teams. For example, an 11-a-side international match between service-user teams from Iceland and Norway was held at the grounds of the Norwegian side Brann FC in May 2018. Perhaps the best example of a regular international service-user football competition is the EASI Cup. The European Association for Sport and Social Integration (EASI) is an organisation that was founded in 2002 with the guiding principle of enhancing social participation through sport and other leisure activities. EASI is a group made up of health and community groups from 12 European countries who promote sport to improve the wellbeing of people with mental health issues and learning disabilities. Each year they hold a football tournament which brings together more than 25 teams. Venues for the competition have included Munich, Manchester, Lintz, Gratz and Barnsley.

The evidence to support the hypothesis that exercise has a positive impact on mental health problems is increasing (Carter et al. 2016; Turner et al. 2017). As football is one of the most popular forms of exercise on offer it appears that this development of programmes that involve playing football can be one piece of a jigsaw of mental health interventions that can have a very positive impact on the mental health of local communities.

Basing mental health programmes in football settings

The idea of placing mental health interventions in football environments has developed extensively in recent years. The positive impact of using such venues has been seen in evaluations of several programmes (Smith and Pringle 2010; Spandler and McKeown 2012; Friedrich and Mason 2017), as has the delivery of mental health interventions by football coaches and other coaching staff (Pringle 2009).

The success of placing interventions in these areas has been in part due to some main aspects that are recurring in the literature.

One is the non-clinical environment that a football-based intervention brings. Respondents in studies frequently site the venue as important stating that they are intimidated by hospital settings and in some cases are afraid that people will see them accessing a mental health unit (Pringle 2009; Smith and Pringle 2010;

Spandler et al. 2013). The stadium often gives a sense of normality; it is a place where people gather whether they are ill or not and irrelevant of age, social status or gender, so going there does not automatically label a person as ill or needing help.

The development of mental health expertise in some organisations has seen some football clubs delivering a whole portfolio of mental health programmes from within the club. For example, Everton in the Community offers programmes like Tackling the Blues for school-age children, Imagine Your Goals for men, Pass on the Memories for older people with dementia and Blue Belles, a project that offers advice and support to mothers who have children with diagnosed conditions such as autism and ADHD.

Another important aspect of engagement is the language of football and football metaphor that is often a foundation of such interventions. The 'It's a Goal!' programme, for example, used sessions broken into a 4–4–2 structure with four defensive sessions identifying skills around building resilience, four identifying linking skills to help build support and two attacking sessions identifying goals to hit. Clinical language often seen in mental health men's groups run in hospital settings was replaced with football metaphor. Ongoing evaluations of the programme (Pringle and Sayers 2004; Smith and Pringle 2010; Spandler et al. 2013) highlighted the importance of language that was not clinical, did not include jargon and was football-based in engaging those who took part.

Partnerships

One of the developing strengths in the football and mental health world is the consolidation of relationships between football clubs and other organisations that can help with the delivery of projects, provide advice education, supervise the projects and help evaluate projects. Bingham et al. (2014) suggest that whilst football interventions have proved to be both popular and enjoyable, they have tended to lack sufficient empirical evidence to confirm their status as a significant facilitator of positive behaviour change.

If we use Everton and Notts County as examples, Everton in the Community has been working closely with Mersey Care NHS Trust since 2007 and they have built a very strong relationship between the two organisations. Similarly, Notts County FitC has developed strong relationships with Nottinghamshire Healthcare NHS Trust and has senior staff from the organisation on their strategic steering group.

Both organisations have also forged strong links with academic institutions to help in the design and facilitation of project evaluations. Notts County works closely with the University of Nottingham, whilst on some projects Everton in the Community works with Edge Hill University. Part of the importance of these collaborations is seen in the robustness and credibility the evaluations can have, and this is reflected in such things as two of the Everton in the Community projects run by Edge Hill University and Everton in the Community being presented as examples of good practice in a UK Government Health Select Committee paper on suicide.

A recurring theme in many of the studies around basing mental health interventions in football clubs highlight the importance of the coaches delivering the sessions to the success of the programmes.

Pringle and Simsey (2010) found in their evaluation of one such project a recurring feeling of coaches at the club being different from clinical staff that participants had met in mental health services, and the most recurring theme was that people 'did not feel they were being assessed or judged by staff on the programme'. This echoed findings from Pringle (2014) and from Mason and Holt (2012) who found non-mental health professionals were viewed positively by users, as they were able to talk openly, without any fear of repercussions. This does raise the question, however, that if coaches with little or no mental health knowledge or experience are delivering mental health interventions, what support and clinical supervision do they need.

Lansley and Parnell (2015) highlight the fact that this is not always taken into consideration when they provide an example from a football-led mental health service that involved the community foundation delivering a 10-month football programme for participants with mental health issues when the staff had little or no experience or any requisite skill for delivering such a programme. Curran et al. (2014) suggest that FitC practitioners need to be trained beyond 'the typical' Football Association Level 2 or UEFA B qualification in order to deal with the increasing demands of FitC schemes and that FitC schemes therefore need to execute relevant professional development and enhanced recruitment procedures to address this.

Responsible programme directors have addressed this issue by developing support and education programmes for staff. Some of these have been ad hoc, but those organisations that have developed good relationships with universities and NHS Trusts have been able to utilise these relationships to develop more robust systems for education and supervision for their staff. One interesting way of developing this has been the creation of a part-time post by Notts County FitC for a mental health consultant. The post holder is a newly retired mental health university lecturer with clinical skills, teaching skills and clinical supervision skills, and is based in the building on days when mental health projects are running to offer support and advice to coaches running these projects.

Watching football

The idea that watching football and being an active football supporter could have a positive benefit on mental health is intertwined with some of the key concepts of the recovery philosophy that underpins the greatest proportion of mental health interventions currently being provided by the NHS, private healthcare companies and the third sector. While as Jacob (2015) suggests there is no single definition of the concept of recovery for people with mental health problems, there are guiding principles which emphasise hope and a strong belief that it is possible for people with mental illness regain and live a meaningful life. Jakob goes on to suggest that a key role for mental health providers is to support people to regain their place in the communities because the act taking part in social activities can support the process of individual recovery.

Bonney and Stickley (2008) suggest that recovery concepts include acknowledgement of the value of social inclusion, the value of social support, the importance of self-esteem, the importance of emotional awareness and safe expression of emotional experience. Pringle (2009) suggests that many of these things that can help people in their recovery journey are already integral parts of the football-supporting experience.

A sense of belonging is an important idea that is central in the promotion of mental health. The feelings generated by the experience of being an outsider and from feeling socially excluded can breed ideas of resentment, isolation and ultimately of depression and despair. Throughout our lives we seek the security of belonging and consistency.

Fans' perception of belonging and consistency in the form of 'being stuck with' their team was a theme to emerge from Pringle's (2008) study in which fans talked about sticking with their club through thick and thin because it was 'their club'. Change creates anxiety, and in a world of constant change one fan of Mansfield Town FC (nicknamed the Stags) encapsulated the sense of belonging and consistency that being a fan can bring when he observed

> It was Stags when I was a boy, Stags when I was single, and when I was married, and when I was divorced, and when I was married again, and when I was divorced again! It's always been Stags. They're rubbish, but they're the one thing you can rely on.

The sense of belonging is heightened by way that the fans behave when attending matches. The Russian scholar Bakhtin described how the sense of belonging for someone who is part of a group can create an experience akin to what he calls the carnivalesque (Bakhtin 1984). Whilst Bakhtin acknowledges that the present day 'carnivals' are pale imitations of the unbridled lusting, binge drinking of alcohol, and even physical mutilation that characteristically occurred in the classic Renaissance carnival environment, some strong common themes link them with these earlier forms. Examples might include the shouts and jeers of a football crowd, the terraces' humour, pie stalls, team heroes and mascots, scarves and banners, all of which provide distinct echoes of the traditional carnival. Why this is important from a mental health perspective is that the carnivalesque helps to create a form of human social configuration that 'lies beyond existing social forms' (Bakhtin 1984, p. 280) and means that any individual can have a genuine sense of belonging, even in a crowd of thousands that they do not know.

Another important concept in recovery is that the ability and opportunity to express emotion which is seen as a very positive thing for promoting mental health and wellbeing. Reeck et al. (2016) suggest that the cathartic release of emotions is often believed to be therapeutic for affected individuals and this is important especially for men who have very limited opportunity for positive cathartic release. Armstrong (2003) acknowledges the importance of emotional release and feels that the opportunities and environments for this to take place in contemporary society are diminishing. Armstrong goes on to suggest that although emotions can, and sometimes do, run riot in the fans, the football stadium is one of the last spectacles in British life offering the chance of intense emotion and social relationships. Central to these ideas is the concept of catharsis.

The cathartic idea began with Aristotle and the idea is defined by Vives (2011) as suggesting it meant that spectators experience an emotional release and cleansing after watching a drama and that this helped to moderate passions and strong emotions, therefore restoring balance. Although a contested idea in psychiatry, the hypothesis has found favour with many practitioners and was described by the majority of participants in Pringle's 2008 study as a positive feature of their supporting experience.

Like other forms of drama football has narrative, shape and discipline with rules, regulations and a clearly defined beginning, middle and end. Yet football, unlike scripted drama, allows for an infinite variety of outcomes and a sense of true surprise, such as the wonderfully unexpected victory of a lower league team over a big club in a cup competition. It is known that the game will end, but not how it will end, so fans find themselves suspended in a state of heightened arousal for the duration of the game. This is, of course, the very essence of drama where we suspend our real life and engage emotionally with the situations unfolding before us. This means that we become part of the experience because of our emotional engagement with the process. This period of escape from the pressures of life and engagement in an all-consuming drama can have very positive outcomes for those involved. Of course, after the drama is finished the crowd steps back into their 'real lives', but the experience has often left them emotional drained and, importantly, connected.

One striking aspect of this in Pringle's (2008) study was that in some ways the result or the team's position was not relevant to the experience. When the team was doing well the connection was elation; when they were doing badly, despair, but fans were still emotionally connected. Of course the other great connection emotionally was hope, primarily the hope that next season it would all come right.

A final idea around the impact of watching football on mental health might be seen in the recovery component that focuses on social support and the development of family relationships.

A study by Flouri and Buchannan (2002) based on 17,000 children who were born in the UK in 1958 followed subjects up at ages 7, 11, 16, 23 and 33. This found that good father-child relationships are associated with an absence of emotional and behavioural difficulties in adolescence and greater academic motivation. It also found that boys who had involved fathers were less likely to be in trouble with the police as they grew older. This echoed McCann (2000) who found that in families where there was little or no involvement with a father there was a marked increase in behavioural disorders, psychiatric diagnosis and suicide.

Football offers an arena within which these positive supportive relationships can flourish. If, as the literature suggests, the relationship between fathers and sons can be a major component in the development of good mental health for young men, the activity of attending matches may offer one of the most accessible ways of helping this relationship find some 'ring fenced' planned time in which to develop.

The shared language and experience of football means that there is a common language and experience to connect a 70-year-old grandfather with his 15-year-old granddaughter or a 30-year-old dad with his 10-year-old son. There are not many areas in communities where this is possible, as across the generational gaps it is less likely to find a shared point of contact with film, music or computer games.

Much emphasis is placed in mental health promotion on the development of relationships between parents and children and the importance of 'quality time' (Hill et al. 2013; Carlson et al. 2014). It may well be that some of this quality time can be found in unlikely places with names such as Sheffield Wednesday, Rushden and Diamonds or Accrington Stanley. In these strange-sounding settings it appears that the elusive goal of parents and children being involved in meaningful dialogue and sharing quality time often starts and continues well after the children are grown up and often well into the time when they have children of their own.

Whist it is, in no way, being suggested that football support already offers all of the components identified as being prerequisites for good mental health, it does appear to offer many of them at a foundation level. As such it may mean that rather than, as fans frequently quip, 'I must be mad to watch this lot', it may in fact be that the opposite that is true and that watching football actually can actually be good for your mental health.

Conclusion

The last 15 years has seen a huge expansion of football and mental health programmes so that such programmes have moved from having a novelty value into becoming embedded into mainstream practice.

Whilst there is no suggestion that these programmes should be used as an alternative to mental health services, many participants who have professionals involved with their lives value their professional input but suggest that football-based programmes offer something that can be complimentary to this. Football-based programmes can also often offer a way in to services that would not have been taken if participants had not attended.

The growing body of evidence to show that football is of great use in mental health interventions suggests the relationship between football and mental health provision can develop further and the development of strong relationships between football clubs, mental health service providers and academic institutions could mean the future for this type of intervention looks very positive indeed.

References

Armstrong, G. (2003) *Football hooligans: Knowing the score*. London: Berg.

Ayala, G. X. and Elder, J. P. (2011) Qualitative methods to ensure acceptability of behavioral and social interventions to the target population. *Journal of Public Health*, 71, Suppl 1, S69–79.

Bakhtin, M. M. (1984) *Rabelais and his world*. Indiana: Indiana University Press.

Biddle, S. J. and Asare, M. (2011) Physical activity and mental health in children and adolescents: A review of reviews. *British Journal of Sports Medicine*, 45 (11), 886–895.

Bingham, D. D., Parnell, D., Curran, K., Jones, R. and Richardson, D. (2014) Fit fans: Perspectives of a practitioner and understanding participant health needs within a health promotion programme for older men delivered within an English Premier League football club. *Soccer & Society*, 15 (6), 883–901, DOI: 10.1080/14660970.2014.920624

Bonney, S. and Stickley, T. (2008) Recovery and mental health: A review of the British literature. *Journal of Psychiatric and Mental Health Nursing*, 15, 140–153.

Brown, H. E., Pearson, N. and Braithwaite, R. E. (2013) Physical activity interventions and depression in children and adolescents: A systematic review and meta-analysis. *Sports Medicine*, 43, 195–206.

Bushman, B. A. (2013) Exercise and sleep. *ACSM's Health & Fitness Journal*, 17 (5), 5–8, DOI: 10.1249/FIT.1240b1013e3182a1205fce

Carlson, D. S., Hunter, E. M., Ferguson, M. and Whitten, D. (2014) Work: Family enrichment and satisfaction: Mediating processes and relative impact of originating and receiving domains. *Journal of Management*, 40 (3), 845–865, DOI: 10.1177/0149206311414429

Carter, T., Morres, I., Repper, J. and Callaghan, P. (2016) Exercise for adolescents with depression: Valued aspects and perceived change. *Journal of Psychiatric and Mental Health Nursing*, 23 (1), 37–44.

Cherry, S. and Munting, R. (2005) 'Exercise is the thing'? Sport and the asylum c.1850–1950. *The International Journal of the History of Sport*, 22 (1), 42–58, DOI: 10.1080/0952336052000314629

Cooney, G. M., Dwan, K., Greig, C. A., et al. (2013) Exercise for depression. *Cochrane Database of Systematic Reviews*, 9, Cd004366.

Curran, K., Bingham, D. D., Richardson, D. and Parnell, D. (2014) Ethnographic engagement from within a Football in the Community programme at an English Premier League football club. *Soccer & Society*, 15 (6), 934–950, DOI: 10.1080/14660970.2014.920627.

Curran, K., Drust, B., and Richardson, D. (2014) 'I just want to watch the match': A practitioner's reflective account of men's health themed match day events at an English Premier League football club. *Soccer & Society*, 15 (6), 919–933.

Curran, K., Rosenbaum, S., Parnell, D., Stubbs, B., Pringle, A. and Hargreaves, J. (2017) Tackling mental health: The role of professional football clubs, *Sport in Society*, 20 (2), 281–291, DOI: 10.1080/17430437.2016.1173910

Darongkamas, J., Scott, H. and Taylor, E. (2011) Kick-starting men's mental health: An evaluation of the effect of playing football on mental health service users' well-being. *International Journal of Mental Health Promotion*, 13 (3), 14–21.

Diaz, A. B. and Motta, R. (2008) The effects of an aerobic exercise program on post-traumatic stress disorder symptom severity in adolescents. *International journal of emergency mental health*, 10 (1), 49–59.

Ekeland, E., Heian, F., Hagen, K. B., Abbott, J. and Nordheim, L. (2004) Exercise to improve self-esteem in children and young people. *Cochrane Database Syst Rev*, 1, Cd003683.

Flouri, E. and Buchannan, A. (2002) What predicts good relationships with parents in adolescence and partners in adult life? Findings from the 1958 British birth cohort. *Journal of Family Psychology*, 16 (2), 186–198.

Friedrich, B. and Mason, O. (2017) 'What is the score?' A review of football-based public mental health interventions. *Journal of Public Mental Health*, 16 (4), 144–154.

Gorczynski, P. and Faulkner, G. (2010) Exercise therapy for schizophrenia. *Cochrane Database of Systematic Reviews* [Online]. Available at: http://onlinelibrary.wiley.com/doi/10.1002/14651858.CD004412.pub2/abstract

Hamer, M., Stamatakis, E. and Steptoe, A. (2009) Dose-response relationship between physical activity and mental health: The scottish health survey. *British Journal of Sports Medicine*, 43 (14), 1111–1114.

Henderson, C., O'Hara, S., Thornicroft, G. and Webber, M. (2014) Corporate social responsibility and mental health: The Premier League football imagine your goals programme. *International Review of Psychiatry*, 26 (4), 460–466.

Heun, R. and Pringle, A. (2018) Football does not improve mental health: A systematic review on football and mental health disorders. *Global Psychiatry*, 1 (1), 25–37.

Hill, R., Tranby, E., Kelly, E. L. and Moen, P. (2013) Relieving the time squeeze? Effects of a white-collar workplace change on parents. *Journal of Marriage and Family*, 75, 1014–1029, DOI: 10.1111/jomf.12047

Holley, J., Crone, D., Tyson, P. and Lovell, G. (2011) The effects of physical activity on psychological well-being for those with schizophrenia: A systematic review. *British Journal of Clinical Psychology*, 50 (1), 84–105, DOI: 10.1348/014466510X496220

Hoskin, A. (2015) *Cultivating and tending social capital: A case study of Arsenal in the Community*. Birkbeck Sport Business Centre Research Paper Series Birkbeck, London, University of London.

Hughes, C. W., Barnes, S., Barnes, C., et al. (2013) Depressed Adolescents Treated with Exercise (DATE): A pilot randomized controlled trial to test feasibility and establish preliminary effect sizes. *Mental Health and Physical Activity*, 6, 119–131.

Hynes, J. (2008) The Positive Mental Attitude (PMA) Football League. *A Life in the Day*, 12 (3), 6–10, https://doi.org/10.1108/13666282200800022

Jacob K. S. (2015) Recovery model of mental illness: A complementary approach to psychiatric care. *Indian Journal of Psychological Medicine*, 37(2), 117–119. DOI: 10.4103/0253-7176.155605

Jenkins, H. and James, L. (2012) It's not just a game: Community work in the UK Football industry and approaches to corporate social responsibility. *The ESRC Centre for Business Relationships, Accountability, Sustainability and Society*, Cardiff University Press, Cardiff.

Lansley, S. and Parnell, D. (2015) Football for health: Getting strategic. *Soccer & Society*, 17 (2), 1–8.

Lubans, D. R., Plotnikoff, R. C. and Lubans, N. J. (2012) Review: A systematic review of the impact of physical activity programmes on social and emotional well-being in at-risk youth. *Child and Adolescent Mental Health*, 17 (1), 2–13.

Malcolm, E., Evans-Lacko, S., Little, K., Henderson, C. and Thornicroft, G. (2013) The impact of exercise projects to promote mental wellbeing. *Journal of Mental Health*, 22 (6), 519–527.

Mason, O. J. and Holt, R. (2012) A role for football in mental health: The coping through football project. *The Psychiatrist*, 36 (8), 290–293.

McCann, R. (2000) *On their own; Boys growing up unfathered*. Sydney: Finch.

McElroy, P., Evans, P. and Pringle, A. (2008) Sick as a parrot or over the moon: An evaluation of the impact of playing regular matches in a Football League on mental health service users. *Practice Development in Health Care*, 7 (1), 40–48.

Moloney, L. and Rohde, D. (2017) Experiences of men with psychosis participating in a community-based football programme. *Irish Journal of Occupational Therapy*, 45 (2), 100–111, https://doi.org/10.1108/IJOT-06-2017-0015

Morgan, W. (1968) Selected physiological and psychomotor correlates of depression in psychiatric patients. *Research Quarterly*, 39, 1037–1043.

Nickell, J. and Pringle, A. (2011) Time to change sport and mental health project evaluation. *Time to change*. London: The English Football Association.

Parnell, D., Stratton, G., Drust, B. and Richardson, D. (2013) Football in the community schemes: Exploring the effectiveness of an intervention in promoting healthful behaviour change. *Soccer & Society*, 14 (1), 35–51. DOI: 10.1080/14660970.2012.692678

Peluso, M. A. M. and Andrade, L. H. S. G. d. (2005) Physical activity and mental health: The association between exercise and mood. *Clinics*, 60, 61–70.

Pringle, A. (2008) I must be mad to watch this lot; a qualitative study examining the effect that supporting a small, local football club has on the mental health of supporters. PhD thesis, University of Nottingham.

Pringle, A. (2009) The growing role of football as a vehicle for interventions in mental health care. *Journal of Psychiatric and Mental Health Nursing*, 16 (6), 553–557.

Pringle, A. (2014) *On the ball: An evaluation of the 'On the ball' programme run by the Notts county FC Football in the Community team Notts county FITC Nottingham.*

Pringle, A. and Sayers, P. (2004) It's a goal!: Basing a community psychiatric nursing service in a local football stadium. *The Journal of the Royal Society for the Promotion of Health*, 124 (5), 234–238.

Pringle, A. and Simsey, R. (2010) *Right Mind; An evaluation of the Right Mind programme delivered by the Notts County Football in the Community team Notts county FITC Nottingham.*

Pringle, A., Zwolinsky, S., McKenna, J., Robertson, S., Daly-Smith, A. and White, A. (2014) Health improvement for men and hard-to-engage-men delivered in English Premier League football clubs. *Health Education Research*, 29 (3), 1–18.

Reeck, C., Ames, D. R. and Ochsner, K. N. (2016) The social regulation of emotion: An integrative, cross-disciplinary model. *Trends in Cognitive Sciences*, 20 (1), 47–63.

Repper, J. and Perkins, R. (2003) *Social inclusion and recovery: A model for mental health practice.* London: Baillière Tindall.

Skinner, J., Zakus, D, H. and Cowell, J. (2008) Development through sport: Building social capital in disadvantaged communities. *Sport Management Review*, 11, 253–275.

Slade, M. (2009) *Personal recovery and mental illness.* Cambridge: Cambridge University Press.

Smith, M. and Pringle, A. (2010) The latest score: An evaluation of the it's a Goal! *Programme It's a Goal Foundation Macclesfield.*

Spandler, H. and McKeown, M. (2012) A critical exploration of using football in health and welfare programs: Gender, masculinities and social relations. *Journal of Sport & Social Issues*, 36 (4), 387–409.

Spandler, H., Mckeown, M., Roy, A. and Hurley, M. (2013), Football metaphor and mental well-being: An evaluation of the It's a Goal! Programme. *Journal of Mental Health*, 22 (6), 544–554.

Sport England (2008) *Engaging hard to reach groups: Lessons from the Active England programme.* London: Sport England.

Stanton, R. and Happell, B. (2014) Exercise for mental illness: A systematic review of inpatient studies. *International Journal of Mental Health Nursing*, 23 (3), 232–242.

Turner, D., Carter, T., Sach, T., Guo, B. and Callaghan, P. (2017) Cost-effectiveness of a preferred intensity exercise programme for young people with depression compared to standard care. *An economic evaluation alongside a clinical trial (accepted) BMJ Open.*

Vives, J. (2011) Catharsis: Psychoanalysis and the theatre. *The International Journal of Psychoanalysis*, 92 (4), 1009–1027.

Walters, G. and Chadwick, S. (2009). Corporate citizenship in football: Delivering strategic benefits through stakeholder engagement. *Management Decision*, 47 (1), 51–66.

White, A., De Sousa, B., De Visser, R., Hogston, R., Madsen, S., Makara, P., Richardson, N. and Zatonski, W. (2011) *The State of men's health in Europe*. Luxembourg: European Commission.

Chapter 16

Tobacco-free stadia

A case study at the 2016 UEFA European Championships in France

Michael Viggars, Kathryn Curran and Matthew Philpott

Acronyms

FCTC	Framework Convention on Tobacco Control
FIFA	Fédération Internationale de Football Association
FSR	Football and Social Responsibility
LOC	Local Organising Committee
UEFA	Union of European Football Associations
WHO	World Health Organization

Introduction

The tobacco epidemic is one of the biggest, and most important, public health issues of our time. Tobacco use is the leading cause of preventable mortality worldwide and one of the main risk factors for several chronic diseases, including cancer, lung disease and cardiovascular disease (Carter et al. 2015). Despite this, tobacco use is common throughout the world. The World Health Organization (WHO 2018) reports that tobacco kills more than 7 million people each year. More than 6 million of those deaths are the result of direct tobacco use, while around 890,000 deaths are the result of non-smokers being exposed to second-hand smoke.

Second-hand smoke is the smoke that fills restaurants, offices or other enclosed spaces when people burn and consume tobacco products such as cigarettes, *bidis* and water-pipes. In adults, second-hand smoke causes serious cardiovascular and respiratory diseases, including coronary heart disease and lung cancer. In infants, it causes sudden death and in pregnant women, it causes low birth weight. Almost half of children regularly breathe air polluted by tobacco smoke in public places (WHO 2018). Indeed, implementing effective strategies to reduce the harm caused by tobacco use and second-hand smoke is of paramount concern for international public health agencies, national governments and health insurance companies.

To address the tobacco epidemic, several countries have implemented legislation restricting tobacco advertising, regulating who can buy and use tobacco products, and where people can smoke (WHO 2018). Currently, over 1.4 billion people, or 20% of the world's population, are protected by comprehensive national smoke-free laws (WHO 2018). National smoke-free laws make it illegal for anyone to smoke in an enclosed public place and within the workplace. Smoke-free legislation has already served to improve the health of those previously at risk from second-hand smoke as well as smokers themselves who may have cut down or quit smoking altogether following the ban (Department of Health and Social Care 2011).

However, across the world, not all enclosed and semi-enclosed public spaces are protected by national smoke-free laws. It is therefore important that we consider how tobacco use, and harm caused by tobacco, can be reduced by implementing innovative public health initiatives in a variety of different settings.

In countries without comprehensive smoke-free legislation, football supporters are often exposed to second-hand smoke inside sports stadiums. In seated areas, on concourses, around concessions, on stairwells and in toilets there is often ample opportunity for smoke to accumulate, elevating the risks of acute adverse health events. This chapter provides a detailed account of the rationale, development, implementation, delivery and outcomes of a tobacco-free sport stadia policy at the 2016 UEFA European Championships in France. The chapter closes with recommendations for future implementation of tobacco-free policies within similar settings.

Healthy settings

Settings-based health promotion has become a prominent feature in efforts to tackle the burden of non-communicable diseases and reduce health inequalities. The 'healthy settings' approach, developed following the World Health Organization's (WHO) Ottawa Charter, is based on the notion that investment in and modification of social environments is more effective than placing emphasis on the individual to change their behaviour (WHO 1986). Action to promote health through a settings-based approach can include, but is not limited to, considering the implications of the physical environment; changing organisational structures, administration and management; analysing the impact, or lack of policy or national legislation; and, targeting hard-to-reach populations.

The idea of utilising a 'setting' to promote health has seen success in several everyday contexts including schools, workplaces, hospitals and prisons. Indeed, over the last two decades, there has been increasing recognition that sports stadia, as sites for large gatherings of people, represent a unique opportunity to apply a settings-based approach to public health and health promotion (Parnell, Curran and Philpott 2016).

Healthy stadia

During the mid-2000s, a cluster of sports clubs and venues in the North West region of the United Kingdom began implementing a range of policies, practices and programmes in support of health to a cross-section of population groups, including fans, visitors, players, local communities and stadium staff. This nascent 'healthy stadia' movement, coordinated by cardiovascular disease prevention charity Heart of Mersey, supported sports clubs and venues to trial new schemes using the following definition of 'healthy stadia':

> Healthy Stadia are . . . those which promote the health of visitors, fans, players, employees and the surrounding community . . . places where people can go to have a positive healthy experience playing or watching sport.
>
> (Crabb and Ratinckx 2005)

Following a 30-month project funded by the EU's Public Health Programme, the healthy stadia movement developed a European footprint and, owing to the success of the project, a social enterprise was formally established: the European Healthy Stadia Network (hereon Healthy Stadia). The overarching role of Healthy Stadia is to advocate for sports stadia to become health-promoting environments and has three primary areas of concern:

1 Stadium-based policies and practices
2 Community and fan health
3 Health and wellbeing policies and practices for stadium and club workers

Within these three priority areas, Healthy Stadia has since developed dozens of projects helping to tackle physical inactivity, sedentary behaviour, alcohol and drug misuse, poor diets and consumption of tobacco; the latter most notably through advocating for tobacco-free sports stadia in Europe.

Smoke-free and tobacco-free sports stadia

According to the World Health Organization, tobacco use is the leading global cause of preventable death (WHO 2013). There has, therefore, been increasing international emphasis on implementing measures to reduce the harm caused by tobacco use, including protecting people from exposure to tobacco smoke. The WHO Framework Convention on Tobacco Control (FCTC) is the key policy driver for smoke-free sports stadia (WHO 2005).

The FCTC Article 8 obligates parties to enforce 'Protection from Exposure to Tobacco Smoke'. This article commits signatories to adopt and implement 'effective legislative, executive, administrative and/or other measures, providing for protection from exposure to tobacco smoke in indoor workplaces, indoor public places, public transport and as appropriate, other public places' (p. 8). The World Health Organization have developed the definition of 'other public places' describing them as 'outdoor or quasi-outdoor places such as patios, entryways or crowded outdoor venues such as sports stadia' (WHO 2007, 2011).

Since the FCTC came into force, sporting mega-events have been increasingly viewed as presenting key opportunities to influence public opinion and shift social norms towards tobacco-free environments. The 'WHO guide to Tobacco-Free

Mega Events' (WHO 2010) defined such an event as: 'an organised planned event normally hosted by a city, governed by a parent organisation, and involving or influencing large numbers of people . . . they can be social, sporting, cultural, religious and political'. The guide included a sample tobacco-free venue policy using sports venues as the working example. This focus on sports stadia is consistent with the WHO's 'healthy settings' approach (WHO 2014). In this context, the healthy settings are sports stadia.

This development of smoke-free sports stadia has been assisted by WHO's increasing focus on the implementation of smoke-free policies at national level. The WHO established and now monitors national performance against six MPOWER measures, a package of the most effective tobacco control policies, of which the 'P' measure is P *rotect people from tobacco smoke* (WHO 2008). In the WHO's 2013 progress report on global implementation of the MPOWER measures, the key findings included that: 'the creation of smoke-free public places and workplaces continues to be the most commonly established measure at the highest level of achievement' (WHO 2013, 45). However, although progress has been made in the national adoption of such policies, how legislation is constructed affects where the regulations apply.

Smoke-free or tobacco-free policies have been adopted at several recent major football tournaments. In 2012 for example, the Union of European Football Associations (UEFA) adopted a tobacco-free policy at the 2012 UEFA European Championships held in Poland and Ukraine (UEFA 2011). In the years following, the 2013 FIFA Confederations Cup and 2014 FIFA World Cup, both hosted by Brazil, were smoke-free (FIFA 2013). However, there is known to be variation in the definition and implementation in practice of such policies, both at national, regional and tournament/competition level. For example, there are examples of sports stadia which allow smoking in open stands without a roof, or in designated smoking areas within the stadium complex. Therefore, even where smoke-free policies are in place, there is considerable variation in how they operate in practice.

UEFA and tournament context

The Union of European Football Associations (UEFA) is the governing body for association football in Europe, consisting of 55 national association members. UEFA represents the national football associations of Europe, runs nation and club competitions including the men's and women's UEFA European Championship and UEFA Champions League, and controls the prize money, regulations and media rights to these competitions.

At a time when professional sport is coming under increasing pressure from government, fans and other stakeholders to contribute to social agendas (Anagnostopoulos and Shilbury 2013; Parnell et al. 2013), UEFA continues to develop an innovative and pragmatic approach to social responsibility and sustainability at all their tournaments. UEFA cooperates with several expert non-governmental organisations on a range of social, environmental and humanitarian issues as part of their Football and Social Responsibility (FSR) portfolio under the banner of 'Respect'.

Social responsibility and health

As part of their commitment to social responsibility, UEFA has consulted with both Healthy Stadia and the World Heart Federation on how best to leverage the power of football and the reach of their member associations to promote health to football fans.

Alongside their commitment to implement tobacco-free stadia policies at its club competition finals and national tournaments, UEFA is also committed to taking a holistic approach to healthier stadium environments. As such, UEFA currently partners with Healthy Stadia in order to maximise provision of active travel (walking and cycling) to stadia, encourage stadium operators to provide healthier catering options from concessions, and support UEFA Member Associations to implement grassroots and community-orientated programmes in support of the health of various population groups.

UEFA EURO 2016

The 2016 UEFA European Championship, commonly referred to as UEFA EURO 2016, was the premier football competition contested by the senior men's national teams affiliated with UEFA. Held every four years since 1960, the tournament determines the continental champions of Europe. The tournament was hosted in France from 10 June to 10 July and was contested by 24 teams for the first time in 2016. The Respect Your Health project, coordinated by Healthy Stadia, was one of UEFA's eight priority areas under the banner of social responsibility and sustainability at UEFA EURO 2016.

Building upon policy work implemented at previous editions of the UEFA European Football Championships (UEFA EURO) and UEFA's club competition finals, in 2015 UEFA announced that a 'Tobacco-Free Policy' prohibiting the use, sale and promotion of tobacco and e-cigarette products would operate across all internal and external areas of the ten French stadiums staging UEFA EURO 2016 – the most ambitious tournament policy to date. This chapter outlines the reasons why this policy was implemented at UEFA EURO 2016, the role Healthy Stadia played in the delivery of the project, the primary communications and enforcement mechanisms used, and the main results, learning and recommendations to be taken from this project.

Smoke-free legislation and legal context in France

France formally ratified the WHO's FCTC on 19 October 2004 and is one of a growing number of countries that have introduced comprehensive smoke-free regulations that cover most indoor workplaces and public spaces. Subnational jurisdictions do not have the authority to implement smoke-free laws, leaving national government to effect such changes. National smoke-free laws were implemented in two phases (Fong et al. 2013):

- Phase 1 was realised in February 2007 prohibiting the use of tobacco products in workplaces, shopping centres, airports, train stations, hospitals and schools;
- Phase 2 was completed in January 2008 and extended the smoke-free ban to hospitality venues including cafés, bars, restaurants, hotels, casinos and nightclubs.

Prior to the launch of each phase of smoke-free legislation, media campaigns were coordinated in order to inform the public of the incoming policies and in order to raise awareness of the health harms of second-hand smoke.

Despite the relatively comprehensive legislature, smoking is still permitted in recreational spaces such as cafes, restaurants and indeed sports stadia in France if they are not covered, or the main façade is open; i.e. they are considered only semi-enclosed spaces (Article L. 3511–7 of the Code of Public Health). Therefore, use of lit tobacco products is permissible in many aspects of French sports stadia, including seated areas. Current legislation only prohibits the use of lit tobacco products in indoor sports arenas (Article L. 3511–7 of the Code of Public Health). This seemingly minor discrepancy contrasts strongly with national legislation in many parts of northern and eastern Europe including the United Kingdom, Republic of Ireland, Sweden and Russia, which prohibits smoking even in semi-enclosed spaces, making it illegal to smoke in seated areas of sports stadia.

Tobacco use and smoking behaviour

Smoking is the leading cause of preventable death in France and is responsible for 73,000 premature deaths annually, which corresponds to about 13% of recorded deaths in Metropolitan France every year (Bonaldi et al. 2016). Between 2000 and 2013, while the number of deaths attributable to tobacco decreased slightly for men, it more than doubled for women, from approximately 8,000 deaths in 2000 to more than 17,000 deaths in 2013 (Bonaldi et al. 2016).

Survey data from 2016 suggests that smoking prevalence in France remains high with 38.1% of men and 31.2% of women aged between 15–75 currently classified as either an occasional or daily smoker (Pasquereau et al. 2017). A total of 32.1% of men and 25.5% of women in 2016 were estimated to smoke daily. E-cigarette usage was much lower, with 3.3% of all adults using a device occasionally or daily (Pasquereau et al. 2017).

Compliance with the introduction of smoke-free national legislation in France is high. An evaluation by Fong et al. (2013) of the effectiveness of France's smoke-free law reported decreases in observed smoking from almost 100% of bars and approximately 60–71% of restaurants to about 4% of bars and 2–3% of restaurants one year after phase 2 of the legislation was introduced. Five years after implementation, smoking was recorded at 6–8% for bars and 1–2% for restaurants – a significant success story.

Fong et al. (2013) also reported increased support for indoor smoke-free legislation post-introduction amongst smokers and non-smokers in restaurants, bars and workplaces. Interestingly, support fell from 56% to 50.6% amongst smokers for the introduction of smoke-free football stands after national legislation was introduced, perhaps suggesting that football fans would be reluctant to relinquish an age-old custom of smoking at football matches. However, amongst non-smokers, there was a small increase in support.

Development of no-tobacco policy for UEFA EURO 2016

UEFA's ambition to implement a complete tobacco-free tournament at UEFA EURO 2016 was somewhat undermined by France's national smoke-free legislation which does not explicitly prohibit smoking in semi-enclosed spaces. Therefore, the No Tobacco Policy for UEFA EURO 2016 would need to *exceed* existing national legislation. This led to the creation of a partnership between UEFA, the Local Organising Committee (LOC) and Healthy Stadia to develop a No Tobacco project that would protect all stadium users, including fans, staff, volunteers and contract workers, against the health and safety dangers presented by tobacco use. Of upmost concern was protecting all stadium users from the health harms of second-hand smoke, in all aspects of host stadia, including areas not currently covered by national smoke-free legislation. Therefore, the policy would operate as follows:

- The no smoking regulation would apply without exception to all spaces within a designated 'No Tobacco' perimeter at each stadium, including all internal and external aspects of host venues.
- The policy would apply to all stadium users, including fans, very important persons (VIPs), staff, volunteers, media personnel and contractors.
- Any individuals using tobacco or e-cigarette products beyond the No Tobacco perimeter would be asked to extinguish their product or cease usage.
- Designated smoking areas would not be made available for fans or staff, with staff asked to move off-site if they wished to smoke.
- The policy would come into effect at host stadia at 08.00 the day before match day and would cease 4 hours after completion of each match.

In addition to regulations on smoking inside stadium environments, the policy would also prohibit the sale of tobacco and e-cigarette products, including sale through cigarette vending machines, and the promotion and advertising of tobacco or e-cigarette products within the perimeter of host stadia, which is forbidden as part of the France's commitment and ratification of the WHO's FCTC. All ashtrays and smoking-related paraphernalia would need to be removed from all areas of host venues include general access, VIP and media areas. Research suggests that the presence of ashtrays if often regarded as tacit approval of smoking and could therefore hinder enforcement of the smoke-free regulation (Moore et al. 2006, 2009).

Key challenges

The lack of legislation covering semi-enclosed spaces inside host stadia presented several specific obstacles to the successful implementation of a complete tobacco-free stadia policy, including:

- Low levels of awareness and poor compliance with smoke-free stadia policies amongst host nation fans
- Inability to use penalty fines as a key enforcement tool
- A lack of prior training amongst stadium stewards and security staff on how to enforce such a wide-reaching policy without recourse to 'hard' penalties enshrined in national law
- Minimal pre-existing No Smoking signage at host stadia (only internal office spaces had no smoking signage)
- How to adequately communicate such a policy to fans travelling from 24 nations, many of whom would not be used to smoke-free policies applying to public spaces

Taking the above considerations into account in advance of the tournament, it was apparent that taking a 'hard approach' to enforcement would be extremely difficult to achieve, with such an approach likely leading to heightened tensions amongst fans and the possibility of crowd control issues. As such, UEFA took the strategic decision to maximise communication of the policy to fans both pre-tournament and at host venues on matchdays, whilst taking a 'soft approach' to enforcement of the policy at matches through a cohort of specially trained volunteers and basic training for stewards. It should be noted that taking a soft approach did not compromise the protective value of the No Tobacco policy but was simply a pragmatic and effective strategy for implementing such an ambitious policy for a mega event of this scale that had no grounding in tobacco control legislation.

Implementation of no tobacco policy on matchdays

UEFA recruited a team of volunteers that would help to communicate the policy to fans and intervene in instances of non-compliance. Volunteers were recruited based on having a background in a health-related discipline, were non-smokers and were fluent in both French and English language. The volunteers received specialist training and were equipped with yellow and red information/enforcement cards, with a team of 11 volunteers operating at each host venue. A dedicated team of Sustainability Managers coordinated all social responsibility and sustainability activities and were in regular contact with Healthy Stadia throughout the tournament.

Training for stewards and volunteers

To help volunteers communicate the policy, in particular its protective health benefits, to fans and members of the tournament workforce, Healthy Stadia developed content for a detailed online training programme. The training programme covered the following key areas:

- Health and safety dangers of tobacco use in stadium environments and acute dangers to health from second-hand smoke
- Restricted products and behaviours covered by the policy
- Primary communications tools used pre-tournament and at host venues
- Use of yellow and red information/enforcement cards and how to engage fans
- Understanding likely areas of non-compliance and protocol for graduated enforcement plan
- Monitoring, reporting and staying safe

Healthy Stadia also delivered a 'train the trainer' programme for the tournament's Sustainability Managers. This training module was delivered prior to the tournament and equipped managers with the skills and materials to deliver face to face training sessions with their volunteers, with a focus on role-play, the enforcement process and conflict resolution. Stadium stewards also received situational briefings from operations staff at each venue to support volunteers on matchday. Furthermore, the entire tournament workforce received a short online module briefing staff on all of UEFA's sustainability projects, including the No Smoking policy.

No smoking signage

Owing to a lack of pre-existing No Smoking signage at host stadia, a signage placement strategy was developed to: 1) sensitise fans to the No Tobacco policy at key stages of a supporter's journey from the first security cordon to their seat; and, 2) cover likely 'hotspot' areas such as entrances to toilets, concourses, catering areas, stairways and entrances/exits to seating areas where smokers were likely to gather, particularly at half-time.

All tournament stadia used A2 size signage boards incorporating an internationally recognised No Smoking and No E-cigarette pictogram with the following wording in both English and French:

- No Smoking: Use of tobacco and e-cigarette products are prohibited in any part of this stadium.
- Interdiction de Fumer: Le tabac et les cigarettes électroniques sont interdits dans l'enceinte du stade.

Supplementary No Smoking, No E-cigarette stickers were also used to bolster communication of the policy in areas such as toilet facilities and placed on fixed ashtrays in VIP areas. The stadium regulations that were placed along the perimeter of all host venues also provided information about the policy.

Pre-tournament and matchday fan communications

In keeping with their commitment to a 'soft approach' to enforcement, UEFA took advantage of several key communications channels to sensitise fans to the No Tobacco regulation in operation at the tournament. In addition to signage, the No Tobacco policy was communicated to fans through the following mechanisms:

- UEFA media releases were distributed to major news outlets, participating UEFA Member Associations and fan groups ahead of the tournament
- UEFA published an article on their website detailing the policy (UEFA 2015a) and communicated the regulation via multiple UEFA-affiliated social media channels
- Public address announcements outside and inside of host stadia at key intervals
- 'Big Screen' and concourse screen messaging (where available) at host stadia prior to kick-off and during half-time
- The dual No Smoking, No E-cigarettes pictogram appeared on all match tickets with accompanying wording
- Notice of the policy appeared in official programmes for each tournament fixture
- Yellow and red information/enforcement cards distributed by volunteers

Enforcement of policy

Volunteers were equipped with a set of yellow and red cards which contained basic information on the No Tobacco policy including where it operated and its overarching objectives. The yellow cards where primarily deployed as an 'ice-breaker' in order to help initiate conversations with fans in breach of the policy. This allowed volunteers and stadium stewards to set a non-confrontational tone, in keeping with UEFA's soft approach to enforcement. With repeat offenders, volunteers could the issue a red card with additional information. If any given fan continued to disregard the policy, volunteers would refer the incident to stadium stewards or security personnel that would then take appropriate action.

Matchday monitoring

Whilst the yellow and red cards were primarily used as an information/enforcement tool, they simultaneously acted as a monitoring mechanism. Volunteers documented instances of non-compliance in a bespoke diary, recording the type of card issued (yellow or red), what product the card related to (tobacco or e-cigarette), and where each card was issued (e.g. seated areas, toilets, concourses).

After each match a designated team leader aggregated the data collected by volunteers and delivered a monitoring report via e-mail to Healthy Stadia. Sustainability Managers and personnel from Healthy Stadia could then provide timely feedback on hot spot areas at host venues and reprioritise volunteer positioning before the venue's next fixture.

As smoking rates and indeed national tobacco legislation varies from country to country, Healthy Stadia identified 'high priority' group stage fixtures where compliance and enforcement could be an issue. Staff from Healthy Stadia attended several of these fixtures, providing on-the-ground support to Sustainability Managers and volunteers on signage placement, likely hotspot smoking areas and deployment of volunteers.

Impact and key results

The No Tobacco policy was well received and well observed by fans across all host stadia. Volunteers reported that most fans cooperated with requests to extinguish lit tobacco products or cease use of their e-cigarettes, often in an apologetic manner. Volunteers stated that smokers were in the vast minority amongst supporters and a combination of the communications campaign, stadium signage and interventions by volunteers themselves discouraged the use of tobacco products, thereby protecting stadium users against exposure to second-hand smoke. Fans from individual nations were not singled out for enquiry, however, volunteers did report that French fans, who likely attended host stadia on a regular basis for domestic fixtures, were among the more difficult supporters to convince of the benefits of the No Tobacco policy.

The monitoring data reveals there was a total of 13,964 recorded interventions by volunteers over the course of the 51-match tournament, captured through the distribution of yellow and red cards. In total, 12,805 yellow cards and 1,159 red cards were issued, indicating that 0.57% of the total tournament attendance (n = 2,427,303) received a direct intervention from volunteers.

The monitoring data also suggests that once a volunteer had intervened in an instance of non-compliance, most fans were then happy to observe the No Tobacco policy, as detailed by comparably few red cards being issued for both tobacco and e-cigarette products. The relatively few interventions concerning use of e-cigarettes is reflective of the prevalence of e-cigarette usage in France and many European countries.

Less than a fifth (18.9%) of yellow and red cards were issued in seated areas in view of the pitch and over half of interventions (54%) occurred on concourses or in stairwells. Volunteers indicated that those wishing to smoke or use an e-cigarette product often wanted to do so at half-time, and would leave their seats to enter the concourse, often via a stairwell, after the first 45 minutes. This correlates with the quantitative data captured, and although volunteers and stadium stewards were made aware of this during the tournament, the task of discouraging smoking behaviour at half-time was a constant issue throughout the UEFA EURO 2016.

Table 16.1 Aggregated monitoring data collected through the recording of yellow and red card interventions by volunteers.

Smoking Hotspot Area	*Yellow Cards distributed for Tobacco Usage*	*Red Cards distributed for Tobacco Usage*	*Yellow Cards distributed for E-cigarette Usage*	*Yellow Cards distributed for E-cigarette Usage*	*Total*
Seated Areas	2251	223	156	9	2639
Toilets	459	112	19	2	592
Concourse/Stairs	6711	616	270	17	7614
Catering Areas	2430	130	70	25	2655
VIP Areas	205	18	8	0	231
Media/Offices	212	6	14	1	233
Total	**12268**	**1105**	**537**	**54**	**13964**

Limitations

- At key points during fixtures, particularly half-time, volunteers were unable to record all interventions due to the volume of fans on concourses and therefore they took the pragmatic decision to prioritise intervening over recording data. Therefore, the data here likely underestimates the true number of interventions and fans using tobacco and e-cigarette products.
- At certain stadia, volunteers could not access VIP and media areas and therefore occurrences of smoking in these areas were not recorded.
- Host stadia varied massively in terms of their capacity and physical structure. For volunteers working at larger stadia, such as Stade de France, the burden of responsibility was much greater which could have impacted their effectiveness on the ground.
- Whilst there were several instances were individual stadium stewards had taken ownership of and responsibility for the policy, others remained unconvinced and were largely disinterested in its enforcement. This undermined the authority of volunteers and could have led to supporters disregarding the policy.

Discussion

The tobacco-free policy developed and operated for UEFA EURO 2016 is significant in that the operator of a major international football tournament implemented a no-smoking policy at host stadia in a country where there was no national legislation to assist in the enforcement of such a policy. In addition to this positive outcome, there are wider public health benefits that can be taken from this and previous implementation of tobacco-free policies at UEFA tournaments.

Whilst UEFA had previously implemented a no-smoking policy at its 2012 edition of the EURO in Poland and Ukraine, both host countries had adopted smoke-free legislation ahead of the tournament, a political act that the French government was not willing to follow in advance of hosting UEFA EURO 2016.

It is also worth reflecting on the 2008 edition of the EURO that was jointly hosted by Austria and Switzerland, where the LOCs of both host countries pushed back on a *request* from UEFA to operate no-smoking policies at host venues for the tournament. Consequently, UEFA took the unprecedented step of inserting new requirements for countries bidding to host future editions of the EURO to operate tobacco-free stadia, a step that also now features as part of the bidding requirements for UEFA's club competition finals.

There are several learning and discussion points that can be taken from this historical arc on policy development. Firstly, in addition to the obvious public health benefits of host stadia being declared tobacco-free, the hosting of such mega events can (in some cases at least) be used to influence wider tobacco-free policy changes at national level in host countries. This is evidenced in the example of UEFA EURO 2012 illustrated above, but also from the 2018 hosting of the FIFA World Cup in Russia (FIFA 2017). Hosting of such high-profile competitions should be noted by public health advocacy organisations working in the area of tobacco control as a significant point of leverage. In the cases of Poland, Ukraine and Russia, the strengthening of tobacco-free legislation in public spaces had far greater reach than simply sports stadia, with public transport, hotels, restaurants and bars also covered.

Secondly, in order to ensure that international sports events operate tobacco-free stadia, it is imperative that this is clearly set out as a mandatory requirement in the bidding criteria for host countries. Outside of football, there is also an opportunity for public health advocacy organisations to work with governing bodies of sport and operators of events to ensure this requirement is included in bidding criteria to host the competition (UEFA 2015b).

Finally, in cases such as UEFA EURO 2016 where the French government did not adopt a more rigorous form of tobacco-free legislation covering stadium environments, the operation of a tobacco-free policy at the tournament has already acted as a strong example of good practice that has inspired some of the host venues in France to adopt similar protective policies at a domestic level. Healthy Stadia has used a combination of good practices from UEFA EURO 2016 and Tobacco-Free Stadia Guidelines published in 2016 to work with stadium operators, football clubs and wider stakeholders in France to help further this objective. This can be evidenced by la Ligue de Football Professionnel and French professional clubs supporting the Mois Sans Tabac (month without tobacco) campaign in 2017 and 2018, where stadia operated as tobacco-free environments for the month of November (Ligue de Football Professionnel 2016).

Learning and recommendations

The soft approach to enforcement combined with a comprehensive communications plan proved highly effective in protecting fans from the dangers of second-hand smoke, particularly in the internal aspects of host stadia. However, there are several areas where significant learning can be taken. We present a set of recommendations that will further assist the implementation of pragmatic tobacco-free policies at future UEFA events and indeed other sporting events including major international tournaments hosted in countries with relatively weak tobacco control legislation.

Recommendations for LOCs and UEFA events

Communications

Yellow and red information cards should be used as a soft enforcement tool at all of UEFA's signature events including club competitions finals and national competitions such as the EURO. In-stadia infrastructure such as advertising hoardings and concourse television screens should also be used to communicate the policy to fans. Big Screen announcements would benefit from a 'human element' to compel fans to observe the policy.

UEFA should commit to producing non-branded No Smoking signage for all major events. The donation of this signage post-event could then act as a stimulus to encourage tenant club(s) and stadium operations teams to implement comprehensive tobacco-free policies for domestic fixtures where no national legislation does not already exist.

No-tobacco perimeter

For UEFA EURO 2016, it was decided that all internal and external aspects of host stadia would be declared smoke-free. For stadia with large external concourses beyond the turnstiles, enforcing this aspect of the policy became problematic given the relatively small volunteer base. Therefore, we recommend that No Smoking policies should only apply within the main stadium structure.

Designated smoking areas

We recommend that UEFA consider the operation of designated smoking areas in completely open-air spaces external to the main stadium structure. The operation of designated smoking areas is dependent on a number of legal and practical factors including, but not limited to: the legality of their operation in the country in which the event is taking place, the amount of open-air space immediately outside of the main stadium structure, the likelihood of second-hand smoke accumulating; the presence/absence of outer perimeter fencing that would prevent non-ticketed individuals from entering the complex, and the additional capacity required in terms of stewarding to maintain the safety and security of the event.

Additional steward training and enforcement

The No Tobacco policy would have gained much greater traction through uniform enforcement by stewards and security staff. For future tournaments, UEFA stewarding and security should be engaged at a much earlier stage of planning with the aim of achieving binding agreements on enforcement protocol and greater support for volunteers.

However, regarding the tobacco-free policy at UEFA EURO 2016, we would include the caveat that the tournament took place during a period of great upheaval in France with heightened tensions due to the threat of terrorism, and this was rightly prioritised by UEFA, the local organising committee and security forces.

Extending the volunteer base

It became apparent very early on in the tournament that the volunteers dedicated to enforcing the No Smoking policy were insufficient, and indeed for larger venues such as Stade de France, the volunteers struggled to cover all tiers and concourses effectively, particularly at half-time. At future events the wider volunteer workforce should receive online and situational No Tobacco training and be equipped with yellow and red cards to aid enforcement and boost compliance.

Enforcement of policy in VIP and media areas

There was clear evidence of non-compliance with the No Smoking policy in some VIP and media areas. At future events, UEFA should endeavour to remove all loose and fixed ashtrays, which could be regarded as tacit approval to smoke, and provide specific briefing and training for stewards and other staff operating in these areas.

Recommendations for other sporting bodies

Bidding criteria

Include a commitment to implementing a tobacco-free policy at all host venues, training facilities and athlete accommodation as part of the bidding criteria for all tournaments irrespective of existing national legislation.

Political support

Sporting bodies and LOCs should endeavour to engage with both local municipalities (who may hold subnational or regional powers) and national government to sensitise them of their aspiration to provide smoke-free environments with a view to encouraging them to adopt smoke-free legislation covering stadia.

Partnership working

Information and support from charitable and other civil society organisations tackling the tobacco issue will be able to add a much-needed local perspective on barriers and facilitators to implementing such a policy. These organisations may also be able to help galvanise political support.

Stadia assessments

No two stadiums or sports venues are alike, and every facility has its own quirks. It is essential that venues are assessed prior to an event to provide an initial insight into existing policies and practices, signage placement, likely hotspot areas and their potential to operate designated smoking areas.

Conclusion and legacy

It is particularly pleasing to report the effectiveness of the tobacco-free policy at UEFA EURO 2016 that was implemented through a 'soft approach' surpassing tobacco control legislation applying to sports stadia in France. One should also consider that the policy operated at a tournament with heightened security concerns, and with fans from 24 different nations, the majority of which do not have tobacco-free stadium policies. As such, the No Tobacco policy at UEFA EURO 2016 should be held up as a significant success story and provides a strong case study for future mega-events, particularly those hosted in countries with tobacco legislation that does not cover stadium environments.

It is anticipated that the operation of a tobacco-free policy at the tournament will act as a strong example of good practice which will inspire host venues in France and beyond to adopt similar protective policies. In follow-up to the tournament, Healthy Stadia will use a combination of good practices from UEFA EURO 2016, and its recently published Tobacco-Free Stadia Guidelines, to work with stadium operators, football clubs and wider stakeholders in France to advocate for tobacco-free policies to be adopted at domestic matches. Indeed, the opportunity presented by the Respect Your Health: No Tobacco project for spreading smoke-free and broader tobacco control measures should not be underestimated, not least through exposing hundreds of thousands of travelling fans from all over Europe to tobacco-free football environments.

Healthy Stadia recognises that whilst the No Tobacco policy at UEFA EURO 2016 should be regarded a success, it will still take many years of sensitisation amongst fans, staff and even national associations to embed comprehensive levels of compliance with smoking restrictions at UEFA's flagship tournament. It is hoped that the learning from Respect Your Health: No Tobacco in France, and the recommendations detailed, will further enhance implementation of a tobacco-free policy at future editions of UEFA's European Championships, protecting the health of all stadium users against second-hand smoke, and disassociating all links between football and tobacco.

Indeed, Healthy Stadia has been engaged by a number of UEFA's Member Associations and league operators in the months since UEFA EURO 2016 including the

Portuguese Football Federation, the Belgian Pro League and the Dutch Eredivisie for support in advocating and adopting tobacco-free stadia policies that exceed national legislation. We will continue to work with a broad mix of sporting and public health bodies to secure a tobacco-free footballing future in Europe.

Statement of intellectual property

The Healthy Stadia word mark and logo mark are registered as official trademarks to the European Healthy Stadia Network CIC Ltd at EU level.

Acknowledgements

The authors would like to thank UEFA for their progressive and open approach to partnership working, for their commitment to operating tobacco-free football environments and for helping to eradicate any lingering association between football and tobacco.

Disclosure statement

European Healthy Stadia Network CIC received funding from UEFA for development and implementation of the Respect Your Health programme delivered at EURO 2016.

References

Anagnostopoulos, C. and D. Shilbury. 2013. Implementing corporate social responsibility in English football: Towards multi-theoretical integration. *Sport, Business and Management: An International Journal*, 3(4), 268–284.

Article L. 3511–7 du code de la santé publique. Décret no 2006–1386 du 15 novembre 2006 fixant les conditions d'application de l'interdiction de fumer (en particulier aux articles R. 3511–1 à R. 3512–2 du code de la santé publique). Available at: www.tobaccocontrollaws.org/files/live/France/France%20-%202006%20MOH%20SF%20Circular%20-%20national.pdf [Accessed: 9th April 2014].

Bonaldi, C., F. Andriantafika, S. Chyderiotis, M. Boussac-Zarebska, B. Cao, T. Benmarhnia, and I. Gremy. 2016. Smoking-attributable mortality in France. *Latest Estimates and Trend, 2000–2013* [online] Available at: http://opac.invs.sante.fr/doc_num.php?explnum_id=10535 [Accessed: 18th April 2019].

Carter, B., C. Abnet, D. Feskanich, N. Freedman, P. Hartge, C. Lewis, J. Ockene, R. Prentice, F. Speizer, M. Thun, and E. Jacobs. 2015. Smoking and mortality: Beyond established causes. *New England Journal of Medicine*, 372(7), 631–640.

Crabb, J., and L. Ratinckx. 2005. *The Healthy Stadia Initiative: A Report for North West Public Health Team*. Preston, UK: Department of Health.

Department of Health and Social Care. 2011. *Impact of Smokefree Legislation: Evidence Review* [online] Available at: www.gov.uk/government/publications/impact-of-smokefree-legislation-evidence-review-march-2011 [Accessed: 18th April 2019].

FIFA. 2013. *Global Showpieces to Be Smoke-Free Events* [online] Available at: www.fifa.com/aboutfifa/footballdevelopment/medical/news/newsid=2025637/ [Accessed: 8th April 2014].

FIFA. 2017. *The Tobacco-Free Policy for FIFA Events* [online] Available at: https://resources.fifa.com/image/upload/the-tobacco-free-policy-for-fifa-events-2890383.pdf?cloudid=pvi2z8z67qu53cdhm3se [Accessed: 3rd May 2019].

Fong, G, L. Craig, R. Guignard, G. Nagelhout, M. Tait, P. Driezen, R. Kennedy, C. Boudreau, J. Wilquin, A. Deutsch, and F. Beck. 2013. Evaluating the effectiveness of France's indoor smoke-free law 1 year and 5 years after implementation: Findings from the ITC France survey. *PLoS One*, 8(6), e66692.

Ligue de Football Professionnel. 2016. *La LFP Partenaire de #MOISSANSTABAC* [online] Available at: www.lfp.fr/corporate/article/la-lfp-partenaire-de-moissanstabac.htm [Accessed: 3rd May 2019].

Moore, R., J. Lee, T. Antin, and S. Martin. 2006. Tobacco free workplace policies and low socioeconomic status female bartenders in San Francisco. *Journal of Epidemiology & Community Health*, 60(2), 51–56.

Moore, R., J. Lee, S. Martin, M. Todd, and B. Chu. 2009. Correlates of persistent smoking in bars subject to smokefree workplace policy. *International Journal of Environmental Research and Public Health*, 6(4), 1341–1357.

Parnell, D., K. Curran, and M. Philpott. 2016. Healthy stadia: An insight from policy to practice. *Sport in Society*, 20(2), 181–186.

Parnell, D., G. Stratton, B. Drust, and D. Richardson. 2013. Football in the Community schemes: Exploring the effectiveness of an intervention in promoting healthful behaviour change. *Soccer & Society*, 14(1), 35–51.

Pasquereau, A., A. Gautier, R. Andler, R. Guignard, J. B. Richard, and V. Nguyen-Thanh. 2017. Tabac et e-cigarette en France: niveaux d'usage d'après les premiers résultats du Baromètre santé 2016. *Bull Epidémiol Hebd*. 12, 214–222.

Union of European Football Associations (UEFA). 2011. *No Tobacco at UEFA EURO 2012* [online] Available at: www.uefa.org/mediaservices/mediareleases/newsid=1701708.html [Accessed: 8th April 2014].

Union of European Football Associations (UEFA). 2015a. *No Tobacco at UEFA EURO 2016* [online] Available at: www.uefa.com/insideuefa/mediaservices/mediareleases/newsid=2252741.html [Accessed: 1st June 2015].

Union of European Football Associations (UEFA). 2015b. *UEFA European Football Championship Final Tournament 2016: Tournament Requirements* [online] Available at: www.uefa.com/MultimediaFiles/Download/Regulations/uefa/Others/84/03/26/840326_DOWNLOAD.pdf [Accessed: 3 May 2019].

World Health Organization. 1986. Ottawa Charter for Health Promotion. *Canadian Journal of Public Health*, 77, 425–426.

World Health Organization. 2005. *WHO Framework Convention on Tobacco Control* [online] Available at: www.who.int/fctc/text_download/en/index.html [Accessed: 8th April 2014].

World Health Organization. 2007. *Guidelines for Implementation of Article 8: Guidelines on the Protection from Exposure to Tobacco Smoke* [online] Available at: www.who.int/fctc/guidelines/adopted/article_8/en/ [Accessed: 8th April 2014].

World Health Organization. 2008. *WHO Report on the Global Tobacco Epidemic, 2008: The MPOWER Package* [online] Available at: www.who.int/tobacco/mpower/gtcr_download/en/index.html [Accessed: 8th April 2014].

World Health Organization. 2010. *A Guide to Tobacco-Free Mega Events* [online] Available at: www.wpro.who.int/publications/PUB_9789290614982/en/ [Accessed: 8th April 2014].
World Health Organization. 2011. *Building Capacity for Tobacco Control: Training Package: 'Drafting Smoke-Free Legislation' Presentation* [online] Available at: www.who.int/tobacco/publications/building_capacity/training_package/smoke_free/en/index.html [Accessed: 8th April 2014].
World Health Organization. 2013. *WHO Report on the Global Tobacco Epidemic 2013* [online] Available at: www.who.int/tobacco/global_report/2013/en/ [Accessed: 8th April 2014].
World Health Organization. 2014. *Healthy Settings* [online] Available at: www.who.int/healthy_settings/en/ [Accessed: 8th April 2014].
World Health Organization. 2018. *Fact Sheet on Tobacco* [online] Available at: www.who.int/en/news-room/fact-sheets/detail/tobacco [Accessed: 18th April 2019].

Chapter 17

A closing comment on the policy and politics of implementing Football as Medicine

The English context

Daniel Parnell, Søren Bennike, Laila Ottesen and Paul Widdop

Background

Football is one of the most popular sports in the world and given its mass youth appeal and global reach, it provides a potentially invaluable vehicle for promoting health (Smith and Westerbeek 2007). The participative nature of football (whether as a leisure activity, exercise or competitive sport) (see Bennike et al. 2014), as an event and place to attend; or as a hook to engage people appears to be a prudent consideration for policymakers and practitioners who aim to deliver health outcomes (Krustrup and Krustrup 2018; Parnell et al. 2016). Despite the burgeoning evidence that supports Football as Medicine, this chapter argues that in order to capitalise on this evidence, greater consideration must be placed on the policy and politics of countries. This chapter focuses on England in the United Kingdom (UK), given that football is a prominent sport of the country and *should* prove excellent territory to deliver and lead the Football as Medicine agenda. Following this, a brief analysis is provided on the football context in Denmark. These two countries and policies have been chosen given their respective adoption of different welfare models. England having an Anglo-Saxon model and Denmark having a Scandinavian model. This chapter concludes with a call to arms for those involved in Football as Medicine research.

Between the 1970s and 1980s, England engaged in a range of recreation and welfare policies (King 2009). In the 1990s, greater political acclaim was attached to sport endorsing its potential to impact social welfare and regeneration (Coalter 2007). Sport was lauded as an instrument to deliver upon multiple agendas, such as increasing income and jobs, improving education, health and social inclusion (Coalter 2007; King 2009). Given the widespread appeal and reach of sport, some authors have acknowledged that it may provide a more effective vehicle in reaching those at risk who may not be reached by traditional political or civic activities (Mellor 2008; Bloyce and Smith 2010; Collins and Kay 2014; Parnell and Richardson 2014; Parnell et al. 2015a). In contrast, several authors challenged the social impact of sport, claiming a lack of empirical evidence (Smith and Waddington 2004; Bailey 2005; Collins and Kay 2014). Despite this lack of evidence, policies continued to endorse sport as a vehicle to attend to social agendas and change (Coalter 2007).

Football is considered the national game in England and has been a prominent vehicle in the health agenda. Whilst successive governments have used sport policy to deliver policy goals, including youth justice, social inclusion and public health, with limited evidence of effectiveness (Coalter 2007), it is now beyond doubt that regular physical activity during childhood and adolescence is an important part of the foundation of a happy, healthy and longer life. The serious dangers associated with inactive lifestyles are equally clear, such as heart disease, diabetes and obesity (see Bailey et al. 2015). As such, football has been employed in a variety of contexts to deliver public health outcomes for various populations.

Tackling inactivity through a public health position is of particular importance, given its role in the major causes of death and disability, through non-communicable diseases like obesity, heart disease and stroke, cancer, chronic respiratory disease and diabetes. Estimations from the World Health Organization claim the annual worldwide tally of 35 million people per year dying of these chronic diseases, which is double the number dying from all combined infectious diseases, like HIV/AIDS and malaria (WHO 2005). This extends beyond the human cost. In the UK, around 20 million adults are physically inactive, which costs an estimated £7.4bn per year (NICE 2018). As such, sport has increasingly featured as a vehicle for public health (Bailey et al. 2015).

Despite this, Kohl et al. (2012) suggest that contrary to evidence on the benefits of physical activity being available since the 1950s, it is only recently that government action has developed. One of the reasons for this lack of action is the cross-cutting nature of sport development, which makes it difficult to manage. Indeed, whilst there is now an acknowledgement of the link between sport, physical activity and health, strategies to address these issues are underdeveloped. Yet, the importance of football (sports and physical activity) for most policymakers and politicians lies in its status as the least expensive and most effective preventive treatment for combating the increasing worldwide problem of obesity (Bailey et al. 2015). Given the widespread appeal of football, it would be remiss for policymakers and governments not to explore the potential of the game as a vehicle of public health.

Football has received much attention in recent years for its contribution to society via corporate social responsibility strategies, which have been delivered through a variety of methods. One approach in England has been Football in the Community (FitC) programmes, the community arms and often registered charities of professional football clubs. Some examples of interventions delivered by FitC programmes include those engaging hard-to-reach groups (Curran et al. 2014), social inclusion (Parnell et al. 2015a) and health (Parnell and Richardson 2014) across the lifespan and with men and women (Parnell et al. 2013; Bingham et al. 2014; Parnell et al. 2015b) and in football stadia as a setting to promote health (Parnell et al. 2016). Football has even entered educational domains and is now seen as a major contributor to the delivery of Physical Education and

School Sport, as sport policy in England ultimately encouraged schools to outsource this aspect of the curriculum (Parnell et al. 2016). Despite this, football is under enhanced scrutiny for what has been observed as grassroots and community failure (see O'Gorman et al. 2018).

To understand the present context, it is worth offering a brief historic perspective. Evidence suggests that there has been a historic mismanagement of sport facilities, most notably playing fields – and resultantly football pitches, which are a vital resource for community participants to play the game (King 2009). This previous policy disorganisation has resulted in lost playing fields and lack of maintenance, certainly over the past six decades. Subtle changes over times such as shifting the protected area from 6 hectares to 0.2 hectares at present can have a significant impact on practice (see King 2009). This would suggest that despite the political hyperbole around sport in England, little genuine value has been placed on sport locally and nationally, historically and geographically over time.

Evidence points towards a combination of both an absence of collaboration between central government, national governing bodies for sport, Sport England, other major stakeholders and local government, alongside the absence of (real) power nationally to prevent local decisions. Ultimately, local government can make local agreements to sell playing fields (King 2009). This exists due to the absence of rigid, coherent and extensive statutory laws related to playing fields, a manifestation of political devolution. This decline in playing fields has developed overtime, despite many local governments previous support for football (and sport). Indeed, many local governments remain inclined to support the benefits of football today. However, in England, the current political and fiscal climate suggest that over the past decade this decline has heightened and worsened the state of play for community and grassroots football, despite the best intentions of some local governments.

In May 2010, a Conservative Party-led coalition government assumed political leadership of the UK. This was in response to (real and perceived) debt incurred by the previous Labour administration, so the new government initiated considerable cuts to public spending, including a raft of austerity measures in its 'Comprehensive Spending Review', which outlined £81 billion cuts to government departments. This meant that public spending was reduced on a national scale, leaving few government departments untouched. By the end of 2013, almost three and a half years after the introduction of austerity-driven policy measures, it was estimated that £64 billion had been wiped from public expenditure. Austerity was rolled out across the UK, spreading to all tributaries of public spending. Later, the then Chancellor scheduled a further 20% expenditure cut between 2014 and 2018 (Croucher 2013). The cuts impacted upon provision including services being reduced, reorganised or disposed of. This included services such as libraries and clubs for disabled children, to leisure centres and community sport facilities (Blyth 2013; Parnell et al. 2015; Parnell et al. 2018). Importantly, these cuts were primarily focused on social benefits and local government budgets.

Local governments were charged with delivering these expenditure reductions (Audit Commission 2011). The Department of Communities and Local Government's funding was cut by 51% between 2010 and 2015, resulting in grants to local government falling by 27%. As a consequence, discretionary services, such as sport, leisure and culture faced funding uncertainty (Collins and Haudenhuyse 2015; see Parnell et al. 2018).

During 2015, David Cameron, the Prime Minister of the UK at the time, stated that there is a need for 'a leaner, more efficient state' in which 'we need to do more with less. Not just now, but permanently' (quoted in Krugman 2012), ensuring austerity would continue. Indeed, in the UK, the economy was set to face a continued period of what scholars would describe as 'super austerity' (i.e. further cuts upon already financially constrained services) (Lowndes and Gardner 2016).

In terms of local government expenditure, the annual spending commitment to services categorised by the Chartered Institute of Public Finance and Accountability as 'sport development and community recreation' are important to consider, as these services primarily aim to raise and widen participation among socio-economic groups considered to be the most excluded and tend to be subsidised in order that income is not a barrier to participation (King 2009). It is recognised that the Chartered Institute of Public Finance and Accountability category for expenditure on 'indoor and outdoor facilities' is also critical for participation as is the expenditure on 'parks and open spaces'. In fact, research undertaken by the Association of Public Service Excellence (APSE 2012) noted that although reductions in expenditure on maintaining and servicing facilities have occurred and were likely to continue, it is community-based programmes that have been disproportionately affected, whether these services are a component of direct local authority provision, funded from local budgets and delivered by local authority staff, or are funded by central government agencies and delivered in a partnership arrangement locally.

The impact of these funding cuts is relatively under-researched in scholarly circles. However, recent evidence of the impact on a range of contexts and services is starting to emerge, including the third sector (Walker and Hayton 2017, 2018; Kenyon et al. 2018; Parnell et al. 2014; Parnell et al. 2018), public sector services (Ramchandani et al. 2018; Reid 2018) and sports participation (Widdop et al. 2018). This is of particular importance for football, as playing fields and football pitches often fall under the leadership of local government or third sector organisations. Moreover, football, as the nation's game, is an important contributor to sport participation and physical activity, but its grassroots facilities are often at the mercy of local governments working in an environment of austerity.

Widdop et al. (2018) noted that sport participation among socio-demographic groups defined as 'hard to reach' has not altered significantly by comparing the Active People data in 2008–09 with 2013–14. The study revealed that only marginal differences can be identified across the 5-year timespan (during the period of intense austerity), which is perhaps unsurprising given the difficulties of raising and widening participation among the low-income and socially excluded in a context of disinvestment through austerity policies.

Furthermore a recent government strategy (Cabinet Office 2015) has specifically focused on 'social and community development', implying that a commitment of resources to raising and widening participation among 'hard-to-reach' groups is needed. However, in a period of austerity and public spending reductions, it appears that investment has not followed these policy aspiration to date, in that participation has not increased in these priority groups (Widdop et al. 2018). Indeed, central government has a commitment to, 'distribute funding to focus on those people who tend not to take part in sport, including women and girls, disabled people, those in lower socio-economic groups and older people' (Cabinet Office 2015, p. 10). In order to achieve this, local governments are viewed as critical in delivering policy in this respect. However, it appears investment needs to follow policy statements for any tangible change of participation to result.

As a consequence of funding cuts (whether austerity policy-related directly or not), discretionary services such as sport have faced uncertain times and ultimately an uncertain future, especially as trends suggest further regression of funding for local authority services up until 2020 (Collins and Haudenhuyse 2015). This has created challenges for community sport facilities who have had to manage both their financial viability and sustainability during this fiscal constraint (Parnell et al. 2018). An Association for Public Service Excellence report (2012) anticipated falling revenue budgets, staff cuts, increased charges, reduced opening hours, facility closures and reduced commitments to parks and pitches utilised for organised and casual participation in the light of changes to public funding levels. Some of these predictions have been reported through case studies on reductions to sport and leisure services and its impact on a range of sports from swimming facilities to municipal golf courses. The question remains how this may impact upon the potential for football to deliver upon the health agenda.

Despite austerity, football remains one of the most popular sports in England, with a reported 1.8 million participants on a weekly basis (Sport England 2017). Whilst there is an absence of longitudinal data, evidence suggests a decline in the number of people playing 11-aside competitive football (The FA 2004, 2015; Lusted 2009). The data suggests that this decline accelerated between 2005 and 2015, showing the number of people playing affiliated 11-aside football fell by 180,000 (The FA 2015). A recent analysis on contemporary issues in grassroots and community football suggests we should anticipate a further reduction in the quality of football playing facilities, increased costs, overuse of pitches, more matches cancelled, and potentially poorer experiences for players and, subsequently, less players involved in the game (O'Gorman et al. 2018).

Given the cost of lifestyle-related diseases and inactivity alongside the abundance of evidence for the role football can play towards the health agenda, it would make a reduction in funding for grassroots and community football appear questionable. Given the relatively low estimated costs for community football pitch development, whether grass or artificial grass surfaces, it appears to offer an opportunity to design and deliver programmes to reduce inactivity and increase sport participation. The cost of upkeep and enhancing grassroots and community football could be argued as insignificant when compared to the potential public health benefits of football, especially when compared with the financial burden of inactivity. Given the potential ongoing threat of austerity-driven policies in England, alongside the absence of rigorous protection for sport and leisure services and playing fields, it would appear that we may be missing out on an opportunity to capitalise on the evidence for Football as Medicine.

In the spirit of this book, and beyond merely the geography of the co-editors, it appears pertinent to offer a comparison with a European neighbor country, Denmark. Both countries adopt quite different approaches to a welfare model, which stimulates interest and analysis. Moreover, Denmark is a country in which the national football associations are specifically incorporating football for health in their strategy and activity profile.

Denmark has a population of 5.7 million citizens and a GDP of $286 billion, operating as a universal welfare state, also referred to as the Scandinavian or Nordic model (Esping-Andersen 1990; see also Ibsen 2017). It is beyond the scope of this short text to further unfold the complex model of governance you will find in Denmark. The country is among the healthiest countries in the European Union with a high level of sports participation. According to the Eurobarometer (European Commission 2014), Denmark is the 2nd most 'active' country and the 2nd most 'sport club active' country. The total number of sport clubs in Denmark is estimated to be around 16,000, corresponding to one per 350 inhabitants (Ibsen et al. 2015), making Denmark among the countries in the world with the highest number of sports facilities per capita (Rafoss and Troelsen 2010). In this case, Ibsen and Ottesen highlighted in 2003 that there is a football pitch for every 1,000 people. According to the national database of facilities, Denmark has, at present, approximately 4600 pitches, most of which are grass outdoor pitches, funded by the government (IDAN and LOA 2019). In terms of activity, a national survey estimates 61% of the adult (16+) population is active, of which 39% are active in sport clubs (Pilgaard and Rask 2016). The latter is more than doubled when considering children (age 7–15), as 83 % are active, of which between eight and nine out of every ten children will have participated in sports in a sport club setting (Laub 2013; Pilgaard and Rask 2016). The same survey concludes that 7% of the adult population (16+) and 37% of children (7–15) regularly play football, of which a majority play in local clubs under the wings of the Danish Football Association (DFA), making football the most popular sports-club-based activity in Denmark.

An important aspect of understanding the relative success in sports participation numbers, and more specifically participation in sport clubs, is the relation between the state and voluntarily organised sport clubs functioning as associations, being formal (formal democratic structures), private (self-governed) and non-profit. Building on these characteristics, the clubs are placed in the voluntary (third) sector (Pestof 1992), which plays a unique role in the Scandinavian welfare state model (Klausen and Selle 1996). Overall, Denmark has been progressive with their prioritisation of sport, which is delivered through a state-supported model in which the sport clubs holds a relatively strong autonomy. Please note that this autonomy is not functioning clearly separated from the state, on the contrary it is sphere of social life dependent on the state (Kaspersen and Ottesen 2001).

Of great importance to the development of sport clubs is the School Law of 1937, which required the municipalities to provide public schools of a certain size with a playing field (Ibsen and Ottesen 2003). And more importantly, to make these facilities available to local sport clubs after school hours. This secured available and playable football pitches to football clubs all over the country, which before that time stood as a major issue. Furthermore, in 1948, the Danish parliament adopted a State Football Pool, which secured the Sports Confederation of Denmark (SCD) a relatively large part of the national monopolistic betting profits (including the national lottery profits in 1989), bringing funding to the DFA. Importantly, this funding is earmarked for activities related to grassroots football alone (including the 'football for health' initiatives). In 1968, another law was passed, the Danish Leisure Act, which provided favorable conditions for the clubs, as it obligated the municipalities to support all leisure-time activities organised in associations, including football, by means of grants and access to facilities. By this time, a subsidised structure was created that remains within grassroots football today; the state supports the work of the DFA, and the municipalities support the work of association-based football clubs functioning relatively autonomously on democratic principles. And lastly, the citizens pay membership fees to clubs, and many are involved with voluntary work (see Bennike et al. 2017). Ibsen et al. (2015) argues for the volunteers to be the resource securing the survival of sport clubs, of which especially football clubs have a high number of volunteers. In relation to sport clubs, and thereby also football clubs, about half the income (facilities included) of the sport clubs are based on local government support (Ibsen and Ottesen 2003). In addition, membership fees do likewise stand as a strong financial income for sport clubs (Ibsen et al. 2015). The financial support and state recognition of sport clubs creates an 'associative democracy' as a parallel form of government to 'representative democracy', forming a dual strategy called 'the double democratic principle' (Kaspersen and Ottesen 2001).

Building on the above it becomes clear that the sport clubs of Denmark, including the ones organizing football, are deeply dependent on the government having favorable conditions. Further Ibsen and Eichberg (2012) argue that the sports organisations of today have become a sector in the government intervention. The perspectives in this book stand as an important point to understand how and why the health outcomes of football are receiving an increased focus from politicians and administrative policymakers. In the present time in Denmark, the welfare state does not have the same amount of financial capacity as in previous times, due to numerous factors related to expenditures and the global economic recession. As a result, in a time of austerity policy, the support for sport club activities is being questioned and challenged under a lens of greater scrutiny (see KUM

2014; Bennike et al. 2017). This holds a tendency in which the support for sport clubs is debated according to criteria of cost-utility (Ibsen and Ottesen 2003). In this case, policymakers are increasingly recognizing the value of advocating sport and football as a means of enhancing the overall health of the population (Thing and Ottesen 2010; Bennike 2017). In the public health programme 'A healthier life for all' (Danish Government 2014), the government sets the scene for increasingly involving the voluntary sector, such as football clubs, in addressing issues 'normally' expected to be a state or municipal responsibility. This applies to tackling issues such as health. This goal can be pursued either through infrastructural power (as is currently the case) or through despotic power (Mann 1990). Central to infrastructural power is the state's ability and desire to exercise its power in dialogue with society's institutions, such as sports organisations (e.g. the DFA). Conversely, despotic power is used by the state when it intervenes directly in society without entering into dialogue with the society's agents (Mann 1990). If the state chooses to keep working in the infrastructural way, it will entail that the DFA and the clubs are able and willing to voluntarily participate in working with health. Bennike (2016) shows how health has progressed to a relatively central position in the latest strategy of the Danish Football Association (DFA 2012). The creation and introduction of Football Fitness, which is an initiative coming from the DFA, is an illustrative example. If the concept proves sustainable in the long-term, it will become self-governing as an activity managed by local clubs and with state funding pursuant to the legislation benefitting the associations, especially in regard to facilities.

This short commentary is intended to stimulate the similar yet contrasting aspects of the welfare state model. For a fuller insight, we recommend that readers examine Bennike et al. (2017), which helps reveal the evidence-based collaborative policymaking and strategic support of Denmark against a more splintered and under-funded approach in England. This should serve to stimulate considerations for policy and practice transfer.

In summary, England has seen a historic mismanagement of sporting facilities, which has resulted in lost playing fields and lack of maintenance. There has been little political power or will nationally to prevent local decisions – ultimately, to sell playfields, a strategy which requires greater scrutiny. Austerity has appeared to heighten the decline in football participation and the general experience, resulting in people turning away from the sport. This could be a false economy given the need to get the nation active. It appears important for collaboration across football stakeholders and government departments to tighten legislation and turn the tide on declining playing fields, football pitches and declining football participation – if football is to play a part in creating an active and healthy nation.

The state-funded model observed in Denmark offers a perspective of consideration for researchers, practitioners and policymakers not only in the UK but globally. It prompts us to reflect on the Football as Medicine model (see Krustrup and Krustrup 2018; Figure 17.1). In doing so, we have adapted the Krustrup and Krustrup model to go beyond our current focus on personal and interpersonal

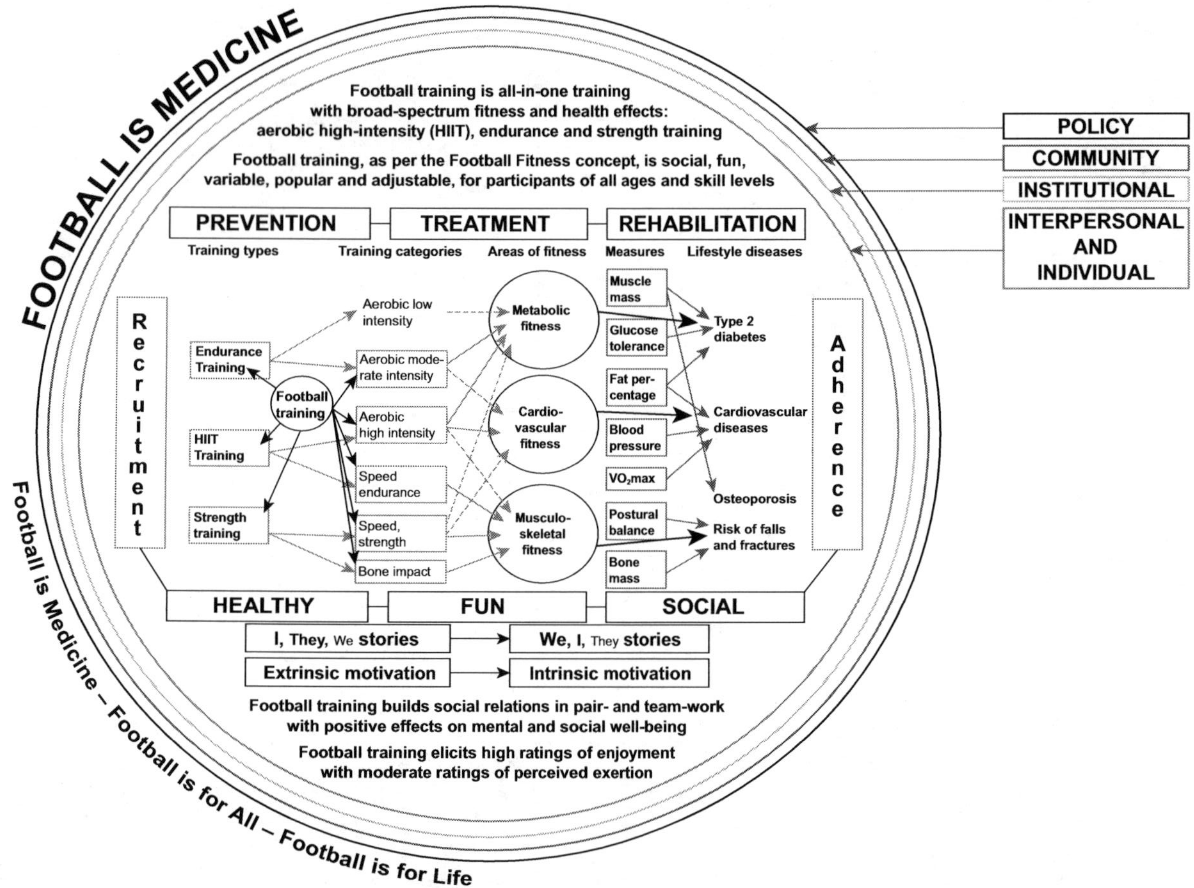

Figure 17.1 *An expanded version of the Football is Medicine model, emphasising that the policy, community and institutional levels are important when using the football as a vehicle to promote world health.*

Source: Adapted from Krustrup & Krustrup, BJSM, 2018.

examination in greater detail. To do this, we have incorporated aspects of ecological theory, i.e., institutional, community and policy to develop the model. Despite evidence that football is medicine (and does work for health promotion and delivering on public health outcomes), broader forces are at play in enabling what we know to be implemented.

Canadian medical sociologist Arthur Frank stated that new evidence does not necessarily help us make better, more ethical decisions for our communities: 'More knowledge may be less important than a clearer sense of value' (Frank 2000, p. 363). As many scholars operate in the knowledge economy of universities on a day-to-day basis, exchanging and discussing new findings and analysis, evidence in England points to either lack of information, willingness to listen and/or action. Our rally call would be for Football as Medicine scholars to take on these bigger policy and government challenges. To work with politicians and policymakers to crow bar the evidence into decisionmaker narratives. Ultimately, this case serves to highlight that despite growing evidence for football's potential role in the health agenda, evidence alone pales in significance against public policy. More needs to be done within policy domains if we are to aspire to share the evidence to strengthen communities and society to be resilient to attend to the health (and social) challenges we face.

References

Association of Public Service Excellence, and King, Neil. 2012. *Local authority sport and recreation services in England: Where next?* Manchester: APSE.

Audit Commission. 2011. *Tough times: Council's responses to a challenging financial climate.* London: Author.

Bingham, David. D, Daniel Parnell, Kathryn Curran, Rob Jones, and David Richardson. 2014. "Fit Fans: Perspectives of a Practitioner and Understanding Participant Health Needs within a Health Promotion Programme for Older Men Delivered within an English Premier League Football Club." *Soccer & Society* 15, no. 6, 883–901. Curran, Kathryn, Daniel. D. Bingham.

Bailey, Richard. 2005. "Evaluating the relationship between physical education, sport and social inclusion." *Educational Review*, 57, no 1, 71–90.

Bailey, Richard, Ed Cope, and Daniel Parnell. 2015. "Realising the benefits of sports and physical activity: The human capital model." *Materializando los beneficios del deporte y la actividad f'sica: El modelo de capital humano: Retos*, 28, 147–154.

Bennike, Søren. 2016. Fodbold Fitness – implementeringen af en ny fodboldkultur. PH.D. Afhandling. University of Copenhagen. Faculty of Science. [Football Fitness – the implementation of a new football culture. PH.D thesis]. SL grafik, Frederiksberg C, Denmark.

Bennike, Søren, Lone Friis Thing, and Laila Ottesen. 2017. Health through state supported voluntary sport clubs. In: *Sport and Health: Exploring the Current State of Play*, 1st edition, edited by Daniel Parnell and Peter Krustrup. London: Routledge.

Bennike, Søren, Johan M. Wikman, and Laila Ottesen. 2014. "Football Fitness: A new version of football? A concept for adult players in Danish football clubs." *Scandinavian Journal of Medicine & Science in Sports*, 24, no 1, 138–146. doi: 10.1111/sms.12276.

Bloyce, Danny, and Andy Smith. 2010. *Sport policy and development: An introduction*. London: Routledge.

Blyth, Mark. 2013. *The history of a dangerous idea*. New York: Oxford University Press.

Cabinet Office. 2015. *Sporting future: A new strategy for an active nation*. London: Cabinet Office.

Coalter, Fred. 2007. *A wider social role for sport: Who's keeping the score?* New York: Routledge.

Collins, Mike, and Rein Haudenhuyse. 2015. "Social exclusion and austerity policies in England: The role of sports in a new area of social polarisation and inequality?" *Social Inclusion*, 3, no 3. doi: 10.17645/si.v3i3.54

Collins, Mike, and Tess Kay. 2014. *Sport and social exclusion*. London: Routledge.

Croucher, Shane. 2013. "Osborne's budget 2013: Beer duty cut can't mask UK's slashed growth forecasts." *International Business Times*, March 20. Accessed 10 January 2019. www.ibtimes.co.uk/uk-budget2013-george-osborne-austerity-beer-448408

Curran, Kathryn, Daniel. D. Bingham, David Richardson, and Daniel Parnell. 2014. "Ethnographic engagement from within a football in the community programme at an English Premier League football club." *Soccer & Society* 15, no. 6, 934–950.

Danish Government (2014). Et sundere liv for all – Nationale mål for danskernes sundhed de næste 10 år. [A healthier life for all – national goals for the health of the Danes in the coming 10 years].

DFA. 2012. *Passion Udvikling Fællesskab: Strategi for videreudviklingen af dansk fodbold frem til 2015*. [Passion development community: Strategy for further development of Danish football until 2015] Brøndby: DBU. Accessed 10 January 2019. www.dbu.dk/~/media/Files/DBU_Broendby/publikationer/PUF_folder.pdf

Esping-Andersen, Gøsta. 1990. *The three worlds of welfare capitalism*. Cambridge: Polity Press.

European Commission. 2014. *Sport and Physical Activity*. Conducted by TNS Opinion & Social.

Frank, Authur. 2000. "The standpoint of storyteller." *Qualitative Health Research*, 10, no 3, 354–365.

Ibsen, Bjarne. 2017. Denmark: The dissenting sport system in Europe. In: *Sport policy systems and sport federations*. A cross-national perspective, edited by Scheerder et al. Palgrave Macmillan. London.

Ibsen, Bjarne, and Henning Eichberg. 2012. "Dansk idrætspolitik: Mellem frivillighed og statslig styring." In: *Idrætspolitik i komparativ belysning: National og international (s. 147–209)*, edited by H. Eichberg. Syddansk Universitetsforlag. Odense.

Ibsen, Bjarne, Karsten Østerlund, and Trygve Laub. 2015. "Sport clubs in Denmark." In: *Sport clubs in Europe: A cross-national comparative perspective*, edited by Breuer et al. Switzerland: Springer, 85–109. doi: 10.1007/978-3-319-17635-2.

Ibsen, Bjarne, and Laila Ottesen. 2003. "Sport and Welfare policy in Denmark: The development of Sport between state, market and community." In: *Sport and Welfare policies: Six European case studies*. The Club of Cologne, Vol. 3, edited by K. Heinemann. Hofmann, Reinheim, 31–86. Cologne.

IDAN, and LOA. 2019. *Facilitetsdatabasen: Idrætsanlæg I Danmark* [Facility database: Sports facilities in Denmark]. https://facilitetsdatabasen.dk/

Kaspersen, Lars Bo, and Laila Ottesen. 2001. "Associationalism for 150 years and still alive and kicking: Some reflections on Danish civil society." *Critical Review of International Social and Political: Philosophy*, 4, 105–130. doi: 10.1080/13698230108403340

Kenyon, James Andrew, Carolynne Mason, and Joel Rookwood. 2018. "Emerging third-sector sports organisations and navigating uncertainty in an 'era of austerity': A single ethnographic case study from Liverpool." *International Journal of Sport Policy and Politics*, 10, no 1, 25–42. doi: 10.1080/19406940.2018.1425732

King, Neil. 2009. *Sport policy and governance: Local perspectives*. Oxford: Butterworth-Heinemann.

Klausen, Kurt Klaudi, and Per Selle. 1996. "The third sector in Scandinavia." *Voluntas: International Journal of Voluntary and Nonprofit Organizations*, 7, no 2, 99–122.

Kohl, Harold, Cora Craig, Estelle Lambert, Shigeru Inoue, Jasem Alkandari, Grit Leetongin, and Sonja Kahlmeier. 2012. "The pandemic of physical inactivity: Global action for public health." *The Lancet*, 380, no 9838, 294–305.

Krugman, Paul. 2012. "The austerity drive in Britain isn't really about debt and deficits at all; it's all about using deficit panic as an excuse to dismantle social programs." *New York Times*, May 31. Accessed 20 January 2019. www.nytimes.com/2012/06/01/opinion/krugman-the-austerity-agenda.html

Krustrup, Peter, and Birgitte R. Krustrup. 2018. "Football is medicine: It is time for patients to play!" *British Journal of Sports Medicine*. 52, 1412–1414. doi: 10.1136/bjsports-2018–099377

KUM. 2014. Udredning af idrættens økonomi og struktur. Analyse. [Clearing sport economy and structure. Analysis]. Kulturministeriet, Idrættens analyseinstitut og KPMG.

Laub, Trygve. 2013. *Sports participation in Denmark 2011: National survey: English version*. Copenhagen: Danish Institute for Sports Studies.

Lowndes, Vivien, and Alison Gardner. 2016. "Local governance under the conservatives: Super-austerity, devolution and the 'smarter state'." *Local Government Studies*, 42, no 3, 357–375. doi: 10.1080/03003930.2016.1150837

Lusted, Jim. 2009. "Playing games with 'race': Understanding resistance to 'race' equality initiatives in English local football governance." *Soccer & Society*, 10, no 6, 722–739.

Mann, Michael. 1990. *The rise and decline of the nation-state*. Oxford: Blackwell.

Mellor, Gavin. 2008. "The janus-faced sport: English football, community and the legacy of the 'third way'." *Soccer and Society*, 9, no 3, 313–324.

National Institute for Health and Care Excellence. 2018. *Physical activity and the environment NICE guideline [NG90]*. London: NICE.

O'Gorman, Jimmy, Danny Fitzpatrick, Jon Sibley, Matthew Hindmarsh, Zora Saskova, and Daniel Parnell. 2018. Contemporary issues in the management of grassroots football. In: *The Routledge handbook on the business of football*, edited by Simon Chadwick, Daniel Parnell, Paul Widdop, and Christos Anagnostopoulos.

Parnell, Daniel, Ed Cope, Richard Bailey, and Paul Widdop. 2016. "Sport policy and English primary physical education: The role of professional football clubs in outsourcing." *Sport in Society*, 20, no 2, 292–302. doi: 10.1080/17430437.2016.1173911

Parnell, Daniel, Kathryn Curran, and Matthew Philpott. 2016. "Healthy stadia: An insight from policy to practice." *Sport in Society*, 20, no 2, 181–186.

Parnell, Daniel, Anthony May, Paul Widdop, Ed Cope, and Richard Bailey. 2018. "Management strategies of non-profit community sport facilities in an era of austerity." *European Sport Management Quarterly*, online. doi: 10.1080/16184742.2018.1523944

Parnell, Daniel, Peter Millward, and Karl Spracklen. 2015. "Sport and austerity in the UK: An insight into Liverpool 2014." *Journal of policy research in tourism, leisure and events*, 7, no 2, 200–203. doi:10.1080/19407963.2014.968309

Parnell, Daniel, Andy Pringle, Paul Widdop, and Stephen Zwolinsky. 2015a. "Understanding football as a vehicle for enhancing social inclusion: Using an intervention mapping framework." *Social Inclusion* 37, no. 2, 200–203.

Parnell, Daniel, Andy Pringle, Stephen Zwolinsky, Jim McKenna, Zoe Rutherford, David Richardson, Lizzie Trotter, Mike Rigby, and Jackie Hargreaves. 2015b. "Reaching older people with physical activity delivered in football clubs: The reach, adoption and implementation characteristics of the extra time programme." *BMC Public Health* 15. doi: 10.1186/s12889-015-1560-5. www.biomedcentral.com/1471-2458/15/220

Parnell, Daniel, and David Richardson. 2014. "Introduction: Football and inclusivity." *Soccer & Society*, 15, no 6, 823–827.

Parnell, Daniel, Gareth Stratton, Barry Drust, and David Richardson. 2013. "Football in the Community schemes: Exploring the effectiveness of an intervention in promoting positive healthful behaviour change." *Soccer and Society*, 14, no 1, 1–17.

Pestoff, Victor. 1992. "Third sector and co-operative services: An alternative to privatization. *Journal of Consumer Policy*, 15, 21–45.

Pilgaard, Maja, and Steffen Rask. 2016. *Danskernes motions-og sportsvaner 2016*. [Sports participation in Denmark 2016]. Idrættens Analyseinstitut. København.

Rafoss, Kolbjørn, and Jens Troelsen. 2010. "Sports facilities for all? The financing, distribution and use of sports facilities in Scandinavian countries." *Sport in Society*, 13, no 4, 643–656. doi: 10.1080/17430431003616399

Ramchandani, Girish, Simon Shibli, and Shia Ping Kung. 2018. "The performance of local authority sports facilities in England during a period of recession and austerity." *International Journal of Sport Policy and Politics*, 10, no 1, 95–111. doi: 10.1080/19406940.2017.1420676

Reid, Gavin. 2018. "Managing budget cuts in Edinburgh's sport and recreation services: Progressive localism in a resilient local authority?" *International Journal of Sport Policy and Politics*, 10, no 1, 113–129. doi:10.1080/19406940.2018.1427127

Smith, Andy, and Ivan Waddington. 2004. "Using "sport in the community schemes" to tackle crime and drug use among young people: Some policy issues and problems." *European Physical Education Review*, 10, 279–298.

Smith, Aaron, and Hans Westerbeek. 2007. "Sport as a vehicle for deploying corporate social responsibility." *Journal of Corporate Citizenship*, 25, 43–54.

Sport England. 2017. *Parklife football hubsnational programme*. London: Sport England.

The Football Association. 2004. *Annual review 2004–2005*. London: The Football Association.

The Football Association. 2015. *The FA national game strategy for participation and development, 2015–2019*. Burton: The Football Association.

Thing, Lone Friis, and Laila Ottesen. 2010. "The autonomy of sports: Negotiating boundaries between sports governance and government policy in the Danish welfare state." *International Journal of Sport Policy and Politics*, 2, 223–235. doi: 10.1080/19406940.2010.488070

Walker, Catherine M, and John W. Hayton. 2017. "Navigating austerity: Balancing 'desirability with viability' in a third sector disability sports organization." *European Sport Management Quarterly*, 17, no 1, 98–116. doi: 10.1080/16184742.2016.1210190

Walker, Catherine M., and John W. Hayton. 2018. "An analysis of third sector sport organisations in an era of 'super-austerity'." *International Journal of Sport Policy and Politics*, 10, no 1, 43–61. doi: 10.1080/19406940.2017.1374296

Widdop, Paul, Neil King, Daniel Parnell, David Cutts, and Peter Millward. 2018. "Austerity, policy and sport participation in England." *International Journal of Sport Policy and Politics*, 10, no 1, 7–24. doi: 10.1080/19406940.2017.1348964

World Health Organization. 2005. *Facing the facts #1: Chronic diseases and their common risk factors*. Geneva: WHO.

Index

Note: Page numbers in italics indicate figures; page numbers in bold indicate tables.